OPHTHALMOLOGY
Just the Facts

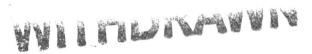

OPHTHALMOLOGY
Just the Facts

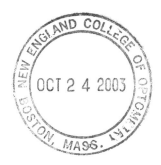
John I. Loewenstein, MD
Assistant Professor of Ophthalmology
Harvard Medical School
Program Director, Ophthalmology Residency
Massachusetts Eye and Ear Infirmary
Boston, Massachusetts

Scott Lee, MD, MPh
Resident in Ophthalmology
University of California, San Francisco
San Francisco, California

McGraw-Hill

Medical Publishing Division

New York   Chicago   San Francisco   Lisbon   London   Madrid   Mexico City
Milan   New Delhi   San Juan   Seoul   Singapore   Sydney   Toronto

Ophthalmology
Just the Facts

1 2 3 4 5 6 7 8 9 0   KGP/KGP   0 9 8 7 6 5 4 3

ISBN 0-07-140332-9

This book was set in Times New Roman by Macmillan India.
The editors were Darlene Cooke, Kathleen McCullough, and Mary E. Bele.
The production supervisor was Richard Ruzycka.
The cover designer was Aimee Nordin.
The index was prepared by Andover Publishing Services.
Quebecor World Kingsport was printer and binder.

This book is printed on acid-free paper.

Library of Congress Cataloging-in-Publication Data

Ophthalmology : just the facts / [edited by] John Loewenstein, Scott Lee.
    p. ; cm.
  Includes bibliographical references and index.
  ISBN 0-07-140332-9 (softcover)
    1. Eye–Diseases–Outlines, syllabi, etc. I. Loewenstein, John, II. Lee, Scott, 1974-
    [DNLM: 1. Eye–Diseases—Outlines, 2. Ophthalmology—methods—Outlines, WW 18.2
O597 2004]
RE50.O627 2004
617.7–dc21   2003046450

ISBN 0-07-121908-0 (International Edition)
Exclusive rights by the McGraw-Hill Companies, Inc., for manufacture and export. This book cannot be re-exported from the country to which it is consigned by McGraw-Hill. The International Edition is not available in North America.

To Louise, for all her support.
JL

To my family: Apa, Ama, and Grant, with the sincerest of gratitude.
SL

CONTENTS

Color Plates appear between pages 178 and 179.

CONTRIBUTORS

Dimitri Azar, MD, Director, Cornea and Keratorefractive Services, Massachusetts Eye and Ear Infirmary, Harvard Medical School, Boston, Massachusetts

Lini S. Bhatia, MD, Research Fellow (Research Assistant), Massachusetts Eye and Ear Infirmary, Harvard Medical School, Boston, Massachusetts

Teresa C. Chen, MD, Glaucoma Service, Massachusetts Eye and Ear Infirmary, Harvard Medical School, Boston, Massachusetts

Kathryn Colby, MD, PhD, Director, Joint Clinical Research Center, Massachusetts Eye and Ear Infirmary, Harvard Medical School, Boston, Massachusetts

Sandra Lora Cremers, MD, FACS, General Eye Service, Massachusetts Eye and Ear Infirmary, Harvard Medical School, Boston, Massachusetts

Daniel M. Laby, MD, Attending Physician and Surgeon, Massachusetts Eye and Ear Infirmary, Harvard Medical School, Boston, Massachusetts

Michael S. Lee, MD, Cole Eye Institute, Cleveland Clinic Foundation, Cleveland, Ohio

Scott Lee, MD, MPh, Resident in Ophthalmology, University of California, San Francisco, San Francisco, California

Don Liu, MD, Professor of Ophthalmology, University Hospital, University of Missouri, Columbia, Missouri

John I. Loewenstein, MD, Assistant Professor of Ophthalmology, Harvard Medical School, Program Director, Ophthalmology Residency, Massachusetts Eye and Ear Infirmary, Boston, Massachusetts

Anh Nguyen, MD, Cornea Service, Massachusetts Eye and Ear Infirmary, Harvard Medical School, Boston, Massachusetts

Harsha S. Reddy, Candidate for Degree in Medicine, Harvard Medical School, Boston, Massachusetts

PREFACE

Ophthalmology is no longer a required rotation in most medical schools. The paucity of texts in our field that serve as medical school literature or review books reflects this. This book was therefore borne out of the need for a concise, yet complete text that would encompass the major topics of Ophthalmology for medical students. We hope that it can serve as a companion text for students on electives, as well as those who want to learn on their own.

Each chapter in *Ophthalmology: Just the Facts* covers the most salient "facts" with regard to the clinical presentation, pathophysiology, diagnosis, differential, and treatment of each disease entity. Since we tend to remember stories much more readily than dry facts, each entity is preceded by an illustrative case. The information is then presented in bulleted form to allow for rapid retention and review. We hope that this format will make the information easy to assimilate.

We would like to express our gratitude to the numerous contributors that made this text possible. Each of these sub-specialists is an expert in their field, and they provided the most current thinking on their subject. We would also like to acknowledge the efforts of the students who assisted with the project, David Goldenberg and Harsha Reddy. We are also indebted to Drs. Jose Cortes, Todd Darmody, Armand Fulco, Jonathan Kaunitz, Edward Livingston, Arun Patel, and Wilfredo Talavera for their consideration, kindness, mentorship, and facilitation of the project. Audrey Melanson and David Walsh kindly helped us collect and prepare illustrative slides.

John I. Loewenstein, MD
Scott Lee, MD, MPh

OPHTHALMOLOGY
Just the Facts

1 VISUAL FUNCTION

Harsha S. Reddy
John I. Loewenstein

When most of us think of having an eye test, we recall having our vision measured with a Snellen chart. This is a test of visual acuity, in a high contrast setting, for distant objects. Although most of the case examples in this book will refer to a patient's visual acuity, it is important to recognize that there is much more to visual function and its assessment. Our ability to function successfully and meaningfully in a visual world depends on more than acuity alone. The term *visual function* encompasses this broader conception of vision, signifying the coterie of mechanisms by which a person images and interprets his or her visual environment. This chapter will discuss visual function introducing the concepts of visual acuity, visual fields, color perception, depth perception, dark adaptation, accommodation, and contrast sensitivity. Examples from the visual systems of animals will be used to illustrate the wide range of mechanisms employed to facilitate vertebrate visual function. These examples show that often a gain in one aspect of vision comes at a loss in another aspect, but over time each species has developed a visual system optimized for survival in the ecological niche to which it is adapted. Human visual function too demonstrates a balanced adaptation to demands placed by the multiple visual environments in which we live. Disorders of human vision can therefore be understood by the aspects of visual function that they compromise, and this chapter will provide examples of associated eye diseases for each of the aspects of visual function introduced.

VISUAL ACUITY

ANIMAL EXAMPLE

- The ability to distinguish detail over large distances is critical for the successful hunting of hawks, eagles, and other diurnal birds of prey. It is no surprise, then, that raptors have the most developed acuity of all vertebrates, nearly two to three times sharper than human distance vision. This ability is due to their eyes' large size and long focal length which enable maximal magnification and resolution. In addition, raptors have two foveas and specialized cone photoreceptors containing oil droplets that act as filters to enhance acuity and reduce aberration. Neurally, raptors have fewer photoreceptors giving input to any one ganglion cell (low summation), thereby enhancing fine discrimination. The high acuity provided by foveal vision, however, comes at a cost of decreased sensitivity under low-light conditions (rod photoreceptor-dependent function).

DEFINITION

- Measure of the eye's ability to distinguish object details and shape.
- Assessed by smallest identifiable object that can be seen at a specified distance (e.g., 20 feet for the Snellen visual acuity test).
- In the United States, legal blindness is defined as distance visual acuity of 20/200 or worse in the better-seeing eye after best conventional correction (i.e., eyeglasses, contacts, intraocular lens).
- In humans, the area of the retina along the eye's central axis called the *fovea* (contained within a larger area called the *macula*) is the region of maximum visual acuity.
- Acuity is primarily a function of cone photoreceptors. The human fovea is composed entirely of cones.

CLINICAL EXAMPLE—AGE-RELATED MACULAR DEGENERATION

- Chronic progressive degeneration of the macula in elderly patients. (See Chap. 10.)
- In the United States, age-related macular degeneration (AMD) is the most frequent cause of blindness in people older than 65.
- Characterized by drusen, i.e., hyaline deposits beneath the retinal pigment epithelium (RPE), proliferation and geographic atrophy of the RPE, choroidal neovascularization, and in severe cases, serous retinal detachments and fibrous scar formation.

- Patients usually notice a gradual loss of visual acuity as the breakdown of the macula progressively disrupts central vision. If subretinal fluid is present, the patient may notice image distortion (metamorphopsia) and a sudden loss of vision.
- The peripheral retina usually appears normal, and the patient typically has full visual fields.

VISUAL FIELDS

ANIMAL EXAMPLE

- Snakes have very narrow visual fields. This is due to the small size and posterior position of their eyes in the orbit. They cannot compensate for these limited fields with eye movements, because they have limited extraocular muscle function. Snakes overcome these difficulties by constantly moving their head from side to side, bringing the areas outside their peripheral visual fields into their central vision. Many species also move their head up and down to bring superior visual fields into better view, especially when confronted by much larger animals. Despite their poor visual acuity and restricted peripheral fields, snakes have developed mechanisms to be highly efficient predators throughout the world.

DEFINITION

- Extent of space visible to an eye that is fixated straight ahead.
- Visual fields are measured in degrees from fixation.
- In the United States, legal blindness is also defined as a visual field less than or equal to 20° at the widest point.

CLINICAL EXAMPLE 1—PRIMARY OPEN-ANGLE GLAUCOMA

- A disease of the optic nerve associated with high intraocular pressures. (See Chap. 9.)
- Leading cause of irreversible blindness in the world.
- Leading cause of blindness among African Americans and Latinos in the United States.
- Pathophysiology: progressive damage to the optic disk and surrounding areas by largely unknown mechanisms.
- Clinical disease is manifested by an enlarged blind spot, scotomas, decreased peripheral visual fields, and ultimately, compromised central vision and blindness.

- Patient may not notice loss of visual fields until the central visual field is disrupted and only a small peripheral residual field of vision remains.
- Patients may compensate for limited visual fields by head movements and off-center (eccentric) fixation of an image on their retina.

CLINICAL EXAMPLE 2—HEMIANOPIC VISUAL FIELD DEFECT

- Patients with lesions that compromise the vasculature that supplies the visual processing portion of the nervous system may display characteristic visual field deficits. These lesions include lumen-obstruction (e.g., emboli, atheromatous plaques) and masses that externally compress the vasculature (e.g., tumors). (See Chap. 11.)
- One can predict the location of the lesion based on the type of visual field defect manifested. For example, a loss of temporal visual fields in both eyes (bitemporal hemianopia) suggests a lesion at the level of the optic chiasm such as a pituitary tumor. By contrast, a loss of the right nasal and left temporal fields (a left homonymous hemianopia) suggests a lesion in the visual system posterior to the optic chiasm on the right side. A stroke, or cerebrovascular accident (CVA) would be a possible etiology.
- Such field defects may have different functional effects for readers of different primary languages. For example, readers of English with bilateral inferior visual field loss may be able to read without difficulty since they can keep the reading material in the superior half of their visual field as they read from left to right. However, readers of Chinese with the same defect may have more difficulty reading text because the script is read from top to bottom and the reading material moves from the superior visual field into the inferior area of no vision. English readers with a left homonymous hemianopia have difficulty finding the beginning of the next line of text. Those with a right homonymous hemianopia often miss the text on the right side of a line.

COLOR PERCEPTION

ANIMAL EXAMPLE

- Mammals with color vision are rare. Only treedwelling (e.g., squirrels) and fruit-eating species (primates, man) have a strong sense of color. These species have retinas containing both cones and rods, the former being responsible for color perception. All remaining mammals, including cats, dogs, rabbits, and raccoons, have very weak or no color vision. A dog trained to fetch a red ball will just as eagerly fetch a gray ball of similar brightness. Not surprisingly, the retinas of most mammals are dominated by rods, allowing these animals to function more effectively under low-light conditions. Both predators and prey have sacrificed some color vision to see better during dawn and dusk when most hunting occurs.

DEFINITION

- The ability to perceive and distinguish between colors, i.e., varying wavelengths in the spectrum of visible light.
- Results from stimulation of red, green, and blue cone photoreceptors in the retina and the subsequent neural processing of these cone outputs.

CLINICAL EXAMPLE 1—RED-GREEN CONGENITAL COLOR DEFICIENCY

- X-linked recessive condition affecting one or more genes.
- Affects 8% of all males and 0.5% of all females in the United States.
- Pathophysiology: defect in red-sensitive cone pigment (protan defect) or green-sensitive cone pigment (deutan defect) or in both pigments.
- Clinically manifested by a range of diseases. In most patients, pastel pinks, yellows, and greens look similar. Few patients confuse pure red with pure green.
- There are many color vision tests. The ones in common clinical use include Ishihara plates (diagrams of red numbers on green backgrounds) and the Farnsworth Panel D-15 test (consists of colored disks). The Farnsworth D-15 is a less sensitive test than the Ishihara plates, but can be used in subjects with limited central vision.

CLINICAL EXAMPLE 2—COLOR AGNOSIA

- Damage to the visual association area of the cerebral cortex preventing the patient from recognizing and identifying colors.
- The optical elements of the eye and the photoreceptors are working normally, and the patient may have a normal electroretinogram (ERG) and electrooculogram (EOG).

ACCOMMODATION

ANIMAL EXAMPLE 1

- The aquatic turtle, *Emys orbicularis*, can see equally well underwater and on land. As light does not travel far in aquatic media, the turtle is focusing on nearby objects while underwater. On land, however, it must be able to see predators and other far away objects. Somehow its visual system must allow both these kinds of vision despite the great difference between the refractive indices of water and air. The aquatic turtle manages both because of its soft, easily deformable lens. While on land, the relatively undeformed lens allows good distance vision. Underwater, however, an extreme deformation of the lens by the iris sphincter muscle allows the maximal refraction necessary to focus on nearby objects.

ANIMAL EXAMPLE 2

- The European lamprey uses a different mechanism to allow both distance and near vision. The lamprey has a firm, spherical lens that does not change its refractive power easily. Very myopic at rest, the lamprey has evolved a special muscle that flattens the cornea to decrease its refractive power and thereby allow better distance vision. In addition, by contracting its six extraocular muscles, the lamprey can elongate its optical axis, aiding in the resolution of distant objects.

DEFINITION

- Increase in optical power by the eye to maintain a clear image (focus) as objects are moved closer.
- In humans, near focusing occurs through ciliary muscle contraction, which leads to zonular relaxation and causes the elastic lens to become more convex, increasing its optical power.

CLINICAL EXAMPLE—PRESBYOPIA

- "Old age vision"—a refractive condition in which there is a diminished power of accommodation arising from loss of elasticity of the crystalline lens.
- It is a normal feature of aging that is usually noticeable by the age of 45.
- Patients notice difficulty in discriminating small close details, e.g., reading newspaper print. Such tasks are managed by holding the object farther from the eyes or by using magnifying lenses or bifocals.

DARK ADAPTATION (SCOTOPIC VISION)

ANIMAL EXAMPLE

- The teleost fishes have evolved an interesting mechanism to respond to changes in illumination. These fish have reflective surfaces within their photoreceptors, and in the light-adapted state, pigment granules migrate between these reflective spheres, screening off reflections. In the dark, however, these pigment granules change position to expose the reflective spheres to the incoming radiation. The spheres then reflect the light back onto the photoreceptors, increasing their eyes' sensitivity to light.

DEFINITION

- Process by which an eye adjusts to decreased illumination and becomes more sensitive to light.
- In humans, scotopic vision is primarily a photoreceptor-mediated process. Dark adaptation (and low-light vision) is primarily accomplished by the photoactivation of rods, and light adaptation (as well as bright-light vision) is achieved by cones. Dark adaptation in humans takes much longer than light adaptation because the rod pigment, rhodopsin, requires a longer time to regenerate than the cone pigments do.

CLINICAL EXAMPLE—CONGENITAL STATIONARY NIGHT BLINDNESS

- Lifelong stable abnormality of scotopic vision.
- Genetic transmission with multiple patterns of inheritance. This condition is clinically diagnosed by electroretinogram (ERG).
- Pathophysiology: failure in communication between the proximal end of the rod photoreceptor and the bipolar cell resulting in varying degrees of diminished scotopic adaptation.
- Patients typically take longer to adapt to low-light conditions than normal patients do. In most types, they do not achieve as low a final dark-adapted threshold as normals even after prolonged adaptation. The markedly reduced vision under these circumstances is sometimes called *nyctalopia*.
- Many patients are not aware of nyctalopia, even though they have had the condition their entire lives. This is because many urban dwellers are rarely in

truly scotopic (very dark) conditions. They are nonetheless severely limited in their ability to function outdoors at night or under dimly lit conditions. Driving at night is a particularly risky behavior.

CLINICAL EXAMPLE—FUNDUS ALBIPUNCTATUS

- A disease of visual pigment regeneration in which recovery of normal rhodopsin levels after intense light exposure takes hours in a dark environment.
- Patients experience "night blindness" until they have spent several hours in the dark environment. Rhodopsin is regenerated after this long adjustment period, and their dark vision stabilizes near levels found in normal patients. Electroretinograms done after a normal period of dark adaptation (30 min) are abnormal. After 3 or more hours in the dark, however, their ERG responses are near normal.

DEPTH PERCEPTION

ANIMAL EXAMPLE

Most animals have laterally directed eyes on the sides of the head with little overlap between the visual fields of the two eyes. Even most mammals, including bovids and horses, have panoramic vision rather than binocular vision. The overlap of the two visual fields is also correlated with the degree of decussation of the optic nerve fibers in the optic chiasm. In addition, there are animals such as the chameleon that are even capable of moving each eye independently. This illustrates that binocular stereoscopic vision is not the only mechanism of depth perception that exists. Moreover, very fine degrees of depth perception may not be critical to the visual function of species preoccupied with only nearby objects or only far away objects.

DEFINITION

- Appreciation of the relative spatial location of objects with respect to distance from the observer.
- In humans, depth perception is accomplished by multiple mechanisms.
- One mechanism is stereoscopic vision, which requires binocularity. The overlap of the two eyes' visual fields produces retinal images of the same object from

slightly different angles in each eye. Objects at different distances from the viewer produce different degrees of disparity between the images on the two retinas. The brain interprets these disparities to perceive the distance of an object from the viewer and to distinguish the relative depths of multiple objects in the visual field.

- For objects beyond a few feet away from the viewer, stereoscopic vision is not critical for depth perception. At this distance, monocular mechanisms take over. Humans interpret the apparent decrease in size of objects with distance as a means of estimating the distance of that object. This mechanism is dependent on visual experience, i.e., our familiarity with the size and shape of objects in our visual world.

CLINICAL EXAMPLE

- Patients who lose vision in one eye must rely on monocular depth perception in their functioning eye. Many will initially have difficulty with activities requiring even gross depth perception such as walking up steps or pouring liquids. Most will eventually learn to use other clues of depth for such tasks. While most patients will be able to function without impairment in most daily activities, they may be limited in activities that require fine or rapid depth discrimination. For example, playing certain sports such as tennis or baseball will usually be difficult. Performing near tasks requiring fine depth perception, such as intraocular surgery, will be very difficult. Interestingly, patients who do not have stereopsis in early childhood, such as those with strabismus or those with good vision in only one eye, tend to function very well except in the most demanding tasks.

CONTRAST SENSITIVITY

DEFINITION

- Ability to detect detail having subtle gradations in grayness between test target and background.

CLINICAL EXAMPLE—DIABETIC MACULAR EDEMA

- Pathophysiology: patients with diabetic retinopathy may develop edema of the macula secondary to leakage from retinal capillaries and microaneurysms. (See Chap. 10.)
- Many of these patients have relatively good acuity on a Snellen chart, which has a high contrast between the letters and the background. Nevertheless, many will have great difficulty reading newspapers where the contrast between letters and background is not as pronounced.
- Use of a bright reading light and magnification is often helpful.

BIBLIOGRAPHY

Albert DM, Jakobiec FA. *Principles and Practice of Ophthalmology: Basic sciences.* Philadelphia, WB Saunders Co., 1994.

Ali MA, Klyne MA. *Vision in Vertebrates.* New York, Plenum Press, 1985.

Jacobs G. *Comparative Color Vision.* New York, Academic Press, 1981.

Lang GK. *Ophthalmology: A Pocket Textbook Atlas.* Stuttgart, Germany, Georg Thieme Verlag, 2000.

Retina and Vitreous. Basic and Clinical Science Course Section 12 (1999). San Francisco, American Academy of Ophthalmology.

2 PHYSICAL OPTICS AFFECTING VISION AND CORRECTION OF VISUAL REFRACTIVE ERRORS

Dimitri Azar

FREQUENCY AND WAVELENGTH OF LIGHT

The frequency of light refers to the number of times a particular position on the wave passes a fixed point in a fixed interval of time. The frequency of the visible part of the spectrum is in the $10^{14}–10^{15}$ cps (cycles per second) range. As light waves travel from one medium to another, the frequency of light does not change. However, the wavelength and velocity of light waves decrease in the denser medium. Electromagnetic radiations in the visual spectrum have wavelengths of 380–760 nm in a vacuum that range between the short wavelengths of cosmic rays, x-rays, and the ultraviolet and the long wavelength of radio frequency and the infrared portions of the electromagnetic spectrum.

Light travels at a speed of 3×10^{10} cm/s (186,000 miles per second) in a vacuum, and its speed is slower in denser media. The ratio of the velocity in a vacuum (C) to the velocity in another medium$_1$ (V$_1$) is referred to as the index of refraction for that medium (n$_1$ + C/V$_1$). As illustrated in Fig. 2-1, the wavelength in a medium$_2$ is less than it is in a vacuum and is proportional to the change in velocity. The wavelength of light in the region around 460 nm results in blue color sensation, and around 520 nm in green, around 575 nm in yellow, and around 650 nm in red sensation. White color sensation results from a mixture of several of these. Each medium, therefore, has a different refractive index for each frequency of light. Blue light is slowed and bent more than the longer wavelengths (chromatic aberration).

REFLECTION OF LIGHT

When light waves strike a smooth polished surface they are reflected according to the rule of reflection: the angle

Relationship	Explanation	Illustration
Index of Refraction		
$n = c/v$ $n_1 = c/v_1$	n = index of refraction n$_1$ = index of refraction in medium 1 c = speed of light in vacuum v = speed of light in medium v$_1$ = speed of light in medium 1	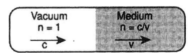
Wavelength-Frequency Relationships		
$c = \lambda \cdot v$ $v_\top = \lambda \cdot v$ $v_2 = \lambda_2 \cdot v$ $\frac{n_2}{n_1} = \frac{v_1}{v_2} = \frac{\lambda_1}{\lambda_2}$	λ = wavelength of light λ_1 = wavelength in medium 1 v = frequency of light wave (does not change as light travels from medium 1 to medium 2) n$_2$ = index of refraction in medium 2 v$_2$ = speed of light in medium 2 λ_2 = wavelength in medium 2	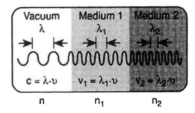

FIGURE 2-1 Relationship of the index of refraction (n) in vacuum vs. various media (n$_1$, n$_2$). The frequency of light wave does not change as light travels from vacuum through medium 1 to medium 2. The wavelength and speed of light decrease as the index of refraction increases. [From Albert DM, Jakobiec FA: Principles and Practice of Ophthalmology, 2nd ed. Philadelphia: WB Saunders, 2000, p 5330.]

of reflection and the angle of incidence measured relative to the normal to the surface at the point of impact are equal.

A plane mirror reverses the direction of the light rays without changing the bending power or vergence. Convex and concave reflective surfaces can change image magnification by altering the vergence of light rays. The cornea, being convex, can act like a mirror, reflecting light and causing image magnification. This is employed in keratometry and topography to measure the curvature of the cornea for refractive surgery, for contact lens fitting, and for diagnosing corneal irregularities such as keratoconus.

REFRACTION OF LIGHT

SNELL'S LAW

When a light ray strikes a surface at a right angle (normal to the surface), it does not deviate from its course. When oblique rays of light strike a surface, however, they are refracted (bent). As the speed of the light is reduced, the oblique light rays proceed at a different angle relationship between the angle of incidence and the angle of refraction. The angle of incidence is the angle between the ray of light striking the surface and the normal to the surface. The angle of refraction is the angle between the ray exiting the surface and the normal

to the surface. This relationship is governed by Snell's law: $n_i \sin_i = n_r \sin r$, where i = angle of incidence, r = angle of refraction, and n = index of refraction.

When the rays are incident perpendicular to the surface, the velocity of the light is reduced but the direction of the light is unchanged (i = r = 0).

When light passes from a medium of low density to a medium of high density, light rays are bent toward the normal (Fig. 2-2). Conversely, when light passes from a high-density to a low-density medium (such as out of the eye into air), the angle of refraction is greater than the angle of incidence (Fig. 2-3).

REAL AND VIRTUAL OBJECTS AND IMAGES

Light rays from real objects are divergent, but their direction can be altered by introducing a lens or an optical element of a different refractive index and they can be made less divergent, parallel to one another, or convergent, depending on the shape and refractive index of the optical system. The image is *real* if the pencil of light rays emerging from the optical system is convergent to a point in space (Fig. 2-4). The image is *virtual* if the new pencil of light rays is divergent (Fig. 2-5).

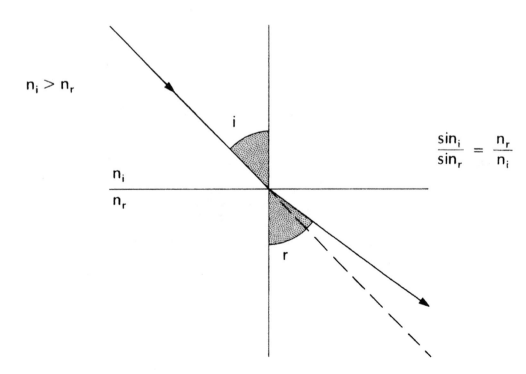

$$\frac{\sin_i}{\sin_r} = \frac{n_r}{n_i}$$

FIGURE 2-2 When light travels from one medium to another with a lower index of refraction, the rays are bent away from the normal to the surface. A critical angle of incidence (i) may be reached if the angle of refraction (r) reaches 90°. Light rays striking the surface with an angle of incidence greater than the critical angle are completely reflected. [From Albert DM, Jakobiec FA: Principles and Practice of Ophthalmology, 2nd ed. Philadelphia: WB Saunders, 2000, p 5330.]

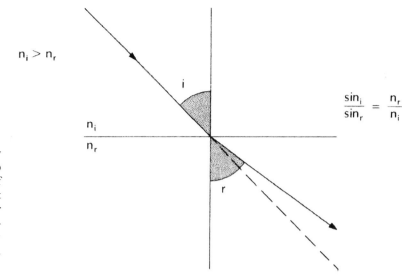

FIGURE 2-3 When rays strike a surface, they may be refracted, as shown, or reflected. The relationship between the angle of incidence (i) and the angle of refraction (r) is governed by Snell's law. When light travels from one medium to another with a higher index of refraction, the rays are bent toward the normal to the surface. [From Albert DM, Jakobiec FA: Principles and Practice of Ophthalmology, 2nd ed. Philadelphia: WB Saunders, 2000, p 5329.]

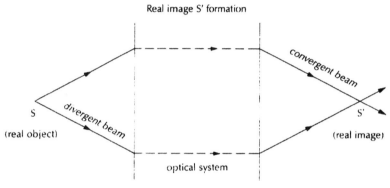

FIGURE 2-4 A real image S′ is formed when light rays emerging from the optical system converge to S′. In general, a screen can be placed at S′ and a luminous point will appear on it. [From Albert DM, Jakobiec FA: Principles and Practice of Ophthalmology, 2nd ed. Philadelphia: WB Saunders, 2000, p 5330.]

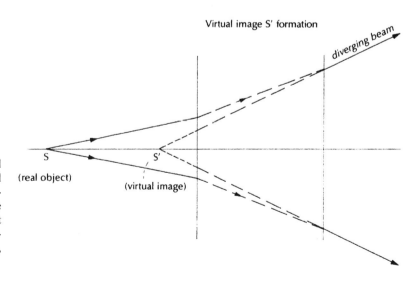

FIGURE 2-5 Optical system forming a virtual image S′. The light rays emerging from the optical system are diverging. The light rays do not converge to S′. However, S′ may be seen by an eye located behind the optical system. [From Albert DM, Jakobiec FA: Principles and Practice of Ophthalmology, 2nd ed. Philadelphia: WB Saunders, 2000, p 5330.]

SPHERICAL AND ASTIGMATIC LENSES

MEASUREMENT OF LENS POWER

Spherical lenses have equal curvature in all meridians. Lenses are measured in diopters (D). The D power of a lens is the reciprocal of its focal length (f) in meters: $d = 1/f$. For example, a lens that focuses light from an object at infinity (parallel light rays or 0 vergence) at a plane 2 m beyond the lens has a focal length of 2 m and a power of 0.5 D.

TYPES OF CORRECTIVE LENSES

CONVERGING (CONVEX OR PLUS) LENSES

Convex (plus) lenses refract light rays so as to make them more convergent (or less divergent). Plus lenses of the same power can be made in several shapes, but at least one of the two surfaces must be converging (Fig. 2-6). A meniscus plus lens, in which the front surface is more convex than the back surface is concave, is desirable for spectacles because there is less aberration over a wider area of the lens. Plus lenses are used for the correction of hyperopia, presbyopia, and aphakia. If the lens is moved sideways, the object appears to move in the opposite direction.

DIVERGING (CONCAVE OR MINUS) LENSES

Minus lenses refract light rays so as to make them more divergent. They can be made in many forms (Fig. 2-7). Minus lenses are thin in the middle and thick at the edges. The most common design used in minus spectacle lenses is the meniscus, wherein the back or ocular surface is more concave than the front surface is convex. Minus lenses are used to correct myopia. When an object is viewed through a minus lens, the object appears smaller.

ASTIGMATIC (SPHEROCYLINDRICAL OR TORIC) LENSES

In these lenses one meridian is more curved (steeper) than all of the others, and the orthogonal meridian is the flattest meridian. The meridians of least curvature and of greatest curvature are referred to as the principal meridians. Astigmatic lenses can be plus lenses, minus lenses, or one

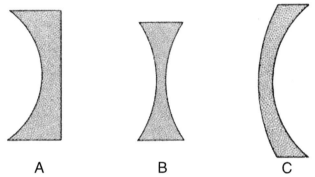

A   **B**   **C**

FIGURE 2-7 Diverging lenses have at least one concave surface. The other surface may be plano (A), concave (B), or convex (C). [From Albert DM, Jakobiec FA: Principles and Practice of Ophthalmology, 2nd ed. Philadelphia: WB Saunders, 2000, p 5332.]

Undeviated Central Rays Passing Through Thin Lens

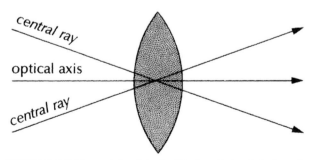

FIGURE 2-8 The nodal point of a thin lens is located along the optical axis connecting the two centers of curvature. A central ray passes undeviated through the nodal point of a thin lens. [From Albert DM, Jakobiec FA: Principles and Practice of Ophthalmology, 2nd ed. Philadelphia: WB Saunders, 2000, p 5331.]

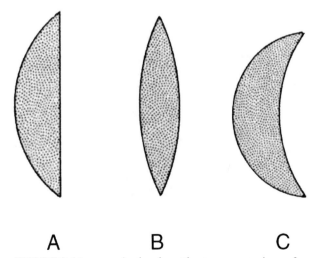

A   **B**   **C**

FIGURE 2-6 A converging lens has at least one converging surface. The other surface may be plano (A), convex (B), or concave (C). [From Albert DM, Jakobiec FA: Principles and Practice of Ophthalmology, 2nd ed. Philadelphia: WB Saunders, 2000, p 5331.]

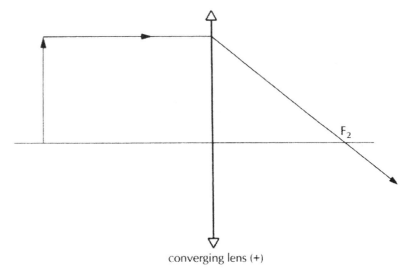

converging lens (+)

FIGURE 2-9 Ray tracing using the secondary focal point of a converging lens. [From Albert DM, Jakobiec FA: Principles and Practice of Ophthalmology, 2nd ed. Philadelphia: WB Saunders, 2000, p 5332.]

principal meridian plus and the other minus. They can be fabricated as meniscus lenses or in a planocylinder form in which one principal meridian is plano (zero optical power) and all other meridians either plus or minus.

GRAPHIC REPRESENTATION

The location of an image can be determined graphically by tracing the cardinal rays as illustrated in Figs. 2-8–12.

PRISMS

A prism is an optical device composed of two nonparallel refracting surfaces that are usually flat. The line at which the two surfaces intersect is the apex of the prism. The greater the angle formed at the apex, the stronger the prismatic effect. An object viewed through a prism appears to be displaced in the direction of the prism apex, but the focus is not altered and no magnification or minification occurs. Prisms are usually prescribed to achieve single binocular vision in a patient with an extraocular muscle imbalance. The strength of a prism is measured in prism D, each prism D displacing a ray of light 1 cm at a distance of 1 m.

VERGENCE FORMULAS

The locations of object and image with respect to an optical system are related by the formula U + D = V,

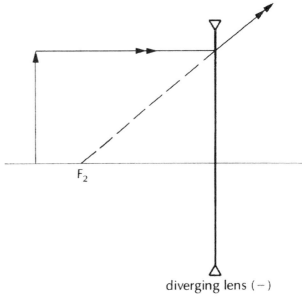

diverging lens (−)

FIGURE 2-10 Ray tracing using the secondary focal point of a diverging lens. [From Albert DM, Jakobiec FA: Principles and Practice of Ophthalmology, 2nd ed. Philadelphia: WB Saunders, 2000, p 5332.]

where U is the vergence of the object rays entering the optical system, D is the power of the optical system, and V is the vergence of the image rays leaving the optical system (Fig. 2-13).

LENSOMETERS

Lensometers are precision instruments used to measure the spherical power, cylindrical power, and axis of astigmatism of a spectacle or contact lens. The lens to be

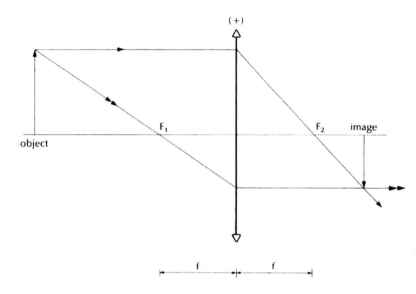

FIGURE 2-11 Ray tracing to determine image size and location using primary and secondary focal points of a converging lens. [From Albert DM, Jakobiec FA: Principles and Practice of Ophthalmology, 2nd ed. Philadelphia: WB Saunders, 2000, p 5333.]

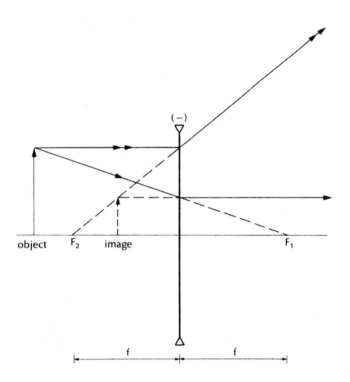

FIGURE 2-12 Ray tracing to determine image size and location using primary and secondary focal points of a diverging lens. [From Albert DM, Jakobiec FA: Principles and Practice of Ophthalmology, 2nd ed. Philadelphia: WB Saunders, 2000, p 5333.]

measured is placed in the lensometer, and the power wheel is turned until the target mires are in focus. If the mires all focus simultaneously at a given power, no cylinder is present and the lens is completely spherical. Otherwise the power wheel is turned twice to line up the principal meridians of an astigmatic lens and determine the power and axis of the lens. This can be performed manually or using an automated lensometer. The lens prescription is the strongest plus-power minus the difference in power between the two principal meridians, and the axis of the cylinder is that of the more minus meridian.

Spectacle lens prescriptions may be written in minus or plus cylinder form. Conversion of minus cylinder prescriptions to plus or of plus cylinder prescriptions to

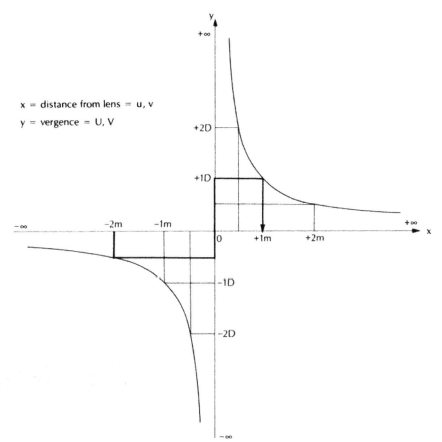

x = distance from lens = u, v

y = vergence = U, V

FIGURE 2-13 The equation $y = 1/x$ governs the relationship between the vergence at the lens of a pencil of light and the distance between the lens and the object or image. According to the vergence equation, light from an object located $-2\,m$ to the left of the lens has a vergence of $-0.5\,D$ at the lens. If the power added by the lens is $+1.5\,D$, the vergence at the lens of the image rays becomes $+1.0\,D$. The image would thus be located at $+1\,m$ to the right of the lens. [From Albert DM, Jakobiec FA: Principles and Practice of Ophthalmology, 2nd ed. Philadelphia: WB Saunders, 2000, p 5334.]

minus is carried out in three steps: (1) Reverse the sign of the cylinder, keeping the same power. (2) Add the difference between the sphere and cylinder to obtain the new sphere. (3) Add 90° to the axis. *Example*: $+3.00$ $-2.00 \times 20°$ converts to $+1.00 + 2.00 \times 110°$.

REFRACTION TECHNIQUES

Refraction is the term applied to the various testing procedures employed to measure the refractive error of the eye to provide the proper correction. Refractive error is by far the most common cause of poor vision but is easily correctable.

RETINOSCOPY

A manual retinoscope is a hand-held instrument that is used to shine a light through the pupil to observe the reflex created by the light reflected from the retina. A small aperture in a mirror allows the examiner to view the patient's illuminated pupil, while the mirror reflects the light along the line connecting the examiner's and the patient's pupils. By placing plus or minus lenses in front of the patient's eye, the patient's focal point can be altered until it is brought to the examiner's pupil, which produces a visible end. Moving the light back and forth across a series of lenses held in front of the patient's pupil results in a linear light reflex moving in the same (hyperopia) or opposite direction (myopia) as the light. Plus or minus lenses are placed in front of the patient's eye to achieve a visible end point of filling of the entire pupil with light that does not move, indicating neutralization of the refractive error. In the case of astigmatism, the retinoscope linear light must be sequentially lined up along the two principal meridians and plus or minus lenses put up until movement of light in each principal meridian is neutralized. The amount of ametropia can also be determined using an automated refractor. Although manual and automated retinoscopy are highly accurate and useful, opacities of the media, tiny pupils, poor fixation by the patient, or distortion of the light reflex preclude their use in some cases. Prescribing lenses on the basis of retinoscopic findings alone is frequently inadequate. A subjective refraction is required to refine these results.

SUBJECTIVE REFRACTION

On the basis of old spectacle prescriptions or the retinoscopic findings and in the absence of astigmatism, the subjective refraction involves adding more plus or minus spheres to reach the optimal end point. One method of achieving this end point is to perform the red-green test, which takes advantage of chromatic aberrations of the eye. It is described in greater detail below. In the presence of astigmatism, the subjective refraction involves refining the axis of the cylinder and the powers along the principal meridians. Fogging techniques and use of the Jackson cross-cylinder (JCC) are helpful for refining the results of retinoscopy. These techniques require the cooperation of the patient. In very young children or others who cannot assist in subjective refraction, the retinoscopy or other objective refraction must be given.

CYCLOPLEGIC REFRACTION

The use of tropicamide, cyclopentolate, or similar agents to paralyze the ciliary muscle allows stabilizing the refraction of the eye so that a definitive end point may be measured. It is useful during retinoscopy and subjective refraction, especially in young hyperopic patients with active accommodation.

ABERRATIONS

Optical systems generally contain imperfections referred to as aberrations. (An *aberrometer* is an optical instrument that can quantify the amount of optical aberrations by analyzing the deviation of the wavefront from a planar wavefront. This is often represented by displaying the wavefront Zernike polynomials of various aberrations.) The important aberrations in the visual system and spectacle lenses are chromatic aberration, spherical aberration, coma, astigmatism of oblique incidence, and distortion.

CHROMATIC ABERRATION

The index of refraction for any transparent medium varies with the reciprocal of the frequency of the incident light. When white light is passed through a prism, a rainbow effect (chromatic dispersion) is produced. Blue light is refracted more than red light. In the eye and in a plus lens, green light is focused slightly closer to the lens than red light. (The red-green test is used to refine

spherical corrections within 1D of emmetropia. While the eye is fogged with a plus lens, the patient compares the letters on a half-red, half-green background. The red side should be clearer. Plus sphere is removed in 0.25-D steps until the two backgrounds appear equally clear. If the letter on the green side appears clearer, more plus correction is required.)

SPHERICAL ABERRATION

Light rays that are paraxial, i.e., that pass through the center of the lens, form a single image point by focusing at a single point. However, rays that are parallel to the axis but that pass through the periphery of the lens are usually refracted more than the paraxial rays (Fig. 2-14). Wavefront analysis using an aberrometer is valuable in evaluating the extent of spherical aberration in the eye. Instead of a single image point, the focused image becomes a blur circle. The size of this blur circle can be reduced by restricting the passage of light through the lens to the central portion (as is done when an object is viewed through a small pupil or pinhole aperture) or by modifying the lens shape (aspheric lens design).

ASTIGMATISM OF OBLIQUE INCIDENCE

When light rays pass through a lens obliquely, two linear images form at right angles to one another with a *circle of least confusion* between them. Although this form of aberration is of minimal significance in the eye, it can create considerable blurring of the image formed by tilting spectacle lenses. Tilting a minus lens induces minus spherocylindrical power (the minus cylinder axis being the same as the axis of the tilt).

DISTORTION

Distortion is the result of differential magnification in an optical system. This occurs particularly when high-power plus lenses are used to correct aphakia (*pin cushion* distortion) or high minus lenses are used to correct myopia (*barrel* distortion). In these situations, light from some parts of the object is focused by the central portion of the lens while other parts are focused by peripheral portions of the lens.

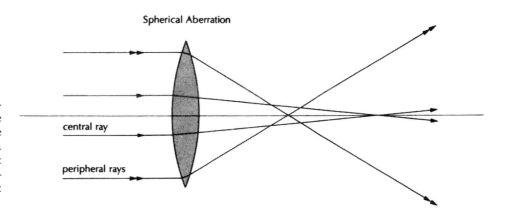

Spherical Aberration

central ray

peripheral rays

FIGURE 2-14 Spherical aberration. Rays of light striking the periphery of a spherical lens are bent more than the central rays. [From Albert DM, Jakobiec FA: Principles and Practice of Ophthalmology, 2nd ed. Philadelphia: WB Saunders, 2000, p 5339.]

THE HUMAN EYE AS AN OPTICAL SYSTEM

The optical system of the eye has camera-like features. The focusing elements of the eye are the cornea and the crystalline lens, the diaphragm is the iris, and the "film" is the retina. The cornea contributes approximately two-thirds of the refracting power of the eye. Light rays undergo the greatest amount of bending at the air–cornea interface because of the large difference in index of refraction between these two media. Although the crystalline lens is a more powerful lens in air, in its natural surrounding media, the difference in refractive index at the aqueous–lens and lens–vitreous interfaces is less than the air–corneal difference of refractive index. Thus, it contributes +18 D as compared to + 43 D contributed by the cornea.

The index of refraction of the cornea is 1.376. The crystalline lens has an index of refraction that increases from the cortex to the nucleus, averaging 1.41. The pupil constricts when illumination is increased, reducing the amount of light that enters the eye. This constriction contributes to reduced aberrations and increased depth of focus.

The retina contains the highly sensitive rods for registering images at very low levels of illumination and the "fine grain" color-sensitive cones for high resolution and discrimination at high levels of illumination. Only one or two quanta of light energy are required to activate the rods. Rapid neural adaptation and the more gradual process of adjusting the balance between bleaching and regeneration of retinal visual pigments enable the retina to function perfectly at extremely high levels of illumination.

REFRACTIVE ERRORS OF THE EYE

EMMETROPIA

The nonaccommodating emmetropic eye brings any pencil of parallel light rays, from an object more than 6 m away to focus at the plane of the retina. An emmetropic eye will have a clear image of a distant object without any internal adjustment of its optics (Fig. 2-15). While most emmetropic eyes are approximately 24 mm in length, a larger eye can be emmetropic if its optical components are weaker, and a smaller eye can be emmetropic if its optical components are stronger. In all these situations, the far point of the emmetropic eye is optical infinity (Fig. 2-16).

MYOPIA

The myopic eye brings a pencil of parallel rays to focus in front of the plane of the retina. The anteroposterior diameter of the eye is too long or the cornea is too steep in myopia or nearsightedness (Fig. 2-17A). There is a point, the far point of the eye, such that rays diverging from this point are brought to focus on the retina in an unaccommodated state (Fig. 2-17B).

TYPES OF MYOPIA

In *axial myopia*, the anteroposterior diameter of the eye is longer than normal, although the corneal and lens curvatures are normal and the lens is in the normal anatomic position. A peripapillary myopic crescent from an exaggerated scleral ring and a posterior staphyloma are associated posterior segment disorders.

Myopia can result from increased corneal curvature (*curvature myopia*). This is more common than axial

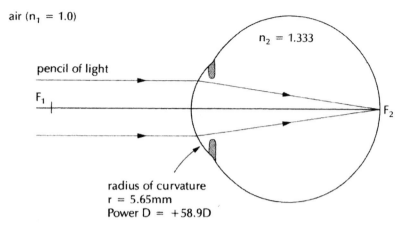

air (n_1 = 1.0)

pencil of light

F_1

n_2 = 1.333

F_2

radius of curvature
r = 5.65mm
Power D = +58.9D

FIGURE 2-15 A pencil of light rays parallel to the optical axis focuses at the secondary focal point of the emmetropic eye (F_2) located on the retina. Pencils of rays parallel to other central rays focus on points of the retina other than F_2 (not shown). In this manner, the image of a distant extended object is formed on the retina. [From Albert DM, Jakobiec FA: Principles and Practice of Ophthalmology, 2nd ed. Philadelphia: WB Saunders, 2000, p 5337.]

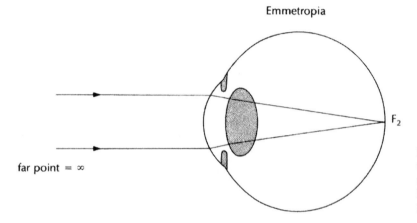

Emmetropia

far point = ∞

F_2

FIGURE 2-16 The plane conjugate to the retina of the emmetropic eye in the nonaccommodating state is at infinity. [From Albert DM, Jakobiec FA: Principles and Practice of Ophthalmology, 2nd ed. Philadelphia: WB Saunders, 2000, p 5338.]

myopia, and may be associated with corneal disorders such as keratoconus or keratoglobus.

Lenticular myopia can result from increased curvature of the lens or increased index of refraction in the lens. The onset of early to moderate nuclear cataracts is a common cause of myopia in the elderly. Many older people find themselves able to read without glasses ("second sight"). Anterior movement of the lens increases the myopic error such as after glaucoma surgery.

Clinical Course. Myopia is rarely present at birth, but often begins to develop as the child grows. It is usually detected during school and increases during the years of the growth spurt until stabilizing around the mid to late teens. Symptoms of myopia include blurred distance vision and squinting to sharpen distance vision (pinhole effect), but headaches are rare.

Progressive myopia is a rare form of myopia that increases by as much as 4 D yearly and is associated with vitreous floaters and liquefaction and chorioretinal changes. The refractive changes stabilize at about the third decade of life. It frequently results in higher degrees of myopia.

Congenital high myopia is usually a high refractive error detected in infants who are unaware of a visual world beyond their immediate surroundings. They develop normal binocular vision focusing on small nearby objects. Once the myopia is corrected, the child can develop normal distance vision.

HYPEROPIA

The unaccommodating hyperopic eye brings a pencil of parallel rays to focus at a point behind the retina (Fig. 2-18). Accommodation of the eye may produce enough additional plus power to bring such a pencil to focus on the retina. Although this condition is also referred to as "farsightedness," persons with hyperopia may have problems seeing objects at distance and near, especially when elderly. Near images are usually blurred. Most children are born with mild hyperopia, but this usually resolves in the second decade of life.

The crystalline lens or the cornea may have a weaker than normal curvature leading to hyperopia. In axial hyperopia, the eye is shorter than normal in its anteroposterior diameter. Hyperopic eyes are more prone to develop angle-closure glaucoma because of the crowding of the angle. The optic nerves are also smaller and

A
Myopia

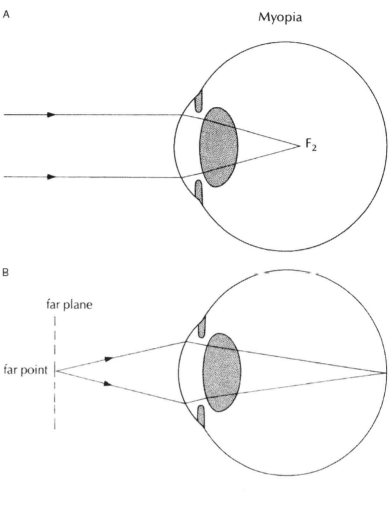

B

FIGURE 2-17 (A) The secondary focal point of a myopic eye. (B) The far point of a myopic eye is a point between infinity and the cornea from which divergent rays focus on the retina without accommodation. [From Albert DM, Jakobiec FA: Principles and Practice of Ophthalmology, 2nd ed. Philadelphia: WB Saunders, 2000, p 5338.]

Hyperopia

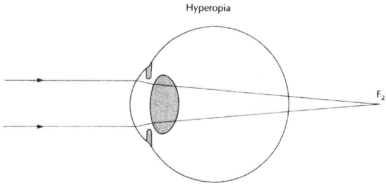

FIGURE 2-18 In hyperopia, the secondary focal point of the eye is located behind the retina (parallel rays striking a hyperopic eye in a nonaccommodating state focus behind the retina). [From Albert DM, Jakobiec FA: Principles and Practice of Ophthalmology, 2nd ed. Philadelphia: WB Saunders, 2000, p 5338.]

more densely packed, as they are crowded at the disk. Physiologic cupping is uncommon, and pseudopapilledema (normal blind spot and no venous congestion) may be noted.

ACCOMMODATION IN HYPEROPIA

Three portions of the hyperopic refractive error can be observed depending on the relative degree of accommo-

dation in hyperopia: latent, manifest facultative, and manifest absolute hyperopia.

LATENT HYPEROPIA Latent hyperopia is that portion of the refractive error completely corrected by accommodation. It is the difference in measurement between manifest hyperopia and the results of the cycloplegic refraction [cycloplegic (total) hyperopia = latent plus manifest].

Manifest Hyperopia Manifest hyperopia could be facultative or absolute. Manifest facultative hyperopia is that portion of hyperopia, measured at distance, that may be corrected by the patient's own powers of accommodation. It is revealed by fogging the eye to relax accommodation without pharmacological cycloplegia. Vision is normal with or without corrective plus lenses, but accommodation is not relaxed without the glasses. Manifest absolute hyperopia is that portion of the distance refractive error that cannot be compensated for by the patient's accommodation. Plus lenses are used to correct this part of the hyperopic refractive error.

Progressive loss of accommodative power with age moves the eye from latent and facultative hyperopia to greater degrees of absolute hyperopia.

SYMPTOMS OF HYPEROPIA

Asthenopia or "uncomfortable" vision is one of the most common complaints of hyperopic patients. It occurs when the patient focus is at a near distance for prolonged periods of time. Frontal headaches may also occur, especially when focusing at near objects.

Blurred distance vision may be the presenting symptom in older patients or in high degrees of hyperopia. Early presbyopia is also seen in patients with hyperopia (before the fourth decade of life).

ASTIGMATISM

The most common etiology of astigmatism is the variation of the corneal curvature in different meridians. Light rays passing through a steep meridian are bent more than those passing through a flatter meridian. This results in the formation of a more complicated image, referred to as the *conoid of Stürm*, wherein a point source of light is represented by an image consisting of two lines that are at right angles to one another with a circle of least confusion in a plane midway between them (Fig. 2-19).

TYPES OF ASTIGMATISM

If the vertical corneal meridian is steeper, the astigmatism is called *with the rule*, and if the horizontal meridian is steeper, it is referred to as *against the rule astigmatism*. When the steep meridian is not along the vertical or horizontal meridians, it is referred to as *oblique astigmatism*.

One meridian may be emmetropic and the other hyperopic or myopic (simple hyperopic and myopic astigmatism, respectively). When both meridians are hyperopic or myopic, the astigmatism is *compound astigmatism*. When one meridian is hyperopic and the other myopic, the condition is referred to as *mixed astigmatism*.

When the principal meridians are 90° apart, the astigmatism is referred to as *regular astigmatism*. Otherwise it is referred to as *irregular astigmatism*. Irregular astigmatism results from an unevenness of the corneal surface such as in corneal scarring or keratoconus. The principal meridians cannot be completely corrected with ordinary astigmatic or toric lenses. The use of corneal topography and keratometry allow measurements of the cornea in cases of irregular corneal astigmatism. Irregular astigmatism is correctable in some cases with hard contact lenses.

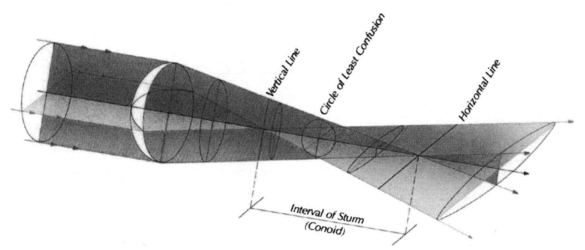

FIGURE 2-19 The three-dimensional image formed by a pencil of light striking a spherocylindrical refractive surface or lens is the conoid of Stürm. This consists of two focal lines that are perpendicular to each other and separated by the interval of Stürm. Cross-sections of the conoid at planes between the two focal lines consist of ellipses that become more round as the dioptric center of Stürm's interval is reached, at which point a "circle of least confusion" is formed. [From Albert DM, Jakobiec FA: Principles and Practice of Ophthalmology, 2nd ed. Philadelphia: WB Saunders, 2000, p 5334.]

The symptoms of astigmatism include blurred vision, asthenopia, head tilt, and squinting. Although treating astigmatism depends on the patient's visual needs and symptoms, the most important determinant of successful outcome is accurate refraction. The use of fogging with plus cylinders, Lancaster-Regan charts, and Jackson cross cylinders (JCC) is most valuable. Fogging is used to relax accommodation. It is followed by refinement with the Jackson cross cylinder to refine the axis and power of the correcting cylinder to correct regular astigmatism. The Jackson cross cylinder is a lens of equal-power plus (white dot) and minus (red dot) plano cylinders with axes 90° apart. If the final cylinder correction is greater than 3 D and the patient has never worn glasses before, giving two-thirds of the correction may avoid the discomfort associated with the full correction.

ANISOMETROPIA

Anisometropia with aniseikonia is a state in which there is a difference in the refractive errors of the two eyes, i.e., one eye is myopic and the other hyperopic or both are hyperopic or myopic but to different degrees. The differences in refractive error may result in differences between the two eyes of visual acuity. With correction at the spectacle plane, there is a difference in size of the ocular image in each eye (possibly causing symptomatic retinal rivalry). This is known as aniseikonia. In children below age 5, suppression scotoma, amblyopia, and strabismus may develop. Refractive correction with spectacles may induce anisophoria and aniseikonia, which may necessitate the use of contact lenses with patching and possible prisms for associated extraocular muscle deviations.

ACCOMMODATION

The crystalline lens increases its plus power when focusing at a near object (accommodation). The lens is suspended in the eye by the zonules that are attached to the ciliary body at one end and the lens capsule at the other end. When the ciliary muscle contracts, the zonules relax, which reduces the tension of the zonules on the lens capsule. The anterior pole, and to a lesser extent the posterior pole, becomes more convex, thereby increasing the power of the lens. This change in power is called accommodation.

The amplitude of accommodation is the range of plus-power the lens can produce. Determining the amplitude of accommodation may be done by several methods: minus sphere test, Lebensohn target, cycloplegic testing, and the push-up method. In the latter, a target is gradually moved toward the patient's eyes until the patient notes onset of blurred vision.

PRESBYOPIA

Symptoms of presbyopia occur as a result of decreased accommodative amplitude in patients over 40 and inability to see clearly at near. The symptoms are aggravated by fatigue, illness, fever, or other debilitating conditions. Presbyopia is a physiologic change in the crystalloids of the lens that results in a decreased elasticity of the lens fibers or a hardening of the lens. When the eye attempts accommodation, the curvature of the lens changes less in a presbyopic patient than in younger patients. By the mid forties, accommodative amplitude decreases to less than 4 D, and objects smaller than 25 cm appear out of focus. Correcting presbyopia is done through supplementing accommodation with plus lenses that do part of the focusing for the eye, i.e., the *add*.

The average eyeglass adds for various age levels are:

45 years: +1.00 D to +1.25 D
50 years: +1.50 D to +1.75 D
55 years: +2.00 D to +2.25 D
60 years: +2.50 D to +3.00 D

Lenses can be made with more than one corrective power to treat presbyopia. If an additional portion is added for intermediate range vision, it is referred to as a *trifocal lens*. Bifocals and trifocals can be manufactured by altering the curvature of the surface to make a one-piece multifocal, or by fusing a smaller piece of higher density glass into the crown portion to make a fused multifocal lens. Progressive lenses are multifocal lenses with no visible line separating the distance from the add. They are visually less satisfactory than bifocals or plain reading lenses because of the progressively narrower field of view as the eye moves down to look through stronger parts of the lens, and because lateral head movement rather than normal eye movement is needed to reduce peripheral optical distortions.

CONTACT LENSES

Contact lenses rest on the surface of the cornea. The same principles of refraction and optics apply to contact lenses as apply to spectacle lenses. Contact lenses replace the corneal curvature with a contact lens surface that is calculated to correct the refractive error of the eye. Contact lenses offer cosmetic benefits and their small diameter and thinness may provide optical advantages in high degrees of ametropia by reducing peripheral distortions. Since most astigmatism is a result of the toricity of the front corneal surface, rigid (hard) contact lenses will usually eliminate that astigmatism. In the case of soft lenses, which mold to the surface of the cornea, the front surface of the soft lens also becomes toric and the astigmatism will persist. This is referred to as *residual astigmatism*. Residual astigmatism is occasionally found with rigid lenses also, especially when the astigmatism is due to lenticular astigmatism. Patients with keratoconus or other irregular corneal contours can achieve better vision with contact lenses as compared to spectacles. The advantages for those engaged in athletics or with special occupational needs are obvious.

HARD LENSES

Hard lenses are made of polymethyl methacrylate (PMMA) and are relatively rigid and durable. They are easy to clean, and may be stored wet or dry. Since oxygen solubility in tears is limited, a satisfactory flow of tears must be maintained to prevent corneal epithelial decompensation [and the resulting overwear syndrome.]

GAS-PERMEABLE LENSES

Lenses made of cellulose acetate butyrate (CAB), silicone, and silicone cross-linked with PMMA exhibit varying degrees of oxygen permeability and interfere less with corneal epithelial metabolism than lenses made purely of PMMA. They result in reduced corneal edema and reduced incidence of overwear.

DAILY SOFT-WEAR LENSES

Daily soft-wear lenses are made of hydroxyethyl methacrylate or related polymers and have the unique characteristic of retaining a large volume of water but still retaining their shape. This high water content contributes to their comfort, easy adaptability, and use for intermittent wear. Oxygenation of the cornea is less of a problem with soft lenses, but still limits the amount of time they may be worn continuously.

EXTENDED-WEAR CONTACT LENSES

The approach of wearing contact lenses continually was originally developed in response to the needs of aphakic patients. However, several problems have been encountered with continuous-wear contact lenses, including tight lens syndrome, corneal edema, corneal molding, corneal vascularization, corneal infections, and iritis. They fall into three categories: (a) 55–80% high water content soft lenses, (b) CAB or PMMA–silicone copolymer rigid lenses, and (c) semisoft pure silicone lenses. The risk of developing ulcerative keratitis was 10 to 15 times greater in extended-wear users who kept them in overnight compared to daily-wear users who removed lenses each night. The FDA has changed its recommendation for extended-wear contact lens use to their being removed and cleaned once weekly as opposed to the originally recommended once-monthly regimen.

DISPOSABLE SOFT CONTACT LENSES

Disposable soft contact lenses are worn for 1 week, discarded, and replaced with a new lens after an overnight without lenses in the eyes. Their advantages include convenience, comfort, less lens tightening, and reduced incidence of giant papillary conjunctivitis and red eye.

TORIC SOFT LENSES

Soft lenses that correct astigmatism are referred to as toric. In order to keep the axes of these lenses in the proper position on the cornea, their rotation must be minimized. Truncation or ballast is used alone to decrease rotation on the cornea. Truncation results in an asymmetric shape, and ballast results in asymmetric weight distribution.

BIFOCAL CONTACT LENSES

Bifocal contact lenses either have a central area to correct far vision and a peripheral concentric area to correct near vision or have a semicircular add area along one edge, combined with truncation or ballast to stabilize the lens when the eye moves down to look at a near object. Many presbyopic patients benefit from a different approach, known as monovision, in which the dominant eye is corrected for distance vision and the nondominant eye is corrected for near vision with conventional single-vision contact lenses.

REFRACTIVE SURGERY

LASIK (LASER IN SITU KERATOMILEUSIS)

Correction of refractive errors may be achieved surgically by altering the curvature of the cornea, the length of the eye, or the index of refraction of the ocular media. Given that the majority of the refractive power of the eye occurs at the air–cornea interface, changing the corneal surface curvature is a very efficient way of surgically correcting ametropia. Only a minimal amount of refraction occurs at the corneal–aqueous interface. A greater amount occurs at the aqueous–lens–vitreous interfaces, given the higher index of refraction of the lens. Changing the lens curvature and implantation of phakic intraocular lenses are additional methods of correcting ametropia.

LASIK is a refractive surgical procedure in which a stromal corneal flap is created with a microkeratome and a refractive ablation is performed in the bed using the excimer laser. This procedure is primarily performed to reduce the patient's dependence on glasses and contact lenses. The exponential growth of LASIK refractive correction makes it the most commonly performed refractive surgery throughout the world today. The excimer or ultraviolet laser is applied to the midstroma after a flap has been lifted from the cornea to modify its radius of curvature. The biomechanical response of the corneal lamellae after creation of the flap may induce peripheral steepening and central flattening of the cornea.

The disadvantages of LASIK include microkeratome malfunction and flap malpositions. Optical aberrations are more frequent for higher degrees of myopia and hyperopia. Postoperative LASIK patients frequently have disturbed tear function for 1 or more months and should be managed with artificial tears and ointments to prevent surface damage. Despite these potential complications which occur in 1–4% of patients, more than 70% of LASIK patients do not need glasses after surgery, more than 90% of LASIK patients achieve 20/40 acuity without spectacles, and less than 2% of patients have one line of loss of spectacle-corrected acuity after surgery.

EXCIMER LASER PRK (PHOTOREFRACTIVE KERATECTOMY) AND LASEK (LASER SUBEPITHELIAL KERATOMILEUSIS)

EXCIMER LASER This procedure directly removes layers of tissue in the central cornea to resculpt the anterior refractive surface of the eye. Ultraviolet photons break molecular bonds, precisely ablating the Bowman membrane and the anterior corneal stroma while causing minimal residual thermal damage. This central area, or ablation zone, altered by PRK, produces corneal flattening over the visual axis, thus reducing myopia. The surgeon achieves the intended change in dioptric power by varying the diameter and depth of the ablation zone. Deeper ablations lead to greater corneal flattening, but may increase the risk of subepithelial haze caused by fibroblastic keratocytes and local collagen synthesis. Postoperative topical steroids are routinely prescribed for 1 to 3 months to limit haze and refractive regression through inhibition of normal wound healing. By changing the pattern of surface ablation, hyperopia and astigmatism can be corrected as well, but to date in a less predictable fashion.

Technique. Treatment of myopia can involve a single ablation or multiple ablations of different diameters, with multizone ablations often performed for higher degrees of nearsightedness. Although larger ablation zone sizes are desirable because they minimize the chance of optical side effects, the depth of the ablation zone varies with the square of the diameter.

Significant corneal haze and loss of best-corrected vision are uncommon complications. Excimer laser PRK for higher levels of myopia and for hyperopia is somewhat less predictable. LASIK has virtually replaced PRK for higher levels of myopia and for hyperopia and higher degrees of myopia.

LASEK By cleaving the epithelial sheet at the basement membrane with dilute alcohol, applying the laser as in conventional PRK, and repositioning the epithelium afterward, there is some decrease in pain, quicker visual rehabilitation, and less haze than after a classic PRK procedure.

RADIAL KERATOTOMY AND ASTIGMATIC KERATOTOMY

RADIAL KERATOTOMY (RK) This procedure refers to the placement of deep paracentral and peripheral incisions in the cornea, producing central flattening and thus reducing central corneal refractive power and myopia. The most accepted theory holds that normal intraocular pressure (IOP) pushes out the peripheral cornea weakened by the incisions, leaving a relatively flatter center. Incisions are ideally 85% to 95% of corneal depth. Deeper incisions give greater flattening effect, but should not extend to the Descemet membrane to avoid the danger of mechanical instability and perforation. Incisions that approach the pupil center produce greater corneal flattening, but any incision breaching a 3-mm optical zone diameter runs a higher risk of producing disabling glare and irregular astigmatism.

Results. The National Eye Institute–sponsored Prospective Evaluation of Radial Keratotomy (PERK) Study began gathering data in 1980 on 427 patients (793 eyes) who underwent a standardized eight-cut RK with 4.0, 3.5, and 3.0 mm optical zones for low, moderate, and high myopes, respectively. The surgical nomogram did not adjust for patient age or astigmatism. There were few subsequent enhancements (12%). The 10-year follow-up results showed an uncorrected visual acuity of 20/40 or better in 855 of all eyes operated on, including 92% of low myopes (-1.50 to -3.12 D), 86% of moderate myopes (-3.25 to -4.37 D), and 77% of high myopes (-4.50 to -8.87 D). Overall, 70% of patients stated they no longer required corrective lenses for distance vision. Three percent of eyes lost two or three lines of spectacle-corrected visual acuity, with the poorest corrected vision no worse than 20/30; 98% of eyes were correctable to 20/20 or better. Forty-three percent of eyes had a $+1.00$ D or greater shift toward a more hyperopic refraction over the 10-year period.

ASTIGMATIC KERATOTOMY (AK) In this procedure transverse or arcuate incisions are placed perpendicular to the steepest corneal meridian to correct astigmatism. The incised meridian flattens while the meridian 90° away steepens by nearly the same amount. Incisions are ideally between 5 and 7 mm from the pupil center. As with RK, deeper, longer, and more centrally located incisions give greater effect, but increase the risk of irregular astigmatism, microperforation, and overcorrection. Irregular astigmatism refers to corneal astigmatism that cannot be corrected by spherocylindrical lenses and requires application of a rigid contact lens to elicit best-corrected visual acuity; irregular astigmatism is generally not amenable to correction by AK.

Examples of irregular astigmatism also include keratoconus and contact lens warpage.

INTRACORNEAL RING SEGMENTS

Intra corneal ring segments (ICRS) are placed in the peripheral cornea and act by compressing the peripheral cornea and changing the radius of curvature of the central cornea. The second mechanism takes advantage of the fact that the arc of the cornea (the distance from limbus to limbus) remains constant at all times, so when the anterior surface is lifted focally over the ring, a compensatory flattening of the central cornea occurs. ICRS are threaded into a peripheral stromal tunnel of 68% depth. A potential advantage of intracorneal segments over other refractive surgical techniques is reversibility. The main drawback is the limited range of correction (up to -3 D in myopia and up to $+2$ D in hyperopia).

PHAKIC INTRAOCULAR LENSES

The iris-claw lens originally devised by Worst for the correction of aphakia was later modified by Fechner et al to correct high myopia in phakic patients. It is enclaved in the midperipheral, less mobile iris and currently requires a 6.00 mm incision for its insertion. The angle-supported phakic IOL was originally used for the correction of myopia and has gone through several modifications. Long-term follow-up has reported progressive pupil ovalization with an older model. The posterior chamber phakic IOL was introduced in 1990. It must accommodate to the space between the posterior iris and the crystalline lens. If it vaults too much, pigment dispersion and even papillary block glaucoma could result. If it lies against the anterior surface of the crystalline lens, cataract could result. Long-term follow-up is needed for all types of phakic IOLs regarding endothelial cell loss, glaucoma, iris abnormalities, cataract formation, and ease of explantation to determine the exact role of this form of optical correction.

3 ORBIT

Scott Lee
Don Liu

ORBIT: AN INTRODUCTION

- The orbit, loosely defined, contains the structures required for ocular function, i.e., the globe, extraocular muscles, blood vessels, fatty tissue, nerves, and extracellular matrix
- With respect to anatomy, the globe and septum divide the orbit into anterior and posterior compartments. The former consists of the external structures, i.e., eyelids and the lacrimal system. The latter is termed the retrobulbar space, and comprises the intraconal (optic nerve) and extraconal spaces. The cone is formed by the extraocular muscles that form a wedge shape.
- Orbital disease can be classified in four major categories: trauma, infection, tumors, and inflammatory/autoimmune disorders.

TRAUMA

ORBITAL HEMORRHAGE

CASE 1

A 27-year-old computer technician came to the emergency department because he could not open his left eye. During a fight in a bar, he was struck in that eye with a fist. Lid retractors were used to gently open the lids, and visual acuity of 20/25 was obtained. There was marked proptosis. Extraocular movements were moderately restricted in all directions. There was subconjunctival hemorrhage. The pupil was normal. The intraocular pressure (IOP) was 25 mm Hg. Dilated fundus examination was limited because of the lid swelling, but no definite abnormalities were seen. An x-ray of the orbits was negative.

PATHOPHYSIOLOGY

- Retrobulbar bleeding is the result of blunt, penetrating, or surgical trauma.

- Blood in the orbit acts like a space-occupying lesion and causes proptosis. Blood may dissect into the lids, causing ecchymoses (Fig. 3-1).

CLINICAL FEATURES

- Patients present with ecchymoses and often proptosis.
- Extraocular movements may be restricted depending on the severity of bleeding.
- Increased IOP may compromise the retinal or optic nerve circulation.

DIAGNOSIS AND DIFFERENTIAL

- Physical examination. Associated eye injuries must be ruled out.

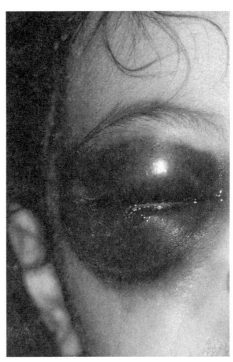

FIGURE 3-1 Orbital or retrobulbar hemorrhage. There is proptosis, severe ecchymoses of the lids, and lid closure. This child is not in acute distress despite the appearance of the external findings. There is no globe injury.

- Orbital x-ray or computed tomography (CT) scan may be indicated to rule out an orbital fracture (see Orbital Fracture below).
- Orbital cellulitis, abscess, and tumor must be considered in the differential.

TREATMENT

- Most cases require no treatment.
- If a markedly elevated IOP and central retinal artery pulsations are observed, a lateral canthotomy and cantholysis are recommended to immediately decompress the orbit.
- Additional treatment with acetazolamide, mannitol, and/or anterior chamber paracentesis may be warranted.

ORBITAL FRACTURE

CASE 2

A 30-year-old professional basketball player was struck in the right eye with an elbow while going up for a rebound. She had immediate pain and blurring. Examination disclosed vision of 20/40 OD (right eye) and 20/15 OS (left eye). The lids OD were swollen, and subconjunctival hemorrhage was present. There was no proptosis. She had hypesthesia of the right cheek. The pupil was normal. Extraocular movements showed restriction of supraduction OD with diplopia. Dilated fundus examination showed possible macular edema. An x-ray of the orbits showed opacification of the right maxillary sinus. A CT scan of the orbits showed a fracture of the orbital floor on the right, with herniation of tissue into the maxillary antrum.

PATHOPHYSIOLOGY

- Direct force to orbital bones may lead to fracture. The more fragile medial and inferior walls of the orbit may "blow out" secondary to increase in orbital pressure from trauma.

- Orbital roof fractures are rare.
- Diplopia may result from muscle entrapment, edema, or neuromuscular damage. The latter may be distinguished from muscle entrapment by the forced duction test (pulling directly on the eye). Entrapped muscles will resist forced movements (Fig. 3-2).
- Enophthalmos and ptosis are other potential sequelae of orbital blow-out fractures.

CLINICAL FEATURES

- Patients present with blunt orbital trauma.
- With muscle involvement or nerve impingement, diplopia will be present.
- A decrease in vision signifies impingement of the optic nerve by hematoma or bony fragment.

DIAGNOSIS AND DIFFERENTIAL

- History and physical examination, CT scan.
- Globe injuries must be ruled out by careful examination, as they are common with orbital fractures.
- Globe rupture is rare with orbital blow-out fracture, probably because pressure is relieved when the orbital wall gives way.
- Orbital hemorrhage must also be considered, i.e., soft tissue injury without fracture.

TREATMENT

- There are three treatment options: observation, high dose corticosteroids, and surgery. Corticosteroid treatment is controversial in compressive optic neuropathy, as many studies show no benefit.
- Indications for surgical repair of blow-out fractures include: (1) early enophthalmos, (2) persistent diplopia with muscle entrapment, (3) a large fracture likely to cause late enophthalmos.
- Antibiotics are administered judiciously after assessing the immunologic state of the patient. It is often best to wait 2 weeks until periorbital swelling decreases to reassess treatment.

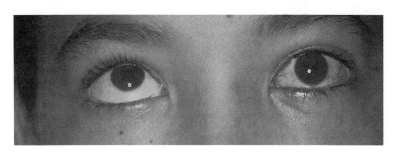

FIGURE 3-2 Blow-out fracture. This is a typical "white-eye" blow-out fracture in youngsters. The involved eye has minimal inflammatory signs, but the motility is limited.

- Fractures that involve the orbital rim generally require repair. Posterior fractures that may injure the optic nerve are uncommon, but serious. If imaging studies confirm bone fragments (or a foreign body) impinging on the optic nerve, then surgery may be indicated.

OPEN GLOBE INJURIES

CASE 3

While fishing with his father and younger brother, a 12-year-old boy was struck in the right eye with a fish hook. He had immediate severe pain. His father reported that he quickly took the hook out of his son's eye, but he could not remember how he did it. Examination disclosed vision of 20/100 OD and 20/15 OS. The pupil OD was teardrop shaped and poorly reactive. There was a 4-mm laceration of the cornea with brown tissue in the wound. The left eye was normal.

At surgery with an operating microscope, the iris that had been incarcerated in the wound was reposited in the anterior chamber. The corneal wound was closed with interrupted 10/0 nylon sutures. The pupil was dilated and the fundus inspected. It was normal. Vision returned to 20/20. The pupil remained slightly oval and poorly reactive to light.

PATHOPHYSIOLOGY

- Open globe injuries may be due to sharp injury (laceration) or blunt injury (globe rupture) or may involve retained foreign bodies.

CLINICAL FEATURES

- Patient presentation can be quite varied.
- Patients generally give a history of some trauma or mechanism of foreign body entry.
- Visual acuity is generally affected with traumatic injury to eye structures.
- A corneal laceration may be present with the entry site of trauma, as well as subconjunctival hemorrhage, a soft globe, and/or non-round pupil (Fig. 3-3).

DIAGNOSIS AND DIFFERENTIAL

- The history is extremely important in ocular injuries. Any patient with ocular pain, decreased vision, extensive subconjunctival hemorrhage, a soft globe, or a

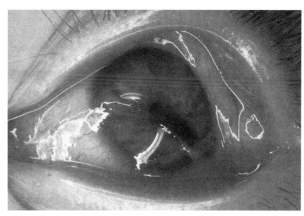

FIGURE 3-3 Ruptured globe. Note flat anterior chamber and oval pupil. (See Color Plate.)

non-round pupil after an injury should be suspected of having an open globe.
- Any patient with these symptoms who was hammering, grinding, using power tools, etc., should be suspected of having an intraocular foreign body.
- X-rays or CT scans are essential in cases of suspected intraocular foreign body.
- In the differential, any of the above signs may occur after injury without an open globe. The index of suspicion should be high, and examination by an ophthalmologist is necessary to rule out an open globe.
- Blunt injuries have a better prognosis than lacerating injuries. Anterior lacerations have a better prognosis than posterior lacerations, i.e., those that involve the retina. With lens injury, additional surgery may be required.

TREATMENT

- Prompt surgery is almost always indicated for open globe injuries.

RETAINED ORBITAL VEGETABLE FOREIGN BODY

CASE 4

A 44-year-old gardener complains of swollen left lower lid with drainage. He also notices some vague discomfort in the left orbit. His vision is 20/20 OD and 20/25 OS. His ocular motility appears full but with signs of discomfort. There is a small draining fistula in the left lower lid.

He was hit in the left eye by a branch 4 months ago. Immediately following the initial injury he was treated by an ophthalmologist. Reportedly, several wooden particles were removed from his left lower lid. The wound was thoroughly cleansed before closure. Postoperatively, he had applied topical antibiotics for 2 weeks. Four weeks later, his left lower lid became swollen and had some discharge. Oral antibiotics helped to quiet it down. A few weeks later his symptoms recurred when he discontinued the antibiotics. Incision and drainage of the left lower lid was performed and no foreign body was identified. A CT scan of the orbits showed no foreign body.

PATHOPHYSIOLOGY

• Infection and chronic inflammation caused by retained vegetable matter.

CLINICAL FEATURES

• Symptoms and signs may vary a great deal. Some may have minimal erythema in the lid, some discharge, little pain on eye movement, and normal vision. Others may present with decreased vision, recent onset of strabismus, eye pain, proptosis, or orbital cellulitis (Fig. 3-4).

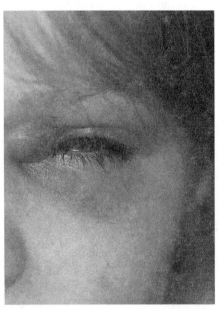

FIGURE 3-4 Retained orbital foreign body. This youngster rode a four wheeler into a bush and sustained facial laceration. Several weeks after the initial repair, the left eye became red and irritated. There is persistent, recurrent drainage in the medial canthus despite antibiotics and surgical debridement.

DIAGNOSIS AND DIFFERENTIAL

• A high index of suspicion is the most important factor in making the correct diagnosis.
• Typically the patient presents with a history of recurring or worsening symptoms despite initial successful treatment or temporary improvement when using antibiotics.
• History is not always clear cut. One needs to elicit from the patient history a seemingly insignificant injury that occurred many weeks or months ago.
• During initial examination, one needs to look for seemingly insignificant wounds in the lid and conjunctiva.
• CT, magnetic resonance imaging (MRI), and ultrasound are not helpful in identifying small vegetable matter.

TREATMENT

• Surgical exploration and removal of retained foreign body is the definitive treatment.

INFECTION

The orbits are predisposed to infection for three reasons:
• Their proximity to paranasal sinuses, which are often infected;
• The thin lamina papyracea is not a functional barrier with infection of the ethmoidal sinuses
• The veins of the orbit do not have valves and serve as another conduit for infection.

ORBITAL CELLULITIS

CASE 5

A 10-year-old boy had rhinorrhea and a low-grade fever. After a few days, his left eye began to swell and his fever was worse. He complained of pain. His pediatrician found a temperature of 39.5°C, lid erythema and swelling, and proptosis. The ophthalmic consultant confirmed these findings, and noted marked decrease in extraocular movements. There was conjunctival chemosis. The vision was 20/20 OU (both eyes), and pupils and fundi were normal. An x-ray showed opacification of the left maxillary antrum and ethmoid. Blood cultures grew *Haemophilus influenzae* (H. flu). Antibiotics were started, but the proptosis became worse. An oto-laryngologist was consulted, and the sinuses were drained. The proptosis and other abnormalities gradually resolved.

PATHOPHYSIOLOGY

- Ethmoidal or paranasal sinusitis spread is the most common cause of orbital cellulitis, although cutaneous trauma, hematogenous spread from bacteriemia, and dacrocystitis are other causes.
- *H. flu, Staphylococcus,* and *Streptococcus* are the most common infective organisms in that order.

CLINICAL FEATURES

- Patients present with decreased vision, proptosis, and restricted eye movement. There is often increased IOP and chemosis (see Fig. 3-5A–D).

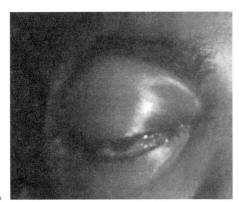

A

FIGURE 3-5A Orbital cellulitis. This teenager has decreased vision, proptosis, and pain on movement. He also looks toxic.

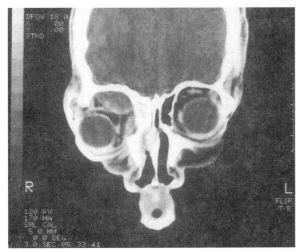

B

FIGURE 3-5B CT scan of the same teenager shows two sub-periosteal abscesses.

- Systemic symptoms include fever, headache, malaise, and rhinnorhea.
- Tenderness of the affected orbit and surrounding areas is present.

DIAGNOSIS AND DIFFERENTIAL

- History and examination, x-ray for sinus evaluation, and CT scan to evaluate for abscesses are essential.
- Blood work includes a complete blood cell count (CBC) and blood cultures.
- On MRI, orbital cellulitis appears hypointense on T1- and hyperintense on T2-weighted images.

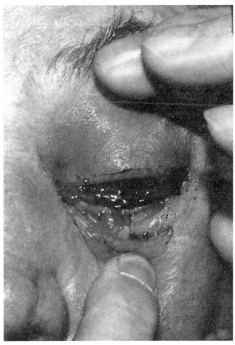

C

FIGURE 3-5C Orbital abscess in an adult with diabetes. (See Color Plate.)

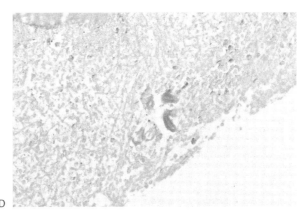

D

FIGURE 3-5D Mucormycosis organisms demonstrated on silver stain.

- Preseptal cellulitis should be monitored for progression to orbital cellulitis.
- Both preseptal and orbital infections present with pain, edema, and erythema. Only the latter will present with proptosis, chemosis, and difficulty with eye movement. Further, with the invasion of pathogens in the intraconal space, impingement of the optic nerve can be observed, and a decrease in vision.
- Other diagnoses to be considered include periorbital cellulitis, dysthyroid exophthalmos (no fever or pain), orbital tumor (no fever or pain), orbital pseudotumor (no fever or pain).

TREATMENT

- Hospitalization with appropriate IV (intravenous) antibiotics including cefotaxime, ceftriaxone with clindamycin.
- Watch for complications, i.e., neurologic symptoms, meningitis, visual loss.
- Surgery is indicated if there is a poor response to antibiotics within 48 to 72 h, or if the CT scan shows the sinuses to be completely opacified.
- Sinus drainage is much more common than orbital abcess drainage.
- HiB (haemophilus influenzae type B) vaccine for prevention.

PRESEPTAL CELLULITIS

CASE 6

A 5-year-old girl was bitten near the right upper lid by an insect. There was mild lid swelling, which initially improved with application of ice. Two days later, lid swelling became worse, and there was considerable erythema. Her temperature was 38°C. An ophthalmologist found normal acuity, full eye movements, and normal pupils. There was no proptosis. Culture of the area of the insect bite grew *Staphylococcus aureus*. The patient improved rapidly on antibiotic therapy.

PATHOPHYSIOLOGY

- Inflammation of structures anterior to the orbital septum, are most commonly by infection with H. flu.
- Causes arise from trauma, insect bites, and, rarely, hordeolum (stye).
- Pupillary reaction, visual acuity, and motility are intact in contrast to orbital cellulitis. Proptosis is not present, in contrast to orbital cellulitis (Fig. 3-6A–B).

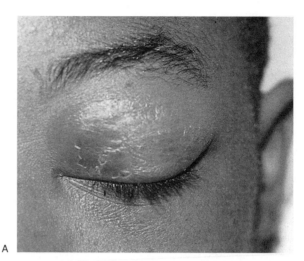

A

FIGURE 3-6A Preseptal cellulitis in a child. There is lid edema and evidence of possible insect bite. Patient is not in distress. (See Color Plate.)

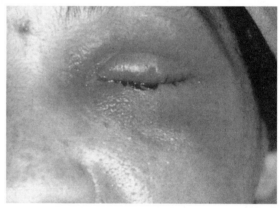

B

FIGURE 3-6B Preseptal cellulitis in an adult. There is diffuse erythema in the periorbital area but there is no proptosis, pain on movement, or decreased vision. (See Color Plate.)

CLINICAL FEATURES

- Patients present with pain, conjunctivitis, epiphora, erythema, and edema of affected regions.
- Patients may have a prior history of hordeola, chalazia, bug bites, upper respiratory tract infection (URI), or trauma.
- Visual acuity changes are generally not present.
- Children are susceptible if not Hib vaccinated. They will then present with concomitant fever and URI.

DIAGNOSIS AND DIFFERENTIAL

- After a thorough history and physical examination, a CT scan is warranted to rule out orbital pathology.

- Preseptal cellulitis on CT imaging appears with a hyperintense signal of swelling of the anterior orbital tissues and obliteration of the fat planes. The septum often functions as a barrier to further spread of infection. With progressive involvement of posterior structures, there will be an increase in the illumination of orbital fat on CT. Further, discrete densities begin to form, and ultimately orbital cellulitis may develop.
- The differential includes orbital cellulitis, conjunctivitis, and contact dermatitis.

TREATMENT

- Children should be managed aggressively, especially if the possibility of systemic infection exists, i.e., hospitalization and IV antibiotics. (ceftriaxone and vancomycin).
- Oral antibiotics are usually sufficient for adults: cefaclor, amoxicillin, or erythromycin.

TUMORS

RHABDOMYOSARCOMA

CASE 7

A 6-year-old boy was brought to his pediatrician because of a "swollen eye." There was nothing to suggest infection, and an allergic reaction was suspected. When his proptosis rapidly worsened, he was referred. The pediatric ophthalmologist noted proptosis and restricted eye movements. CT scan demonstrated an orbital mass.

PATHOPHYSIOLOGY

- Tumor of striated muscle in the orbit.
- Four types in order of commonality: embryonal (two thirds of cases, most often in the superior nasal quadrant) botryoid, alveolar (worst prognosis), and pleomorphic (best prognosis). Growth of tumor leads to rapidly developing exophthalmos, lid edema, and down and out displacement of globe, a palpable mass, and ptosis (Fig. 3-7).
- With rapid growth, destruction of orbital bone and invasion into the cranial cavity is observed.

CLINICAL FEATURES

- Rhabdomyosarcoma is the most common orbital tumor in childhood (but still a rare entity). Usually presents before age 10.

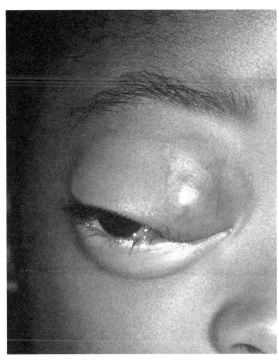

FIGURE 3-7 Rhabdomyosarcoma. This 6-year-old had a lid mass thought to be a chalazion removed 1 week prior to presentation. He now has a large orbital mass with proptosis and downward-outward displacement of the globe. (See Color Plate.)

- In the initial stages of growth of the tumor, patients often present with only proptosis.
- With progression, extraocular eye movements can be affected.
- Loss of vision and pain are uncommon.

DIAGNOSIS AND DIFFERENTIAL

- CT scan may confirm bony destruction and invasion of the tumor.
- Biopsy confirms diagnosis. Examine for metastases throughout the body.
- Other tumors of childhood include orbital pseudotumor, cysts, metastases, lymphangioma, capillary hemangioma, optic nerve glioma, and metastatic neuroblastoma.

TREATMENT

- Treatment includes limited surgical excision, chemotherapy, and radiation.
- Prognosis is good if the tumor has not metastasized; cure rate >90%.

CAVERNOUS HEMANGIOMA

CASE 8

A 34-year-old woman came to the ophthalmologist because her right eye looked prominent. This seemed to be slowly worsening over a year or more. She had her spectacle prescription changed by an optometrist twice during that time, and her prescriptions revealed increasing hyperopia. Examination showed vision with correction of 20/20 OU. The right globe was proptotic. There was a slight restriction of extraocular movement at the extremes of gaze OD. A CT scan revealed an intraconal mass.

PATHOPHYSIOLOGY

- Cavernous hemangioma is the most common adult benign tumor of the orbit.
- These tumors are composed of large endothelium-lined vessels with smooth muscle in their walls. There is a predilection in 30- to 50-year-old women.
- Growth of the tumor may cause increased IOP, optic nerve compression, choroidal folds, and hyperopia. Tumor growth is generally slow and unilateral. Lagophthalmos occurs in advanced disease and is rare.

CLINICAL FEATURES

- Patients present with a slow and progressive bulging of usually one eye, change in visual acuity secondary to mass effect, diplopia secondary to mass effect on extraocular muscles, and fullness or sensation of mass present in the eye.
- On external examination, asymmetry can be observed, as well as resistance to retropulsion of the globe. If a Hertel's exophthalmeter is available, the degree of proptosis can be monitored.
- Color vision or relative afferent pupillary defect changes indicate a possible compressive optic neuropathy.

DIAGNOSIS AND DIFFERENTIAL

- A CT scan will show a well-circumscribed, homogeneous lesion (Fig. 3-8). Ultrasound A-scan will likewise show a homogeneous region of high echogenicity.
- The differential includes other orbital tumors, i.e., neurolemmoma, hemiangiopericytoma, histiofibrocytoma, neurofibroma, as well as other vascular lesions that can present similarly.

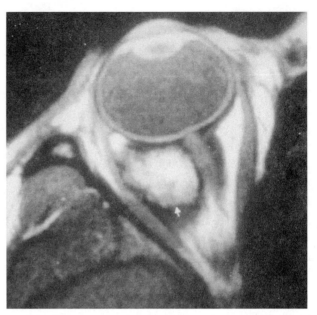

FIGURE 3-8 Cavernous hemangioma. Typically, a well-defined intraconal lesion is demonstrated on CT.

TREATMENT

- Conservative management with observation of symptoms is generally sufficient, unless vision is affected.
- Blunt dissection after a lateral orbitomy is the usual method of tumor excision. Cryoprobe and laser are other less used options.
- Prognosis is good with surgical removal of the tumor.

ORBITAL DERMOID CYSTS

CASE 9

A 65-year-old woman presents with a sensation of fullness around her right eye. An examination reveals no changes in visual acuity or tenderness to palpation. The CT scan demonstrates a small oval radiolucent lesion in the superior temporal aspect of the orbit.

PATHOPHYSIOLOGY

- Orbital dermoid cysts are considered aberrant growths or tumors of epithelial cells which are thought to arise from dermal or epidermal folds that have been cut off by suture lines during embryonic development.
- They may encase blood, fat, extracellular matrix, or serous fluid. These pockets may persist for some duration, and grow intermittently over a period of years.
- There is no known etiology for the induction of growth.

CLINICAL FEATURES

- Patients present with a lesion that has been increasing in size over a long time, sometimes many years.
- Most lesions are nontender and present in the superior temporal aspect of the orbit. Very rarely does the lesion result in a mass effect where vision is affected or proptosis is present, as with other tumors (Fig. 3-9A, B).
- The cyst may rupture, showing a cellulitis pattern of presentation.

DIAGNOSIS AND DIFFERENTIAL

- A CT scan or MRI shows an oval radiolucent lesion, often with the cyst eroding into bone.

TREATMENT

- Management is conservative with observation, as these lesions may regress. Inflammation from a ruptured cyst may be treated with a steroid, although resolution of symptoms will occur without medical treatment.
- Surgical excision is often employed only for cosmetic reasons.

CAROTID CAVERNOUS SINUS FISTULA

CASE 10

A 50-year-old man with longstanding hypertension and diabetes complains of visual changes over the past 2 years. His wife notes that his eyes appear to protrude more. In addition to dry eye and redness, his vision is less acute and he experiences occasional double vision. On examination, the eye appears to protrude outward with every heartbeat.

PATHOPHYSIOLOGY

Two types of carotid cavernous sinus fistula exist. *Direct fistulae* are characterized by a connection of the internal carotid to the cavernous sinus (80% of all lesions). These high-flow lesions are often secondary to trauma. *Dural fistulae* are characterized by a connection of the sinus with any of the meningeal branches of the internal or external carotid. These are low-flow lesions and are often associated with systemic disease, i.e., connective tissue disorders, hypertension, atherosclerosis.

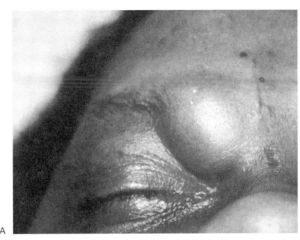

FIGURE 3-9A Epidermoid. A typical clinical picture in an adult.

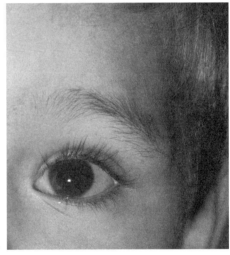

FIGURE 3-9B Dermoid in a child. Note bulge laterally OS, just under the brow.

CLINICAL FEATURES

- Patients present with red eye, bruit, diplopia, decreased visual acuity, proptosis, and, rarely, trigeminal neuralgia (Fig. 3-10A, B).
- On examination, pulsations of the globe with proptosis may be evident, in addition to secondary sequelae of exposure keratopathy, eyelid edema, vitreoretinal hemorrhage, increased IOP, and other manifestations of vascular fistula, such as a bruit.

DIAGNOSIS AND DIFFERENTIAL

- A CT scan or MRI may demonstrate enlargement of the affected cavernous sinuses, vascular dilatation, or muscle involvement.

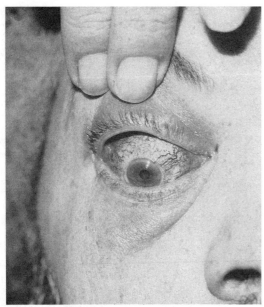

A

FIGURE 3-10A Carotid-cavernous fistula. Note proptosis and dilated episcleral vessels.

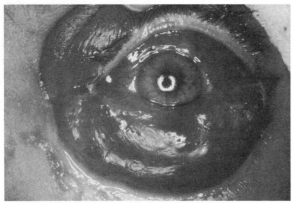

B

FIGURE 3-10B Conjunctival prolapse secondary to longstanding carotid-cavernous fistula.

• Angiography is the gold standard in determining the site of the lesion.

TREATMENT

• Primary care is directed to treating the secondary effects of the fistula, i.e., exposure keratopathy, glaucoma, and retinopathy.
• Direct fistulae are closed by surgical repair of the lesion if possible, or embolization and balloon occlusion.
• Dural fistulae are closed by endovascular balloon occlusion if possible. Cautery or direct surgical closure may also be attempted, but these carry a substantial risk for morbidity.

INFLAMMATORY DISORDERS

THYROID OPHTHALMOPATHY

CASE 11

A 45-year-old loan officer developed foreign body sensation, photophobia, and tearing in his left eye. Visual acuity was normal. Examination revealed proptosis and lid retraction on the left. There was resistance to retropulsion of the globes on palpation through the lids on both sides. Slit-lamp examination with fluorescein staining of the corneas showed superficial punctate corneal erosions inferiorly OS. Past history revealed treatment for Graves' disease 3 years ago.

Frequent use of artificial tears relieved his symptoms for a few months. He then had a recurrence. He also reported diplopia when reading. Reexamination disclosed a slight reduction in visual acuity OS, and increased proptosis. He had limitation of elevation and depression of the left eye. There was a large corneal epithelial erosion inferiorly OS. Medical treatment failed to heal the erosion, and he underwent a partial lateral tarsorrhaphy. The cornea healed.

PATHOPHYSIOLOGY

• Thought to be an autoimmune disease by humoral and cell-mediated components, it primarily affects females by a ratio of 4 to 1. Immunocytic infiltration of orbital tissue results in cytokine release. This triggers a cascade to increase fibroblast production of hyaluronic acid, subsequent osmotic load of muscle fibers, and the clinical presentation of Graves orbitopathy.
• Mild noninfiltrative orbitopathy results in upper lid retraction and proptosis, in contradistinction to other forms of proptosis (e.g., those due to masses) that do not exhibit upper lid retraction. Severe infiltrative orbitopathy can result in lid edema and chemosis, more severe proptosis with corneal exposure, and optic neuropathy (Fig. 3-11A–D).
• A mnemonic for the progression of disease: "NOSPECS," **N**o ocular signs/symptoms, **s**oft tissue swelling, **p**roptosis, **e**xtraocular muscle involvement, **c**orneal exposure, **s**ight loss from optic nerve involvement.[*]

[*]Friedman et al. MEEI Illustrated Manual of Ophthalmology, WB Saunders, 1998.

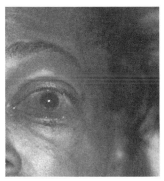

A

FIGURE 3-11A Dysthyroidism. Inflammatory signs may be asymmetric, as in this patient.

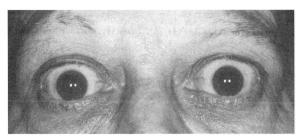

B

FIGURE 3-11B Bilateral upper lid retraction in a patient with dysthyroid eye disease.

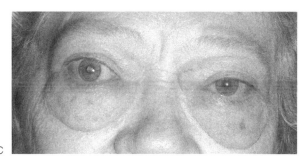

C

FIGURE 3-11C Severe lid edema in a patient with prolonged dysthyroid eye disease.

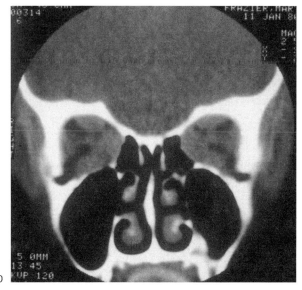

D

FIGURE 3-11D Enlarged extraocular muscles on CT scan.

CLINICAL FEATURES

- Patients may present with any combination of ophthalmic and systemic sequelae from a dysthyroid state.
- Ophthalmic sequelae include proptosis, dry eyes, eyelid edema, visual changes, and pain.
- Systemic hyperthyroidism manifests with anxiety, tachycardia, diaphoresis, and heat intolerance.
- Hypothyroidism manifests with depression, bradycardia, malaise, dry skin, and cold intolerance.
- Scleral show and lid lag on downgaze are prominent physical findings.
- Prolonged corneal exposure gives rise to keratopathies.
- Strabismus may be present secondary to muscle dysfunction, and optic nerve compression and glaucoma may also result from proptosis.
- Hertel exophthalmetric measurements may be useful in the measurement of the progression of the disease.

DIAGNOSIS AND DIFFERENTIAL

- First, a systemic diagnosis of a dysthroid condition is warranted.
- Thyroid lab tests, i.e., T4, T3 levels, and a CT scan to show extraocular muscle involvement are necessary. The CT scan often shows symmetrical and bilateral swelling of extraocular muscles; unilateral involvement is prevalent.
- The medial and inferior rectus muscles are most often involved. The body of the muscle in generally affected, sparing the tendinous attachments, giving a swollen tapered morphology on CT.
- If muscle involvement is unilateral or not symmetric, etiologies other than thyroid ophthalmopathy must be considered.
- Other diagnoses to be considered include: orbital pseudotumor, cellulitis, trauma, sarcoidosis, orbital mass, arteriovenous (AV) malformation, carotid-cavernous fistula, spontaneous or traumatic hematoma.

TREATMENT

- Acute management focuses on corneal protection.
- Thyroid levels should be managed if abnormal. Corticosteroids should be used to control infiltrative myopathy.

- External beam radiation to the orbital apex may also help to control inflammation (if within 7 months of onset).
- Surgical intervention may be necessary for decompression of the orbit and recession of the levator aponeurosis to protect the cornea, once it can be established that the orbitopathy has entered its quiescent phase (Hertel's graph).

ORBITAL PSEUDOTUMOR

CASE 12

A 50-year-old restaurant critic developed foreign body sensation, photophobia, and tearing in his right eye. Visual acuity was normal. Examination revealed proptosis and lid retraction on the right. There was resistance to retropulsion of the globes on palpation through the lids on both sides. Slit-lamp examination with fluorescein staining of the corneas showed superficial punctate corneal erosions inferiorly OS. Past history revealed no history of Graves' disease. CT demonstrated thickening of the extraocular muscles as well as tendons in the right eye.

PATHOPHYSIOLOGY

- Pseudotumor is non-neoplastic idiopathic inflammation of orbital tissue, not related to thyroid orbitopathy.
- Associated vasculidities include Wegener's granulomatosis.

CLINICAL FEATURES

- Presentation depends on affected orbital structures; 25% of presentations of unilateral proptosis are due to orbital pseudotumor.
- Symptoms, generally unilateral, include proptosis, chemosis, lid edema, and rapidly developing pain.
- The Tolosa-Hunt variant causes inflammation of the orbital apex and cavernous sinus leading to decreased visual acuity and painful ophthalmoplegia.

DIAGNOSIS AND DIFFERENTIAL

- The MRI often is best at detecting subtle early manifestations of pseudotumor, such as edema of the retrobulbar fat.
- A CT scan is generally standard procedure and reveals thickening of extraocular muscles and tendons (in contrast to thyroid ophthalmopathy without tendon involvement). The inferior rectus is most often involved (Fig. 3-12A–C).

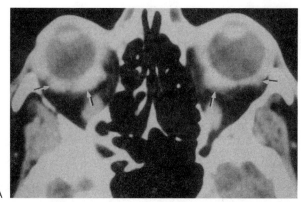

FIGURE 3-12A Orbital pseudotumor. Axial CT of orbits. Rarely, there is uveal scleral thickening, as seen in this patient.

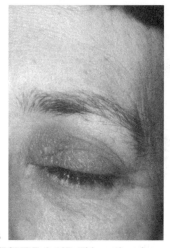

FIGURE 3-12B This patient has complete ptosis and limited ocular motility.

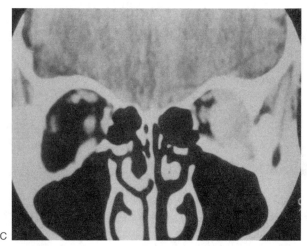

FIGURE 3-12C Orbital myositis, often thought of as a form of orbital pseudotumor. A massively enlarged extraocular muscle is demonstrated on CT scan.

- Other soft tissue densities with poorly defined margins are observed both in the intra- and extraconal spaces. Inflammation of the sclera and edema of the fluid in Tenon's space give rise to apparent scleral margin thickening.
- Pseudotumor must be differentiated from Graves ophthalmopathy and orbital lymphoma. In cases refractory to corticosteroids, a biopsy is warranted after the taper is finished. The histology of non-Hodgkins lymphoma is significantly altered with corticosteroid treatment.

TREATMENT

- Treatment includes systemic NSAIDs, corticosteroids, and, rarely, radiation.
- Surgery often exacerbates the inflammatory reaction.

4 OCULAR MOTILITY AND STRABISMUS

Daniel M. Laby

SENSORY ISSUES—NORMAL BINOCULAR VISION

- The human visual system is designed to use both eyes simultaneously to provide both a clear, well focused image over a wide field as well as information relating to the relative distances between objects.
- The relative distance between objects, otherwise known as *stereovision* or *3-D vision*, differs from other forms of depth perception in that both eyes must be used simultaneously for it to occur. Although depth perception is possible with only one eye (monocular depth perception), fine depth discrimination requires the use of both eyes.
- When both eyes are used simultaneously, identical images of the target fall on **corresponding retinal points** of each eye's retina. For example, when each eye is directed toward the point A (see Fig. 4-1), an image of point A falls on the fovea of each eye, thus each fovea is considered a corresponding point. When the corresponding point of each eye is the same, **normal retinal correspondence** is noted.
- Ideally, each eye, or visual axis, would be perfectly aligned toward a given target of gaze and normal stereovision would be achieved. Unfortunately, this is not the case. In most instances the visual axes are slightly misaligned and similar images do not fall on exactly corresponding retinal points.
- Fortunately, the human visual system is designed to correct these small imperfections in alignment by way of the **fusion** mechanism. There are two main types of fusion. One employs a neural process to correct slight imperfections in ocular alignment (**sensory fusion**), while the second process makes small physical changes in the direction of the visual axes to correct minor misalignments (**motor fusion**).
- **Sensory fusion** is defined as a neural process in which the retinal images from each eye are synthesized and correlated together to form a single visual image, without any change in the visual direction of either eye. For this to occur, the images of the target must fall on corresponding or nearly corresponding retinal points.

- **Motor fusion** requires a change in the direction of one or both eyes designed to physically create the condition where corresponding retinal points are directed toward the same target. Motor fusion can occur by moving one eye alone or both eyes together.
- Both sensory and motor fusion occur as a result of similar visual targets falling on different retinal points (i.e., noncorresponding). Both types of fusion correct this inconsistency by either physically changing the visual direction so that similar images of the target fall on corresponding points (motor fusion) or changing the neural interpretation of the corresponding retinal points (sensory fusion).
- Only when the two eyes are correctly aligned and functioning normally together is the visual system capable of fine depth perception. Fine depth perception, otherwise known as *stereopsis*, is created when almost identical images are seen by each eye, with only a small portion of each image being slightly different. The human visual system interprets this difference as depth relative to the position in physical

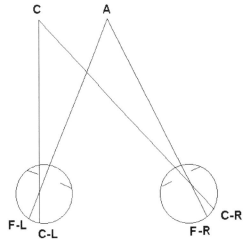

FIGURE 4-1 Diagram illustrating normal retinal correspondence. Both the left (L) and right (R) eyes are directed toward target A. Since the retinal point on which the target's image falls is the same in each eye (F), retinal points F-L and F-R are considered corresponding. In this example, since each eye is directed toward target A, the fovea (F) of the left eye correspond to the fovea of the right eye. A similar argument is made for point C, with corresponding retinal points C-L and C-R.

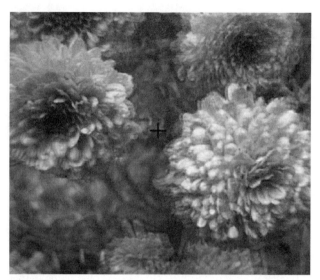

FIGURE 4-2 The centrally located "plus" sign is seen identically by both eyes, not stimulating any sense of three-dimensional depth. The images of the flowers, though, are slightly offset horizontally for each eye, thus stimulating a sense of three-dimensional depth (i.e., stereopsis).

space of that portion of the image, which is identical in each eye.

- Figure 4-2 demonstrates a target (the centrally located *plus* sign) seen identically in each eye. In this case, no depth is noted and the target appears two-dimensional. By adding an image that is composed of two parts, one part viewed only by the left eye and the other part viewed only by the right eye, the image can be made to "float" above the otherwise two-dimensional target. Physiologically, this image stimulates slightly noncorresponding points, allowing the brain to create a special form of sensory fusion called stereopsis. Thus, we learn that fusion is essentially a mechanism to create and maintain single vision, either for an entire image (as in sensory or motor fusion) or for a portion of an image that does not fall on corresponding points (as in stereopsis).

SENSORY ISSUES—ABNORMAL BINOCULAR VISION

- When the fusion system is unable to maintain normal binocular single vision, abnormal binocular vision is said to occur.
- **Diplopia** is the visual condition when two noncorresponding retinal images are stimulated by an identical target and the fusion mechanism is unable to create a single visual image of the target. In this case, the target is seen twice (once by each retinal point in each eye) in two different places.

- When corresponding retinal points are stimulated by different images, the visual condition termed **confusion** is created. In this case, two images, one seen by each eye, appear to be located at the same place in three-dimensional space.

- The human visual system can employ a technique termed **suppression** to deal with the diplopia or confusion created by misalignment of the visual axes. Unfortunately, suppression must be initially employed in youth (before the age of visual maturation), in order to be taken advantage of throughout life. In cases of ocular misalignment commencing after the age of visual maturation, the human visual system cannot employ this technique.

- **Suppression** is the process in which the brain specifically inhibits all or part of the retinal image from one eye when both eyes are simultaneously stimulated. Thus, in cases of diplopia and confusion, the brain can subconsciously ignore one of the abnormal images, thus resolving the diplopia or confusion that is present.

- Suppression is an immediate and constantly changing visual phenomenon, easily adaptable to the instantaneous needs of the visual system. In fact, there are several types of normal suppression, used by the visual system on an ongoing basis. The best example of this is when the visual system suppresses the moving image one might note when the eyes are rapidly moved from left to right horizontally. If physiologic suppression was not present, we would see a quick blur as our eyes scanned horizontally. A fast check will demonstrate that our brain suppresses the images transmitted by each eye until the horizontal saccade is completed and our eyes are directed toward the object of interest.

- Although in cases of ocular misalignment suppression is not binocular, it certainly is adaptable and changeable. When the visual axes are not aligned toward the same target (otherwise known as *strabismus*), suppression can be employed to resolve any diplopia or confusion that may be present. Suppression can be always present in one eye (**monocular suppression**) or can be present in either eye at different times, depending on which eye is aligned toward the target of interest (**alternating suppression**).

- In certain cases, suppression is not employed, and the normal fusion mechanisms cannot correct the disparity between the images formed by each eye. In these cases, known as *horror fusionis*, an intractable form of diplopia occurs that can be especially debilitating. This condition can occur in several clinical settings, such as after fusion has been disrupted for a prolonged period or head trauma has occurred with injury to the visual center.

- In cases of monocular suppression occurring before the age of visual maturation, a condition termed **amblyopia** can develop. Amblyopia is the presence of reduced visual acuity, without any latent or manifest disease responsible for the reduction. In addition, the reduced visual acuity cannot be corrected by refractive means (i.e., glasses or contact lenses).

- Although amblyopia is often present as a result of strabismus (**strabismic amblyopia**), it can be caused by other pathologic conditions. In cases of high refractive errors in one or both eyes, **refractive amblyopia** occurs. If there is a large difference between the refractive error in the right or left eye, where one eye has a chronically blurred retinal image, **anisometropic amblyopia** can occur. Finally, in cases where there is an obstruction to vision, such as in a congenital cataract, **deprivation amblyopia** can occur.

- The treatment for amblyopia, when instituted before the age of visual maturation, can be very effective. In addition to correcting the underlying cause of the

amblyopia (i.e., refractive lenses in refractive and anisometropic cases and surgery in the case of deprivational forms), one must stimulate the previously suppressed eye to be used. Stimulation is often achieved by an ocular occlusive patch over the fellow eye, or by pharmacological agents (e.g., atropine 'penalization') to purposely blur the fellow eye and stimulate use of the previously suppressed eye.

ANATOMY OF THE EXTRAOCULAR MUSCLES

- Each eye contains six extraocular muscles, responsible for moving the visual axis toward any given point of visual interest (Fig. 4-3).

- Two muscles, the medial rectus and the lateral rectus, are able to move the eyes only horizontally; the

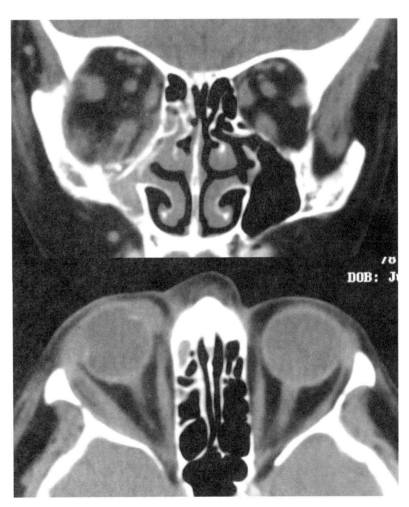

FIGURE 4-3 Axial and coronal computerized tomographs (CT) of the human orbits. Note the extraocular muscles (small circular areas) arranged around the orbital rim. The optic nerve can also be appreciated running from the orbital apex to the posterior portion of the eye.

remaining four muscles are able to move the eyes both horizontally and vertically, as well as circularly around the visual axis (torsion).

- The **medial rectus muscle** starts at the annulus of Zinn in the posterior orbit and courses forward along the medial orbital wall to insert on the eye at a point approximately 5.5 mm posterior to the limbus. The medial rectus muscle has only one possible action, to rotate the eye medially or toward the nose (termed *adduction*).

- The **lateral rectus muscle** also has an origin at the annulus of Zinn and progresses forward along the lateral orbital wall. The lateral rectus muscle inserts on the eye at a point 6.9 mm posterior to the lateral limbal region. The lateral rectus muscle has only one action, to move the eye laterally, toward the ear in a process termed *abduction*.

- There are two simple vertical muscles, the superior and inferior recti, as well as two special vertical muscles, termed the superior and inferior oblique muscles. All of these muscles have a primary action as well as two types of secondary actions.

- The **superior rectus muscle** originates at the annulus of Zinn and moves upward and anteriorly near the roof of the orbit. The muscle inserts on the eye at a point 7.7 mm posterior to the superior limbus. Of note is the fact that the muscle does not align with the visual axis of the eye, but instead forms an angle of 23° between the course of the muscle and the visual axis in the primary position. This difference between the muscle's path and the visual axis is responsible for the additional actions of this cyclovertical muscle. Although the primary or main action of this muscle is elevation, the special anatomic relationship between the muscle's path and the visual axis allows the muscle to act both as an adducting muscle and a rotator of the eye. The superior rectus muscle is able to *incyclotort*, or rotate, the superior portion of the eye medially, while the inferior portion of the eye is rotated temporally.

- The **inferior rectus muscle** follows a course similar to its companion muscle, the superior rectus. The inferior rectus muscle arises from the annulus of Zinn and courses forward along the orbital floor. The muscle inserts on the globe at a point 6.5 mm posterior to the inferior limbus. This muscle also forms a 23° angle between its length and the visual axis in the primary position. In this case, depression is the primary action of the inferior rectus muscle with additional actions of adduction and *excyclotorsion*.

- The **superior oblique muscle** originates from the annulus of Zinn and passes forward along the superomedial portion of the orbital roof. This muscle passes through a special cartilaginous structure termed the *trochlea* before inserting on the eye at a point posterior to the globe's equator in the superolateral quadrant. The superior oblique muscle has a long tendon, with the tendinous portion beginning prior to the passage through the trochlea. The trochlea is located in the anteromedial orbital rim and redirects the tendon of the superior oblique muscle posteriorly much like a pulley. The tendon forms a 51° angle with the visual axis, allowing for the multiple actions of the muscle. The superior oblique's primary action is *incyclotorsion*, while its unique anatomic path allows for depression of the globe as well as abduction.

- The **inferior oblique muscle** course is different from that of all the other muscles owing to its anterior origin. The inferior oblique muscle begins in the periosteum of the maxillary bone in the medial region of the orbital rim. The muscle passes posteriorly and laterally under the lateral rectus muscle, to insert at a point behind the equator in the posterolateral portion of the globe. This muscle also forms a 51° angle between its path and the visual axis in the primary position. The inferior oblique muscle's main action is excyclotorsion with secondary actions of elevation of the globe and abduction.

- The four rectus muscles are noted to insert on the eye in increasing distances from the limbus. The medial rectus inserts at 5.5 mm, the inferior rectus inserts at 6.5 mm, the lateral rectus at 6.9 mm, and the superior rectus at 7.7 mm. This clockwise spiral has been termed the *spiral of Tillaux*.

- There are three cranial nerves (CN) that provide neurologic innervation for the extraocular muscles. Two muscles are innervated by single nerves, and the remaining four muscles are innervated by the third cranial nerve (CN III).

- CN III (oculomotor nerve) is responsible for innervating the medial rectus, inferior rectus, and superior rectus, as well as the inferior oblique muscles. CN IV (trochlear nerve) innervates only the superior oblique muscle. CN VI (abducens nerve) innervates the lateral rectus muscle responsible for abduction.

- The blood supply for the extraocular muscles derives from the ophthalmic artery, a direct branch of the internal carotid artery as it emerges from the cavernous sinus. Many branches of the ophthalmic artery arise in the orbital region, with the medial and lateral muscular branches supplying the extraocular muscles. The lateral muscular branch supplies the lateral rectus, superior rectus, and superior oblique muscles; the medial muscular branch supplies the inferior rectus, medial rectus, and inferior oblique muscles. The muscular branches further subdivide into anterior ciliary arteries. Each rectus muscle has two anterior ciliary arteries, with the exception of the lateral rectus muscle, which has only

Muscle	Muscle Length	Tendon Length	Origin	Insertion	Primary Action	Innervation
Medial Rectus	40	4.5	Annulus of Zinn	5.5 mm from medial limbus	Adduction	CN III
Lateral Rectus	40	7	Annulus of Zinn	6.9 mm from lateral limbus	Abduction	CN VI
Superior Rectus	40	6	Annulus of Zinn	7.7 mm from superior limbus	Elevation	CN III
Inferior Rectus	40	7	Annulus of Zinn	6.5 mm from inferior limbus	Depression	CN III
Superior Oblique	32	26	Orbital Apex	posterior to equator supero-temporally	Intorsion	CN IV
Inferior Oblique	37	1	Anterior orbit	posterior to equator infero-temporally	Extorsion	CN III

FIGURE 4-4 Characteristics of each of the six extraocular muscles. Note that the superior oblique muscle has the longest tendon, while the inferior oblique has almost no tendon at all.

one. After supplying the muscles, the anterior ciliary arteries pierce the sclera to enter the eye and provide blood to the anterior segment structures.

- The venous system parallels the arterial system, with blood emptying into the superior and inferior orbital veins.
- Figure 4-4 summarizes the different actions of the extraocular muscles. Each muscle has a main action—its primary action—as well as possible secondary and tertiary actions. It is the combination of these actions that allows the visual system to finely align each visual axis on a target of interest and follow that target, either quickly or slowly as it moves in relationship to the surroundings. Each muscle has a primary action designed to move the eye in either direction along the x-y-z axis system. The medial rectus moves the eye horizontally (adduction), and the lateral rectus moves it in the opposite horizontal direction (abduction). The superior rectus muscle moves the eye upward (elevation), and the inferior rectus moves the eye down (depression). The superior oblique muscle rotates the 12 o'clock position of the eye nasally (incyclotorsion), and the inferior oblique muscle rotates the 12 o'clock meridian of the eye laterally (excyclotorsion). In addition, the vertical recti and oblique muscles have secondary actions that augment their fellow muscles' cyclovertical actions.

VOCABULARY OF EYE MOVEMENTS

- Ophthalmology, and strabismus in particular, contains a specific set of words that precisely describe physiologic occurrences. Although this list of terminology is not exhaustive, it contains the commonly referenced words in this discipline.
  - **Orthophoria**—The ocular condition where the two visual axes are pointed toward an identical fixation point, without the fusion mechanism being active. Otherwise known as perfect ocular alignment.
  - **Heterophoria**—The ocular condition occurring when the two visual axes are not aligned toward the same fixation point. Heterophoric types of alignment may be corrected via the fusion mechanism (a phoria) or may not be correctable, resulting in a manifest ocular misalignment (a tropia). Depending on the direction of the misalignment, an esotropia, exotropia, hypertropia, or cyclotropia may be present.
  - **Adduction**—Rotation of one eye medially or toward the midline.
  - **Abduction**—Rotation of one eye laterally or away from the midline.
  - **Elevation**—Upward rotation of the eye. Also known as supraduction or sursumduction.
  - **Depression**—Downward rotation of the eye. Also known as infraduction or deorsumduction.
  - **Incyclotorsion**—Also known simply as intorsion, describes the rotation of the eye around the y axis. In this case the 12 o'clock meridian of the eye rotates medially or toward the nose.
  - **Excyclotorsion**—Known simply as extorsion, this action rotates the 12 o'clock meridian of the eye laterally, or toward the ear.
  - **Version**—Conjugate movements of the two eyes in the same direction. Examples of this include dextroversion, where the two eyes move to the right, or infraversion, where the two eyes rotate downward.
  - **Vergence**—Disjunctive movements of the eyes in which the eyes move in different and opposite directions. Examples of this condition include convergence, where the eyes move in opposite directions toward the nose, or divergence where one eye moves left and the other moves to the right.
  - **Comitancy** (Fig. 4-5)—A descriptive strabismus term describing any difference in ocular misalignment occurring as a result of different fields of gaze (i.e., left versus right gaze, or vertical gaze positions). For example, an individual with a 25 prism diopter (D) esotropia in left gaze and 5 prism D of esotropia in right gaze would be considered to have a noncomitant (or incomitant) strabismus.
  - **Emmetropia**—The refractive state of the eye, occurring when accommodation is relaxed, in

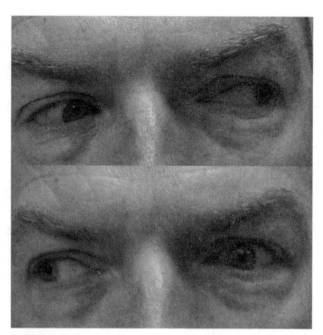

FIGURE 4-5 Restricted movement of the left eye in adduction is the cause for this patient's incomitant strabismus. Note normal ocular alignment in left gaze, with a large exotropia in gaze to the right.

which the eye is focused at infinity. Individuals with pure emmetropia do not require refractive correction in order to achieve normal vision at distance fixation. Although an ideal state, this condition is not often found in clinical practice.

- **Anisometropia**—An ocular condition in which the refractive state of the eyes differ significantly. One eye requires a different lens correction than the other. This can lead to an associated condition (aniseikonia) in which there is a marked difference in the size and/or shape of the images of the two eyes. Both conditions can interfere with a subject's ability to obtain and maintain normal binocular vision.
- Several different physiologic principles guide our understanding of ocular movements. Two of these, Sherrington's law of reciprocal innervations and Hering's law of equal innervation, are valuable in our understanding of strabismus.
  - **Sherrington's law**—This principle states that under normal conditions, the contraction of one muscle is accompanied by a simultaneous and proportional relaxation of its antagonist. If the medial rectus muscle contracts and adducts the eye, the lateral rectus muscle (responsible for the opposite action, i.e., abduction and thus the antagonist of the medial rectus muscle) will simultaneously and proportionally relax to allow the eye to rotate freely.
  - **Hering's law**—This principle states that the neurologic innervation to the extraocular muscles of each

eye is equal. This allows all movements of the two eyes to be equal and symmetrical. In cases where a muscle's movement in one eye is restricted, a secondary deviation may develop manifesting as *strabismus*, in which no misalignment is present when the muscles are at rest in the primary position.

ESODEVIATIONS

PSEUDOESOTROPIA (FIG. 4-6)

CASE 1

A 6-month-old child presents to the office after being referred by his pediatrician for crossed eyes. There is no family history of crossed eyes noted. The patient's birth history was normal, and he is in good physical health. The parents note that their child seems always to have both eyes crossed inward, toward the nose, all of the time, regardless of whether he is looking at near or at distance. Examination reveals normal fix-and-follow behavior, with a normal anterior and posterior segment. The refractive error is minimally hyperopic and the pupillary evaluation is normal. Although the child is able to move each eye normally, the eyes appear to be crossed inward, with less sclera showing in the nasal portions of the eyes as compared with the temporal portions. The Hirschberg corneal light reflex test shows

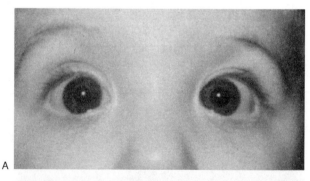
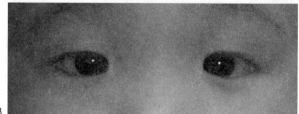

FIGURE 4-6 A, B Despite appearing to have a left esotropia, these young children have normally aligned eyes as demonstrated by the symmetrically placed corneal light reflexes.

equal and symmetrically centered reflexes on each cornea. A cover test, although difficult to perform, shows no movement of either eye on examination.

PATHOPHYSIOLOGY

A condition simulating esotropia, occurring when the visual axes are normally aligned. This condition may be caused by epicanthal folds or a relatively flat bridge of the nose.

CLINICAL FEATURES

An appearance of esotropia, although none is actually present.

DIAGNOSIS

Pseudoesotropia is differentiated from other, true strabismic conditions by the absence of eye movement on the cover test and the presence of symmetrically placed corneal light reflexes created by a hand-held flashlight.

DIFFERENTIAL

This condition is most often confused with infantile esotropia, which occurs in the same age population. In addition, unilateral or bilateral CN VI paresis can create a similar appearance.

TREATMENT

None is needed, since this condition does not represent a truly pathologic condition. The appearance often resolves spontaneously as the child grows and facial changes occur.

INFANTILE ESOTROPIA (FIG. 4-7)

CASE 2

A 6-month-old child presents to the office after being referred by his pediatrician for crossed eyes. There is a family history of crossed eyes in the maternal uncle, who had surgery as a child. The patient's birth history was normal, and his physical health is good. The parents report that their child seems to have one eye crossed inward, toward the nose, all of the time, regardless of

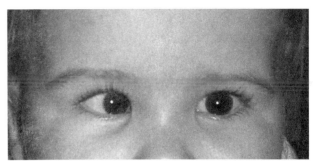

FIGURE 4-7 A true esotropic deviation is demonstrated in this young child whose corneal light reflexes are not symmetrically placed, indicating different direction of the left and right visual axis.

whether he is looking at near or at distance. When questioned further, the parents note that both the left eye and the right eye cross inward, each around 50% of the time. As in the preceding case, examination reveals normal fix-and-follow behavior, with a normal anterior and posterior segment. The refractive error is minimally hyperopic and the pupillary evaluation is normal. Although the child is able to move each eye normally, the eyes appear to be alternating between the left eye and the right eye crossing inward. The Hirschberg corneal light reflex test shows asymmetrically centered reflexes on each cornea. A cover test, although difficult to perform, shows movement of each eye on examination.

PATHOPHYSIOLOGY

Onset of esotropia between birth and 6 months of age. A family history is often present, although a precise inheritance pattern has not been identified. Although not associated with any other physical abnormality, up to 30% of children with cerebral palsy or hydrocephalus have this condition.

CLINICAL FEATURES

- Large-angle esotropia is often noted, frequently larger than 30 prism D. Typically, there is no preference for fixation with either eye, with each eye noted to turn inward about half the time.
- Cross-fixation is sometimes present, with both eyes crossed, allowing for the adducted eye to be used for viewing targets in the contralateral temporal field.
- Amblyopia is often not present, unless fixation is maintained with only one eye. A refractive error is usually normal for the child's age, with no accommodative component noted. The ocular rotations are

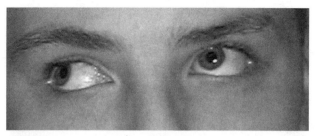

FIGURE 4-8 Overaction of the inferior oblique muscle is best demonstrated in adduction and slightly elevated gaze. This patient's left inferior oblique muscle is overactive as noted in the greater elevation and abduction of the left eye compared to the right.

often normal, although abduction may be limited by cross-fixation.

- Several muscular abnormalities are often associated with infantile esotropia. These include dissociated vertical deviations (DVD), inferior oblique muscle overaction (Fig. 4-8) and rotary or latent nystagmus.
- Dissociated vertical deviation describes a condition in which there is a disconnect between the right and left eye. Normally, when one eye moves upward or downward, the other eye moves in an identical direction. In DVD, the eyes no longer move together; one eye moves up or down while the fellow eye remains stationary.
- Overaction of the inferior oblique muscle is common in infantile esotropia, with the affected eye shooting upward on adduction. This condition may be unilateral or bilateral and may develop many months or even years after the initial onset of esotropia.
- Nystagmus is an often encountered complication of infantile esotropia, presenting as a manifest nystagmus or a latent type. The nystagmus is often rotary, but may be horizontal or vertical. Although this condition does not often require specific intervention, it may significantly complicate visual acuity testing if not noted and accounted for.

DIAGNOSIS

Infantile esotropia is diagnosed based upon a thorough history and physical evaluation. The age of onset and the family history of strabismus is important, as well as the evaluation for normal ocular movements and refractive errors. Care must be taken to ensure normal visual acuity in each eye, since amblyopia in this condition is often overlooked. Typically, a large-angle esotropia with alternate fixation at both distance and near is noted. Cross-fixation may be present as well, depending on the size of the deviation. The ocular rotations are essentially normal, although slightly decreased abduction may be

noted in each eye. The remainder of the ophthalmic evaluation is unremarkable.

DIFFERENTIAL

- Several conditions can mimic the appearance of infantile esotropia and must be excluded in order to make the correct diagnosis. Pseudostrabismus or pseudo-esotropia is often noted in the same age population, and represents a benign condition. The presence of asymmetric corneal light reflexes as well as movement on the cover test eliminates the presence of pseudostrabismus.
- Accommodative esotropia can atypically present in this age group as well. In this condition a higher than normal hyperopic refractive error is noted, as well as a smaller angle of esotropia. Occasionally, the near esotropia is larger than the distance misalignment in an accommodative form of esotropia.
- Congenital CN VI palsy must be considered in every case of infantile esotropia. Although abduction is occasionally limited in cases of infantile esotropia, the eye still is able to abduct (especially following the placement of an occlusive patch over the fellow eye). In cases of true CN VI palsy, the eye cannot abduct past the midline, indicating true lateral rectus underaction. This condition requires a significantly different evaluation plan including cranial imaging studies.

TREATMENT

Recent advances in our understanding of the development of binocular vision have changed the classic treatment plan for infantile esotropia. In the past, the esotropic deviation was surgically corrected after several years of age. Recent research suggests that in order to allow for the development of normal binocular cooperation, ocular misalignment should not be present for more than one year. In cases of infantile esotropia, this suggests correction prior to a child's first birthday. Surgery most often consists of a weakening procedure on the medial rectus muscle of each eye (a bilateral medial rectus recession, or BMR). Alternatively, some surgeons perform monocular surgery, weakening the medial rectus muscle and strengthening the lateral rectus muscle (informally called an "R and R" procedure). Each of these patients requires careful follow-up to be certain that no amblyopia develops and to treat any of the additional components of infantile esotropia that might develop (i.e., DVD and inferior oblique muscle overaction).

ACCOMMODATIVE ESOTROPIA (FIG. 4-9)

CASE 3

A 7-year-old child presents to the office after being referred by his pediatrician for crossed eyes. His mother has noted that the crossing was intermittent in the beginning, but is now more constant. There is a family history of accommodative esotropia in both his sister and his mother. Examination reveals decreased vision in one eye, with an equal refractive error of +4.50 D in each eye. After glasses are prescribed for the child, normal ocular alignment is noted. When the child removes his glasses, his eyes are found to be esotropic. Following a short period of ocular occlusive patching, vision returns to normal in each eye.

PATHOPHYSIOLOGY

All forms of accommodative esotropia share several characteristics. The age of onset is later than that of infantile esotropia, occurring between the ages of 6 months and 7 years. The average age of onset is $2\frac{1}{2}$ years. Often the esotropic deviation is intermittent at the outset only to become more constant as time passes. In addition, there is often a history of a similar condition present in one or more family members. Amblyopia is more common in this form of esotropia because of the smaller angles of deviation and the subject's propensity to use one eye exclusively.

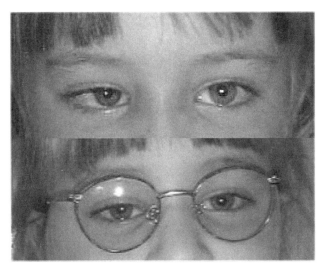

FIGURE 4-9 A young child with accommodative esotropia. The large-angle esotropia noted without glasses (*top panel*), fully resolves when hyperopia correcting glasses are used to limit accommodation (*bottom panel*).

CLINICAL FEATURES

Accommodative esotropia can be subdivided into two major groups. The first group has been termed *refractive accommodative esotropia* and the second group is called *nonrefractive accommodative esotropia*.

- Refractive accommodative esotropia occurs when there is a high hyperopic refractive error. When the subject accommodates to obtain clear vision, a significant esotropic deviation is produced. There exists a natural relationship between accommodation (A) and convergence (AC). This relationship has been termed the AC/A ratio. The average AC/A ratio is approximately 4:1 in young adults and tends to decline slightly throughout life. In cases of refractive accommodative esotropia, the excess accommodation created by the subject is the driving force behind the esotropic deviation.
- In nonrefractive accommodative esotropia, the hyperopic refractive error of the subject is normal and not excessive. In this condition the AC/A ratio is abnormally elevated, resulting in excessive convergence despite a normal amount of accommodation. The excess convergence in this condition is noted clinically as esotropia.

DIAGNOSIS

In cases of refractive accommodative esotropia, the hyperopic refractive error of the subject is usually between +3.00 and +10.00 D with an average refractive error of +4.00 D. The esotropic deviation is equal at distance and near and is usually between 20 and 30 prism D in magnitude. In cases of nonrefractive accommodative esotropia, the refractive errors are normal for age, averaging about +2.25 D. Often there may be little to no esotropia at distance fixation, and an esotropia of 20–30 prism D at near fixation. When the subject is given a small target requiring accommodation at near, the esotropia is often noted to increase. One hallmark of this condition is the resolution of esotropia at near when the subject is asked to use a +3.00 D lens for near fixation.

DIFFERENTIAL

This condition should be differentiated from both the pseudostrabismus condition and infantile esotropia. Often, many features of infantile esotropia overlap with this condition and the clinician is unable to distinguish one condition from the other. In these cases, a provisional diagnosis of accommodative esotropia should be made and treated accordingly. If the subject does not respond properly to this treatment, the final diagnosis of infantile esotropia can be made.

TREATMENT

- If cases of accommodative esotropia are left untreated, an esotropic deviation that may have initially responded to nonsurgical treatments will develop and need surgical correction.
- Treatment of refractive accommodative esotropia is based upon the correction of the abnormal hyperopic refractive error. A careful refraction should be performed, prescribing the minimal refractive correction that allows normal visual acuity as well as a small esophoric deviation. By not correcting the patient fully and leaving a small latent strabismus, the patient is able to gain an ability to control the deviation by means of the fusion mechanism, ensuring continued long-term alignment in the future. Determination of the proper refractive correction may include cycloplegia with either short-acting (cyclopentolate) or long-acting (atropine) agents.
- In addition to correcting any strabismus present, attention must be given to correcting any amblyopia that is coincidentally present. Amblyopia treatment should be initiated as soon as possible, and should be completed as quickly as possible before the age of visual maturation.
- Cases of nonrefractive accommodative esotropia can be treated in two ways. The choice of treatment is usually one of personal preference, with each being equally effective.
  - Bifocals are the main refractive treatment for this condition. By providing an executive type bifocal of +2.50 to +3.00 D strength, accommodation at near can be decreased, resulting in less convergence and normal ocular alignment. Occasionally, a mild hyperopic correction is needed in the upper segment of the bifocal in order to decrease a small distance esotropic deviation that may be present.
  - The other treatment option for this condition entails the use of a long-acting cholinesterase inhibitor. Medications such as echothiophate drops or Difluorophate ointment are placed in each eye daily in order to decrease the effective AC/A ratio, resulting in normal ocular alignment. When using this pharmacologic treatment, care must be taken in administering depolarizing anesthetic muscle-relaxing agents because of the strabismus treatment's effect on pseudocholinesterase and the increased effect of the muscle relaxants.
- In cases of accommodative esotropia where the above treatment is ineffective or not fully effective, strabismus surgery may be needed.

ABDUCENS PARESIS (CN VI PARESIS) (FIG. 4-10)

CASE 4

A 39-year-old woman presents to the office and reports a sudden onset of double vision after being involved in an automobile accident the previous day. The patient was not wearing her seat belt and struck her head on the windshield. There was momentary loss of consciousness, but results of cranial imaging were negative. The patient notes an interesting fact: when she looks to the left she does not experience any double vision, but when she looks to the right, the diplopia is pronounced. In addition, when looking straight ahead, she occasionally is aware of diplopia, especially when tired. Her husband describes also a small face-turn to the right, which was not present before the accident. Examination reveals equal vision in each eye, with a normal pupillary evaluation as well as a normal anterior and posterior segment. A large-angle esotropia is found on right gaze, which diminishes toward left gaze. A 10° right face-turn is noted. Ocular rotations reveal a significantly reduced ability to adduct the right eye, while the remainder of the ocular rotations are full. The patient is followed for several months, and gradually decreasing symptoms are noted. Examination over the same period reveals increased adduction ability of the right eye, although a small adduction deficit permanently remains.

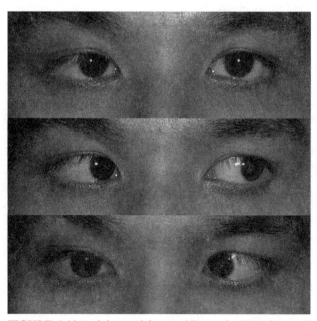

FIGURE 4-10 A right cranial nerve VI paresis. Note the small esotropia in primary gaze, normal ocular alignment in left gaze, and a large esotropia on right gaze.

PATHOPHYSIOLOGY

Abducens paresis can occur congenitally, or as an acquired condition. Causes include intracranial lesions, infection, and immunological processes in addition to head trauma.

CLINICAL FEATURES

This is an incomitant form of esotropia, often associated with a face-turn to maintain fusion. The esotropia is found to increase in ipsilateral gaze, and may be non-existent in the opposite gaze field. Ocular rotations demonstrate significant underaction of the lateral rectus muscle on the affected side, with marked weakness revealed by the active-force–generation test. (In this test, the globe is held in place with a forceps and the patient is instructed to look toward the affected side. In normal cases, the physician notes a significant pulling sensation on the forceps, whereas in cases of lateral rectus weakness, no force is sensed.)

DIAGNOSIS

A new onset of an incomitant esotropia with decreased lateral rectus function and with an appropriate associated preceding event is highly suggestive of this diagnosis. There is often no family history of a similar condition. Given the appropriate setting, bilateral cases are possible.

DIFFERENTIAL

Most commonly confused with Duane's syndrome type I, or with postsurgical restrictive cases of strabismus.

TREATMENT

Although no specific treatment is available to correct the underlying abducens nerve paresis, several techniques may aid in maintaining normal ocular alignment as well as normal binocular cooperation.

- At the very least, alternate patching can be employed to avoid diplopia and maintain vision in each eye. Although patching does relieve diplopia, it, by definition, does not allow for binocular vision.
- A more elegant solution is the use of Fresnel press-on prisms. The Fresnel prism is a thin plastic membrane that is placed over a patient's refractive lens. Despite its thinness, the Fresnel prism is often able to relieve diplopia and allow for normal binocular vision not withstanding the esotropia resulting from the abducens nerve paresis. The Fresnel prism is most often a

temporary solution, until function of the affected nerve returns. In case nerve function does not return, a permanent prism can be ground into the patient's glasses.
- After a minimum of 4 to 6 months, additional treatment may be needed if nerve function does not return. In this case, botulinum toxin or a transposition surgical procedure can be employed to correct the esotropia and resolve the patient's diplopia.

EXODEVIATIONS

PSEUDOEXOTROPIA

CLINICAL FEATURES

Pseudoexotropia is a normal condition in which there is an appearance of exotropia when none is actually present. The appearance can be caused by a variety of normal conditions, including wide interpupillary distance or an ectopic macula due to retinal dragging resulting from retinopathy of prematurity.

DIAGNOSIS

Upon ocular examination with a Hirshberg or cover test, no strabismus is noted despite the appearance of exotropia.

TREATMENT

None is needed. This condition is not directly related to any strabismic abnormality.

EXOPHORIA

PATHOPHYSIOLOGY

Exophoria is a latent tendency for the eye to deviate outward, toward the ear. This condition is controlled by the binocular fusion mechanism, which maintains use of both eyes simultaneously, thus achieving normal ocular alignment.

CLINICAL FEATURES

Under normal conditions, no strabismus is noted. In the event that one eye is covered, the covered eye may obtain an abducted position, only to immediately return to normal alignment once binocular vision is restored.

DIAGNOSIS

In cases of true exophoria, the cover-uncover test does not cause any eye movement, while the alternate cover test produces a characteristic exodeviation.

DIFFERENTIAL

Must be differentiated from intermittent exotropia, which occurs when fusion is not sufficient to maintain normal eye alignment.

TREATMENT

None is required.

INTERMITTENT VS. CONSTANT DEVIATIONS

The ocular fusion mechanism is responsible for maintaining normal ocular alignment. A clinical spectrum exists when exophoria is present and fusion fully corrects any strabismic tendency. Intermittent exotropia exists at times when fusion is not successful in maintaining ocular alignment, and true exotropia exists when ocular fusion is unable to maintain ocular alignment.

CASE 5

A 15-year-old boy presents to the office complaining of a wandering eye. On further questioning, it appears that the left eye wanders in the direction of the ear, mostly when the patient is tired or not feeling well. In addition, the boy's mother reports that he tends to close his left eye when he is in bright sunlight. Examination findings are normal, except that there is normal eye alignment at near testing, with an exotropia of 15 prism D that increases to 30 prism D at distance fixation as the alternate cover test proceeds.

PATHOPHYSIOLOGY

There is a decrease in an individual's ability to maintain fusion, which leads to an intermittent exotropia. Fusion may be disrupted by several factors, including an underlying large exotropia, decreased vision in one or both eyes, illness or fatigue, and bright light that makes clear and comfortable vision difficult.

CLINICAL FEATURES

- A comitant strabismus in which the exotropia is not constant, varying between exophoria and a true exotropia.
- Onset is often between infancy and age 4 to 5 years.
- The periods of tropia may be short or long, depending on the individual's ability to maintain fusion.
- Strabismic deviations can vary, sometimes being moderate in size. The exotropia in intermittent deviations is usually smaller than that noted in constant exotropia. Diplopia may be present at times of exotropia.

DIAGNOSIS

A tropia may be diagnosed by either the subject's history of ocular misalignment or based upon the clinical examination. Often, a subject will have normal alignment when initially examined, only to break down to a more constant exotropia later during the evaluation.

DIFFERENTIAL

This condition must be differentiated from exophoria and constant exotropia.

TREATMENT

- No specific treatment is needed as long as the periods of exotropia are not lengthy.
- In cases where the eye is deviated more than 50% of the time, intervention can be considered. In addition, intervention should be considered in cases where there is disruptive diplopia.
- Treatment consists of improving fusion. This can be accomplished by a variety of techniques, beginning with ensuring best corrected vision in each eye. Additionally, convergence exercises can be used in cases of convergence insufficiency. On occasion, minus lenses are used to stimulate accommodation and accommodative convergence.
- Often surgical intervention is needed. (See Exotropia below for additional treatment options.)

EXOTROPIA (FIG. 4-11)

CASE 6

A 68-year-old woman presents to the office, complaining of difficulty in maintaining a conversation or making normal eye contact with others. The patient reports that she has a right eye that never seems to be aimed presents with a constant and often large strabismic deviation.

CLINICAL FEATURES

- Patients with constant exotropia typically present with a moderate- to large-angle exotropia, sometimes measuring up to 80 prism D.
- These patients never have normal ocular alignment, as the deviation is too large for the fusion mechanism to correct.
- In most cases, there is no diplopia present, since the visual system has learned to suppress the sensory input from the deviated eye. In cases of exophoria, which has been well controlled throughout childhood, if a constant exotropia develops in adulthood, diplopia may be noted.

DIAGNOSIS

A careful patient history is needed to correctly diagnose this condition. In addition, clinical features such as comitancy and the presence of suppression to avoid diplopia aid in identifying these patients as having deteriorated control of an exophoria or intermittent exotropia.

DIFFERENTIAL

In cases of true exotropia (as opposed to intermittent types), patient history is critically important. In cases of sudden onset of an incomitant strabismus, neurologic abnormalities such as CN III paresis should be considered. Otherwise, in cases where the patient's complaint began in the past with an exophoria that progressed to an intermittent exotropia and now is more constant, standard constant exotropia is often the correct diagnosis. In addition, sensory deprivation exotropia (exotropia that develops as a result of longstanding severe visual loss in one eye) should be considered.

TREATMENT

Surgical intervention is most often required to treat this condition. Surgery often consists of a bilateral muscle-weakening technique (i.e., bilateral lateral rectus recession), although some surgeons prefer a monocular approach in cases of exotropia presenting monocularly (i.e., when no alternation between the two eyes is present) or in cases of sensory deprivation exotropia, in which surgery on the normally seeing eye is avoided.

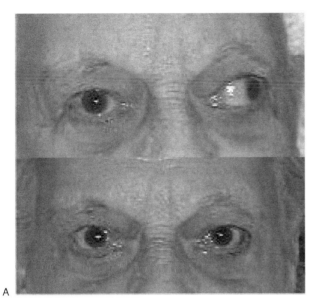

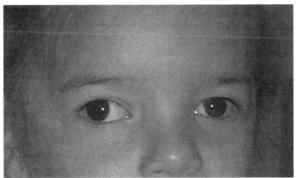

FIGURE 4-11 (A) A large angle exotropia in an adult, both before and after surgical correction. The preoperative deviation measured more than 45°. (B) A young child with congenital exotropia with a left eye preference.

straight ahead. She adds that her right eye has been misaligned since childhood and has never been straight. Recently, the eye has deviated more, and people constantly appear to be looking over their shoulder to see who she is speaking to. In addition, the patient reports a constant pulling sensation in the right orbital region. Examination findings are unremarkable, except for normal visual acuity in each eye with a comitant 80 prism D right exotropia, noted at both near and distance fixation. Despite normal visual acuity, the patient is unable to appreciate any stereoscopic depth perception because of the large exotropia. There also is mild underaction of the right medial rectus muscle.

PATHOPHYSIOLOGY

The most severe abnormality on the *exophoria–intermittent exotropia–exotropia* spectrum, this condition

VERTICAL DEVIATIONS (FIG. 4-12)

HYPERTROPIA VS. HYPOTROPIA

- Both terms refer to a misalignment of the optical axes of fixation in which one eye is fixing on the target of interest and the other eye is aimed either above or below the fixation point.
- Vertical deviations are most commonly named by the vertically nonfixing eye. If, for example, a subject's right eye was used to fix on a target, and the left eye was deviated upward, a left hypertropia would be diagnosed.
- Vertical deviations may be monocular, with the same eye constantly misaligned, or there may be spontaneous alternation between the fixing right or left eye. In the above case, if alternation was present, the subject would have either a left hypertropia (as described above) or a right hypotropia, present when the left eye was used for fixation.

COMITANT VS. NONCOMITANT DEVIATIONS

The concept of comitancy is important in properly diagnosing the etiology of a vertical strabismus. Most causes of vertical strabismus create a noncomitant strabismus pattern, although, over a lengthy period of time, even initially noncomitant vertical deviations will often become more comitant. Commitancy can differentiate a rather harmless small deviation from a recent onset (noncomitant) deviation resulting from a more significant acute neurologic event. Most vertical deviations can be divided into two main categories, those that are due to an innervational abnormality and those that are due to restrictive or mechanical causes.

DISSOCIATED VERTICAL DEVIATION (DVD)

CASE 7

A young child returns to the office after having undergone successful surgery for infantile esotropia at the age of 1 year. The child's mother notes normal horizontal eye alignment, and is very pleased with the surgical result. She also reports that on occasion, one or the other of her child's eyes unfortunately have been noted by friends and teachers to deviate upward. Although the eye does not deviate for long and seems to be easily corrected on request, the mother is concerned about this appearance. The visual examination findings are normal except for the left eye, which rotates upward when covered, and immediately upon removal of the cover, returns to the normal position. Covering the right eye produces no eye movement in either eye.

PATHOPHYSIOLOGY

The precise etiology of this condition is not fully understood.

CLINICAL FEATURES

- A vertical deviation appears to contradict Hering's law of equal innervation, although recent clinical studies suggest that in fact Hering's law is not violated.
- In this condition, either eye may be noted to deviate upward during periods of visual inattention (i.e., daydreaming) or occlusion. When the vertically deviating eye returns to its normal horizontal position, the fellow eye does not move, thus seeming to refute Hering's law. In cases of regular hypertropia, the previously fixing eye rotates in the same direction as the deviating eye when it returns to the horizontal plane to obtain fixation.

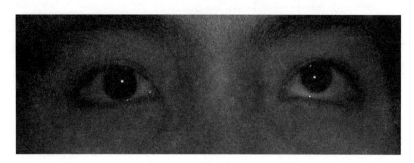

FIGURE 4-12 Left hypertropia. This patient is fixing with the right eye, thus the left eye is noted to be deviated upward. If fixation should change to the left eye, the right eye would then be directed downward (a right hypotropia). Therefore, any vertical deviation can be classified either as a hypertropia or hypotropia as long as the deviating eye is specified.

- The DVD may be latent, occurring only when the eye is covered or the patient is visually inattentive, or may be constantly deviated upward. Also, DVDs, although most often bilateral, are not necessarily symmetrical in presentation.
- Although a DVD can occur in isolation, it is most often noted in cases of infantile esotropia, where latent nystagmus is also present.

DIAGNOSIS

- Observation of the patient as well as clinical evaluation often aids in making this diagnosis.
- A past history of horizontal strabismus, especially at a young age, as well as the characteristic features of the deviation can be used to differentiate this condition from other forms of vertical strabismus.
- Critical to the correct diagnosis is the observation of the fellow eye when the deviating eye returns to the horizontal plane. True DVDs will not demonstrate any compensatory movement in the fellow eye.
- Precise measurement of the DVD is often difficult, with most clinicians turning to a severity scale ranging from *1*, a slight deviation, to *4*, a large deviation.

DIFFERENTIAL

Dissociated vertical deviations must be distinguished from true hypertropia. Also, other conditions, such as weakness of the inferior rectus muscle (often noted following trauma) or fixation with an eye otherwise restricted to vertical movement, may cause a similar clinical presentation. In addition, overaction of the inferior oblique muscles can mimic a DVD.

TREATMENT

Both surgical and nonsurgical means can be used to treat this condition. Nonsurgical methods include changing the subject's fixation pattern by purposely blurring vision in the non-DVD eye as well as using a patch over the nonfixing eye. In some cases, especially those with a large constant DVD, surgical intervention is recommended. Although treatment can frequently improve the condition, it often cannot eliminate it.

SUPERIOR OBLIQUE PARESIS (CN IV PARESIS) (FIG. 4-13)

CASE 8

An otherwise healthy 45-year-old man presents to the ophthalmologist complaining of double vision. The onset of diplopia was noted soon after the patient was aggressively tackled 3 months ago during a touch football game. The diplopia is constant and appears to be present unless one eye is covered. Additionally, the patient's girlfriend reports that he often seems to tilt his head toward his left shoulder. Evaluation findings are normal except for a small right hypertropia, which is larger in left gaze and almost nonexistent in right gaze. Forced head tilt to the right creates a larger right

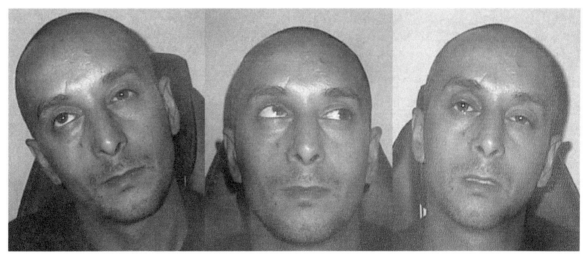

FIGURE 4-13 Right superior oblique paresis. Head tilting is a hallmark of cyclovertical muscle dysfunction. In this case of right superior oblique paresis, head tilt to the left allows for normal eye alignment, while tilt to the right produces a large right hypertropia. The hypertropia is produced by the vertical effect of the now unopposed inferior oblique muscle.

hypertropia, whereas almost no hypertropia is noted on forced left head tilt. Motility evaluation reveals underaction of the right superior oblique muscle with minimal overaction of the right inferior oblique muscle.

PATHOPHYSIOLOGY

Congenital or acquired damage to CN IV causes underaction of the superior oblique muscle. Most acquired cases are traumatic in origin.

CLINICAL FEATURES

- Most patients present with a complaint of either diplopia or hypertropia. Occasionally, a head tilt will be the presenting complaint.
- If the subject is fixing with the unaffected eye, a hypertropia will be present. If the subject fixes with the paretic eye, then a hypotropia will be present in the fellow, unaffected eye.
- If a head tilt is present, it is usually in the direction opposite to the affected eye.
- Amblyopia is uncommon in acquired cases, but may be present in congenital cases, especially those in which a head tilt is *not* noted.
- Most cases are unilateral, although all cases should be considered to be bilateral until proven otherwise. Bilateral cases often have a larger vertical deviation, have a V-pattern esotropia (i.e., the eyes are closer together in downgaze), and usually are associated with greater than 10° of excyclotorsion.

DIAGNOSIS

- Diagnosis is classically based on the *three-step test*. This sequence of three tests is used to systematically eliminate all but 1 of the (8) vertically acting extraocular muscles. The remaining muscle is identified as being weak or paretic.
- Although the three-step test is able to identify a single paretic muscle, it is not able to distinguish between unilateral and bilateral cases; thus, a high index of suspicion must be maintained if these cases are to be correctly identified.
- In addition, a double Maddox rod can be used to measure torsion and to identify bilateral cases.

DIFFERENTIAL

Most commonly, isolated overaction of the inferior oblique muscle must be distinguished from superior oblique paresis. In these cases, there will be no history of trauma and the superior oblique muscle will not underact in its field of action.

TREATMENT

Indications for treatment consist of an abnormal head position (especially in children, in whom craniospinal deformations may be created) as well as large vertical deviations and diplopia. Although prisms and occlusion can be used to ameliorate the symptoms, definitive treatment is surgical. Several different surgical treatment schemes for this condition have been devised over the years. Treatment options include tightening ("tucking") the superior oblique tendon, weakening the opposing inferior oblique muscle, or weakening the vertical rectus to treat hypertropia.

DOUBLE ELEVATOR PARESIS (MONOCULAR ELEVATION DEFICIENCY) (FIG. 4-14)

PATHOPHYSIOLOGY

There are two main types of double elevator paresis, those due to restriction of the inferior rectus, and those thought to be secondary to a supranuclear elevation abnormality.

CLINICAL FEATURES

Limitation of elevation in all positions of upgaze, both monocularly and binocularly. Owing to the limitation, a hypotropia is noted, which increases in upgaze. A chin-up head posture is often adopted as well to alleviate the need for upgaze. Pseudoptosis is also common in the

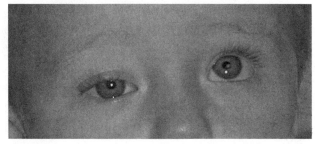

FIGURE 4-14 This young child is unable to elevate his right eye because of double elevator palsy. Both the superior rectus and the inferior oblique muscles are dysfunctional, limiting elevation.

primary position of gaze. In some cases, restriction of the inferior rectus may be noted.

DIAGNOSIS

Careful evaluation of the ocular rotations as well as several specialized tests are helpful in making this diagnosis. Forced duction testing readily identifies any inferior orbital restriction that may be present. In addition, observation of the Bell's reflex can aid in differentiating restrictive cases from those due to a supranuclear etiology. Bell's reflex will be significantly reduced or absent in restrictive cases.

DIFFERENTIAL

In addition to selective abnormality to either the superior rectus or the inferior oblique, Brown's superior oblique tendon sheath syndrome must be considered.

TREATMENT

- Indications for treatment include a large vertical deviation, with pseudoptosis in the primary gaze position. In addition, an abnormal head position, usually chin-up, indicates a need for intervention.
- Treatment is surgical, and depends on the precise etiology for the condition.
  - In cases of inferior rectus restriction, a recession of this muscle is preferred.
  - In supranuclear cases, a transposition of the medial and lateral rectus muscles is performed in order to create the ability to stabilize or move the eye vertically.

A AND V PATTERNS

CASE 9

A 6-year-old boy presents to the office, appearing to have normal eye alignment. The child's father relates that often the child's eyes look fine, although on occasion he appears to lose control of his eyes, resulting in their pointing in opposite directions. Evaluation reveals normally aligned eyes in the primary position, with an exotropia in gaze both to the upper-right side as well as to the upper-left side. Curiously, on downgaze, esotropia is noted. Ocular motility reveals bilateral overaction of the inferior oblique muscles.

PATHOPHYSIOLOGY

- A and V patterns are named based on the formation of those two letters of the alphabet, to signify the ocular position in *up-* and *down*gaze. In an "A" pattern the eyes are closer together (i.e., more convergent) in upgaze and further apart in downgaze, "V" indicates the opposite alignment pattern.
- In addition, an "X" pattern, though uncommon, is possible, in which the eyes are separated in both upgaze and downgaze, only to be normally aligned in the primary position.
- A and V patterns are most often caused by oblique muscle dysfunction, with inferior oblique overaction being associated with V patterns and superior oblique muscle overaction associated with A patterns.
- Additionally, abnormal function of either the horizontal or vertical rectus muscles can produce a V pattern.

CLINICAL FEATURES

- A and V pattern strabismus is characterized by incomitant horizontal strabismus dependent upon vertical gaze.
- Deviations can be either esotropic or exotropic, and vary between greater ocular deviation in upgaze, downgaze, or both.
- The deviation pattern can take the shape not only of the letter A or V, or occasionally X, but also the lower-case Greek gamma, which resembles the letter Y. It may even occur in the shape of a diamond.
- A and V patterns occur in approximately 15 to 25% of cases of horizontal strabismus, and are more easily seen when measured in extreme gaze fields.

DIAGNOSIS

In order for a specific pattern to be clinically significant, there must be a 10 to 15 prism D difference in alignment between 25° of upgaze and 25° of downgaze. As a result of this difference, A and V pattern strabismus is considered to be vertically incomitant.

DIFFERENTIAL

Although there are no other strabismus conditions that mimic this unique pattern of ocular misalignment, several craniofacial abnormalities may be more likely to present with an A or V pattern. Both Apert's and

Crouzon's syndromes frequently demonstrate an A or V pattern form of strabismus.

TREATMENT

In addition to treating any underlying strabismus present, only clinically significant patterns require intervention. In addition to weakening any overacting oblique muscle, the horizontal recti can sometimes be used to correct this unique strabismus pattern.

STRABISMUS SYNDROMES

DUANE'S SYNDROME (FIG. 4-15)

PATHOPHYSIOLOGY

Although the precise etiology is unknown, current thought centers on a congenital abnormality of CN VI. On an autopsy case, CN III was found to innervate the lateral rectus muscle in place of the normal CN VI. This abnormal innervation is thought to be responsible for the clinical signs of Duane's syndrome.

CLINICAL FEATURES

Three types of Duane's syndrome exist.

- Type I is typified by decreased abduction and esotropia, type II by decreased adduction with exotropia, and type III by a decrease in both adduction and abduction with usually normal ocular alignment in the primary position.
- Abduction Duane's syndrome is effected as a result of abnormal enervation of the lateral rectus muscle. Adduction is effected as a result of co-contraction of the lateral and medial rectus muscles in attempted adduction. The normal medial rectus muscle must contract against the contracting lateral rectus muscle, which in the normal case would relax and not act as a restriction to adduction.
- Females are more commonly affected, as is the left eye.
- In addition to the typical decrease in horizontal motility, the eye is often noted to retract within the globe on adduction, with resultant narrowing of the palpebral fissure (likely a result of co-contraction of both the medial and lateral rectus muscle).
- Additionally, some patients demonstrate a typical "upshoot" or "downshoot" of the eye on attempted adduction.

DIAGNOSIS

Although Duane's syndrome usually occurs sporadically, it has been associated with several other systemic conditions (hearing abnormalities, spinal changes) as well as systemic syndromes (e.g., Goldenhar, Klippel-Feil). In addition, an autosomal dominant inheritance

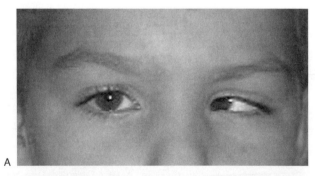
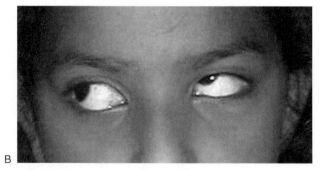
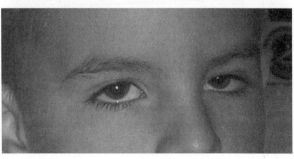

FIGURE 4-15 Typical features of Duane's syndrome include (A) narrowing of the palpebral fissure, (B) upshoots and downshoots of the globe on attempted adduction, and (C) a face turn to allow for normal ocular alignment in a specific field of gaze.

pattern has been noted in up to 10% of the cases. Specific diagnosis is made on clinical grounds, based upon the typical motility disorder present. Occasionally, patients will develop a face-turn to compensate for their motility abnormality, and can thus maintain normal binocular vision.

DIFFERENTIAL

The most commonly confused clinical condition, resembling Duane's syndrome, is paresis of CN VI. Lateral rectus weakness does not demonstrate several typical findings noted in Duane's syndrome; particularly, no globe retraction with pseudoptosis is noted and no upshoots or downshoots are seen.

TREATMENT

Since we are unable to restore normal ocular motility to patients with Duane's syndrome, treatment is limited to cases in which a significant ocular misalignment is noted in the primary position or a face-turn is present. Surgical intervention consists of a weakening procedure for the medial rectus muscle (in an attempt to balance the lateral rectus muscle weakness) with possible transposition of the inferior and superior rectus muscles to the lateral rectus in order to produce abducting forces.

MOEBIUS SYNDROME

PATHOPHYSIOLOGY

Although the precise pathogenesis is unknown, abnormal development of the cranial nerve nuclei during gestation appears to be the cause. The syndrome is characterized by CN VI and VII palsies, although CN V, IX, X, and XII can be involved as well. Many additional systemic abnormalities have been noted, including abnormalities of the extremities, swallowing and speech difficulties, craniofacial abnormalities, dextrocardia, and mild mental retardation in at least 10% of the cases.

CLINICAL FEATURES

- The most common ophthalmic manifestation of Moebius syndrome is esotropia, with decreased function in one or both lateral rectus muscles.
- Occasionally, especially in unilateral cases, a face-turn may be present to allow binocular vision.

- In addition to strabismus, lagophthalmos is often noted as a result of the CN VII paresis. Chronic corneal exposure, resulting from paralysis of the orbicularis oculi, can lead to significant vision-threatening keratitis.
- Systemically, these patients are noted to have a characteristic masklike facies due to the paresis of the facial musculature and the patient's inability to smile.

DIAGNOSIS

The presence of Moebius syndrome is confirmed by the typical clinical presentation of these patients. After ruling out other causes of CN VI and VII palsy, the diagnosis is made based on both systemic and ophthalmic signs.

DIFFERENTIAL

- Infantile esotropia may mimic this condition in younger children, especially if they are not fully cooperative with the examination.
- In addition, any central lesion affecting the brain-stem region and the CN VI and VII nuclei can produce a similar clinical presentation.
- Also myasthenia gravis, thyroid eye disease, orbital inflammatory disease, and Duane's syndrome all can cause limitation of abduction.

TREATMENT

Care must be taken to treat the strabismic as well as the corneal complications of this condition. Aggressive lubrication with possible lid surgery is needed to prevent severe exposure keratitis and resultant vision loss. In cases of large-angle esotropia, or cases with a large face-turn, surgical weakening of the medial rectus muscle with transposition of the inferior and superior rectus to the insertion of the lateral rectus muscle may be indicated.

BROWN SYNDROME (FIG. 4-16)

PATHOPHYSIOLOGY

Although the exact etiology of Brown syndrome is unknown, it appears to be due to a restriction in the area of the trochlea of the superior oblique tendon. The restriction limits the movement of the superior oblique tendon through the trochlea and thus does not allow the superior oblique muscle to obtain its full range of movement. Causes of trochlear restriction include

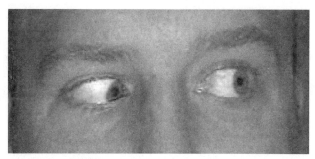

FIGURE 4-16 Brown syndrome. Due to the "leash" effect of the superior oblique tendon, this patient is unable to elevate his right eye to the midline in adduction. The right hypotropia was noted to increase as the patient attempted upgaze.

inflammation of the superior oblique tendon and trochlea (tenosynovitis) as well as abnormalities of the inferior oblique muscle, which can produce a clinical picture similar to the more common tenosynovitis.

CLINICAL FEATURES

- Clinically, Brown syndrome presents as a limitation to elevation of the eye in adduction. In order for elevation in adduction to be accomplished, there must be relaxation of the superior oblique muscle. In cases where there is a physical limitation to the passage of the superior oblique tendon through the trochlea, complete relaxation does not occur and the eye cannot elevate.
- Forced-duction testing is positive, indicating that the eye cannot be elevated with forceps by the examiner.
- Elevation of the eye in other gaze fields is otherwise normal.
- Brown syndrome is bilateral in 10% of cases.

DIAGNOSIS

Clinical signs and symptoms appropriate to Brown syndrome are required for correct diagnosis. In addition, a positive forced-duction test must be present. Additional clinical findings of pain or swelling in the area of the trochlea or recent trauma to the area aid in proper diagnosis.

DIFFERENTIAL

Inferior oblique paresis can produce a lack of elevation in adduction similar to Brown syndrome. Although not technically Brown syndrome, orbital floor fractures with entrapment of the inferior oblique muscle can also limit elevation in adduction. Finally, occasionally a Brown syndrome is created as a necessary byproduct of the surgical intervention for superior oblique paresis.

TREATMENT

Indications for treatment of Brown syndrome include an abnormal head position and a large hypotropia in the primary position. Most acquired cases resolve without surgical intervention, and may require instead a course of anti-inflammatory therapy. Congenital cases most often require surgery consisting of a weakening procedure on the superior oblique tendon.

THYROID EYE DISEASE (FIG. 4-17)

PATHOPHYSIOLOGY

As a result of a systemic autoimmune condition, a lymphocytic infiltrate develops in the orbital region. The extraocular muscles appear to be especially vulnerable, with resulting swelling and loss of function. In addition, the extraocular muscles become inflamed, edematous, and fibrotic. The inferior rectus muscle is affected most often, followed by the medial rectus, superior rectus, and lateral rectus muscles.

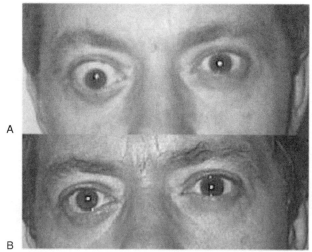

FIGURE 4-17 Proptosis and hypotropia are common findings in thyroid eye disease. The top panel (A) depicts a right hypotropia as well as proptosis in a patient with thyroid eye disease. Panel (B) depicts the same patient postoperatively. Note the well-centered corneal light reflexes as well as the reduced degree of proptosis.

CLINICAL FEATURES

- Most patients with this condition present with hypotropia, although esotropia in combination with hypotropia is often seen as well.
- In addition to strabismus, thyroid eye disease can cause other ophthalmic abnormalities. Additional effects range from mild retraction of the upper lid with a characteristic staring appearance, to the more serious proptosis.
- If allowed to progress, corneal involvement and optic nerve compression can lead to permanent and irreversible vision loss.

DIAGNOSIS

Although most patients will be euthyroid at the time of diagnosis, most will report a history of thyroid disease. In addition to the characteristic ocular clinical appearance, the forced-duction test will be positive, indicating a restriction to eye movement. Orbital imaging studies clearly demonstrate thickening of the extraocular muscles.

DIFFERENTIAL

This condition must be differentiated from inferior orbital floor fracture, with entrapment of the inferior rectus. Also, congenital fibrosis syndrome can present a similar clinical appearance. Lid retraction and lag may be caused in cases of CN III paresis with aberrant regeneration.

Proptosis can be caused by a variety of space-occupying orbital conditions.

TREATMENT

- In addition to many treatments for the general ophthalmic complications of thyroid eye disease, the strabismus component can be treated by several means.
- Prism lenses can often be employed to treat any diplopia present in the primary position of gaze.
- In the event that diplopia persists, or there is an abnormal head position with a large angle of strabismus, surgical intervention may be required. Surgery consists of the recession (weakening) procedure on the rectus muscles. Resections (strengthening procedures) should be avoided in thyroid eye disease. In addition, the use of an adjustable suture technique is often helpful on titrating the final clinical result.

BIBLIOGRAPHY

Millodot M, Laby DM. *Dictionary of Ophthalmology*, Butterworth-Heinemann, Oxford, England: 2002.

Parks MM. Cyclovertical muscle palsy. *Arch Ophthalmol* 60:1027–1035, 1958.

Rosenbaum AL, Santiago AP. *Clinical Strabismus Management—Principles and Surgical Techniques.* Philadelphia, WB Saunders Company, 1999.

von Noorden G. *Binocular Vision and Ocular Motility—Theory and Management of Strabismus*, 5th ed. Mosby, New York: 1996.

Wright KW. *Color Atlas of Strabismus Surgery—Strategies and Techniques*, 2nd ed. Wright Publishing, Irvine, CA: 2000.

5 LIDS, LASHES, AND LACRIMAL DISORDERS

Scott Lee
Don Liu

TRAUMA

MARGINAL LACERATION AND CANALICULAR LACERATION

CASE 1

A 6-year-old girl was bitten near the eye while playing with a dog. Examination showed a laceration through the margin of the left lower lid near the nose. Vision was 20/20 in both eyes (OU) and the eyes were otherwise normal. The consulting ophthalmologist found that the laceration extended through the lacrimal canaliculus of the lower lid. A plastic repair with intubation of the canaliculus was performed.

PATHOPHYSIOLOGY

- Blunt or penetrating trauma to the eyelid or lacrimal apparatus, results in partial or full-thickness tears.
- With bites, a variety of pathogens are implicated. *Streptococcus, Pasteurella,* and *Bacteroides* infections are common. Rabies is also a possibility with wild animals.

CLINICAL FEATURES

- Patients present with pain, ecchymosis, and edema.
- There can be ptosis, decreased visual acuity, and epiphora (tearing).
- Trauma secondary to bite should provide a high index of suspicion for infection. With trauma secondary to a motor vehicle accident, a foreign body should be examined for.
- With penetrating lid laceration, an open globe injury should be suspected.
- With lid eversion, the degree of pathology can be assessed.
- Lid lacerations often present with hyphema, orbital fracture, or other proximal structure involvement.

DIAGNOSIS AND DIFFERENTIAL

- In addition to a history and physical examination, a CT may be warranted if trauma is severe enough, to rule out involvement of other structures and foreign bodies.
- Canalicular involvement in medial lid lacerations must be suspected (Fig. 5-1).
- If one of the lacrimal canaliculi is affected, the other can function to drain the tears.
- If both are affected, an attempt should be made to repair the canaliculi.

TREATMENT

- Surgical repair is dependent on the depth and location of the laceration. Superficial lacerations (involving lid skin only) can be treated with Steristrips and antibiotic ointment.
- Deep lacerations and those involving the margin require sutures left in for 2 weeks. Before surgery, a corneal protector and topical anesthetic should be administered. Lacerations through the lid margin will heal with a notch in the lid if not properly repaired.
- Of primary concern is the prevention of infection. With any laceration, especially secondary to a bite,

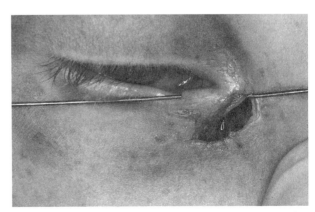

FIGURE 5-1 Canalicular laceration. This can occur with or without lid margin involvement.

sufficient irrigation is mandatory. Bacitracin is often used for prophylaxis.
- The order of repair is generally as follows, if the structures are involved: for ease, the canaliculi are repaired first, followed by canthal and lid margin lacerations. For the best cosmetic appearance and realignment, extracanthal and extramarginal lacerations are repaired last.

PTOSIS

CASE 2

A 72-year-old actor complains of progressive superior field defects for the past 2 years. His wife feels it is secondary to his "droopy" disposition. He is chronically tired and his eyelids are always drooping. He received some plastic surgery about 5 years ago to make his eyes look younger. On examination, the marginal reflex distance is found to be 1 mm and levator function to be 3 mm.

PATHOPHYSIOLOGY

- The function of the lid is dependent on the eyelid muscles, i.e., the levator palpebrae superioris, its aponeurosis, and Mueller's muscle. The former is striated and innervated by the Third cranial nerve (CN III) and the latter is smooth muscle, sympathetically innervated.
- Ptosis results from pathology of any of these components and can be divided into three major etiologies:
- *Structural dysfunction*: Aponeurosis dysfunction or dehiscence is the most common cause of ptosis. Most often in the elderly, the 15–17 mm of levator aponeurosis separates in part or in full from its attachments to the skin or muscle, releasing the lid and resulting in ptosis. Any mass effect impinging of any of the aforementioned structures gives rise to mechanical ptosis. This can be secondary to tumor, infection, or scar formation after surgery or trauma (Fig. 5-2).
- *Muscle dysfunction* is less common. In congenital disease, levator dysgenesis results in ptosis. In adults, myasthenia gravis, myotonic dystrophy, chronic progressive external ophthalmoplegia, and other myoplegias result in ptosis.
- *Neurogenic pathology* is another cause of ptosis. Horner's syndrome, CN III palsies, Marcus Gunn's jaw-winking syndrome (a congenital ptosis where nerve supply is "miswired" so that eyelid movement is in conjunction with the jaw) are all examples of neurogenic dysfunction that can be secondary to congenital, trauma, infections, tumor, or vascular etiologies.

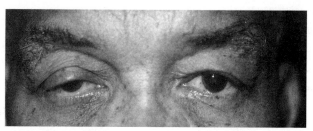

FIGURE 5-2 Ptosis. Note normal brow position and a higher lid crease on the involved side. With normal levator function, this means aponeurotic dehiscence.

CLINICAL FEATURES

- Patients present complaining of droopy eyelids, an appearance of malaise, and superior field defects depending on the degree of ptosis.
- On examination, several measurements can be taken that demonstrate a clinical diagnosis of ptosis: a decreased palpebral fissure distance, marginal reflex distance-1 of less than 2.0 mm (MRD-1 is the distance from the upper lid to the center of the pupillary light reflex; >2.5 mm is normal), and levator muscle function of less than 5 mm of movement.
- Levator muscle function can be assessed by holding the brow and observing the movement of the lid from downgaze to upgaze; <5 mm of movement is considered abnormal.

DIAGNOSIS AND DIFFERENTIAL

- Involvement of the pupil or extraocular muscles must be assessed to rule out a CN III palsy or intracranial process. After a history and physical examination to ascertain the etiology of ptosis, the following tests can be employed if disease is suspected. Otherwise, the diagnosis is often a clinical one.
- A Tensilon test (edrophonium, a cholinesterase inhibitor) to rule out myasthenia gravis is warranted.
- Magnetic resonance imaging (MRI) with gadolinium, as well as cerebrospinal fluid (CSF) testing can be used if multiple sclerosis is suspected.
- Electromyographic studies are rarely used but may be employed to rule out chronic progressive external ophthalmoplegia.
- Chest or brain CT scan and MRI may be employed if acquired Horner's syndrome is suspected.

TREATMENT

- Medical treatment with physostigmine is warranted only with myasthenia gravis.

- If patients do not desire surgery, a crutch can be built into eyeglasses to prevent the lid from drooping; however, drying out of the eyes is a possibility.
- The type of surgical intervention depends on function of structures involved. If the levator has poor function, a frontalis sling can be created. If good Mueller's muscle function is observed, then an internal levator advancement can be used. In most cases, the levator will be resected and reattached from an anterior or posterior approach.
- Phenylephrine drops are used to test sympathetic function of Mueller's muscle. If good function is intact and the eyelid opens up, this muscle can be advanced. Otherwise, the levator must be shortened or its attachment advanced.

ENTROPION

CASE 3

A 70-year-old man complained of a foreign body sensation in his left eye, with discharge and intermittent tearing. Examination revealed vision consistent with early cataracts. The left lower lid turned in, and the lashes rubbed on the globe.

PATHOPHYSIOLOGY

There are five major etiologies of entropion formation:
- *Involutional*: The most common type of entropion is caused by laxity of the canthal tendons. The elderly are particularly prone to involutional entropion.
- *Congenital*: Genetic and/or developmental disorder may contribute to the formation of an entropion. Although rare, dysgenesis of lid muscles or tarsal plate defects give rise to congenital entropion formation.
- *Neurologic*: Trauma, infection, and autoimmune disease can all cause ocular irritation and subsequent spasm of the orbicularis oris muscle, causing inversion of the lid.
- *Cicatricial*: This term derives from the Latin for "scar." Ocular cicatricial pemphigoid, trauma, infection, chemical burns, and Stevens-Johnson syndrome can all induce scar formation of the conjunctiva, creating an entropion.
- *Tumor*: Neurofibromas or any lid or orbital tumor may cause a mechanical inversion of the lid.

CLINICAL FEATURES

- Patients present with an inturned eyelid (Fig. 5-3).

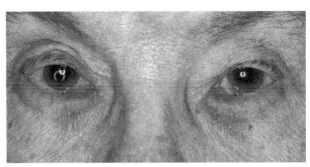

FIGURE 5-3 Entropion. Lid margin rolls inward. This patient has minimal conjunctival injection.

- The eyelashes may appear to have folded inward with the inturned eyelid, causing irritation.
- Patients complain of a foreign body sensation, tearing, and often conjunctivitis. The entropion may have a normal appearance depending on the degree of laxity of the lid.
- Generally the lower lid is affected.

DIAGNOSIS AND DIFFERENTIAL

- An examination is sufficient to diagnose entropion. The specific etiology is important to discern.
- With cicatricial entropion, it is difficult to evert the eyelid because of scarring.
- Further testing is warranted for autoimmune cicatricial entropion, i.e., antibasement membrane antibodies, ANA (anti-nuclear antibody), immunoglobulin testing.
- With involutional entropion, laxity allows for easy eversion.
- The cornea and puncta should be examined for pathology with any suspected ectropion.
- Trichiasis or distichiasis may present with entropion, but are distinct entities.
- Epiblepharon must be considered as well. It is a congenital condition in which the orbicularis muscle forces the eyelashes inward. This resolves on its own, in contrast to congenital entropion.

TREATMENT

- Medical treatment includes lubricants to decrease corneal irritation and taping the eye.
- Botulinum toxin may be injected to paralyze the orbicularis muscle with spastic entropion.
- For most entropion, definitive treatment requires surgery.

ECTROPION

CASE 4

A 68-year-old woman presented with constant tearing and redness of the right eye. Examination disclosed vision of 20/25 OU. The right lower lid turned out, and the lower lacrimal punctum was not in contact with the globe.

PATHOPHYSIOLOGY

The etiologies of ectropion formation are similar to those of entropion. Five major causes are delineated below:

- *Involutional*: Involutional ectropion is the most common. Medial and lateral canthal laxity contribute to eversion of the lid (sagging appearance), which is most common in the elderly.
- *Congenital*: Although rare, it generally affects the lower lid. Associated diseases include Down syndrome and various genetic disorders associated with craniofacial abnormalities.
- *Neurologic*: These ectropions are generally paralytic in nature and can affect CN III or CN VII function. Bell's palsy, herpes zoster, and lesions anywhere along the tracts of these cranial nerves can result in paralysis and laxity of the muscle, resulting in entropion.
- *Cicatricial*: These ectropion are the sequelae of trauma, burns, infection, and autoimmune disease. There is an association of cicatricial ectropion with T-cell lymphoma.
- *Tumor*: Neurofibromas or any lid or orbital tumor may cause mechanical eversion of the lid.
- Sequelae of ectropion include abnormal tear drainage, conjunctival exposure, irritation, and edema, keratitis, and corneal ulceration. Ultimately, vision loss may ensue if ectropion and subsequent corneal exposure are not treated.

CLINICAL FEATURES

- Patients present with a lid eversion (outward). Generally, the lower lid is affected (Fig. 5-4).
- Patients may complain of red eye, irritation, and even vision loss if the cornea has been affected.
- The condition may progress over a period of many years, and patients may not seek medical care until the symptoms or the disfigurement becomes severe. Patients may have had longstanding use of eye drops and lubricants to prevent eye drying with corneal exposure.

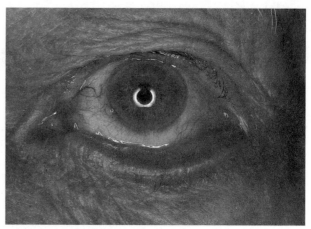

FIGURE 5-4 Ectropion. Lid margin turns outward. This can result in eye irritation and tearing.

DIAGNOSIS AND DIFFERENTIAL

- An examination is sufficient to diagnose ectropion.
- The specific etiology is important to discern through patient history and examination.
- With cicatricial ectropion, there is not the same laxity in the lid as with involutional entropion. With involutional ectropion, the central lid margin everts first.
- With progressive disease, the lateral lid follows.
- The cornea and puncta should be examined for pathology with any suspected ectropion.
- Tumors such as basal cell and squamous cell may have a similar appearance. The specific etiology must be discerned, as well as comorbid systemic disease, i.e., the aforementioned tumors, infection, and Bell's palsy.

TREATMENT

- Medical treatment includes lubricants to decrease corneal irritation and taping the eye.
- Steroids with acyclovir may be used in Bell's palsy if the diagnosis is made within 7 days. Ramsay Hunt syndrome or herpes alone should be treated with acyclovir.
- For most entropion, definitive treatment requires surgery.

TRICHIASIS AND DISTICHIASIS

CASE 5

A 17-year-old girl complains of finding "hair particles" in her eyes. She complains that it causes her to cry continually and to unnecessarily receive the sympathy of concerned onlookers. Eye drops have not worked in getting rid of the redness in her eyes.

PATHOPHYSIOLOGY

- There are four major causes of trichiasis and distichiasis that need to be discerned:
- *Trauma*: Most common postsurgically with lower lid transconjunctival blepharoplasty.
- *Autoimmune and inflammatory disorders* such as Stevens Johnson syndrome and ocular cicatricial pemphigoid (OCP) also give rise to malposition of the eyelashes. In both disorders, posterior lamellar scarring and symblepharon formation give rise to the trichiasis. Distichiasis is associated with Stevens Johnson syndrome.
- *Congenital*: Epiblepharon is prevalent in children of Asian ancestry. It is a horizontal redundant skin fold under the eyelid causing a vertical orientation of the eyelashes, distinct from entropion.
- *Infectious*: Trachoma is the world's leading preventable cause of blindness. Caused by *Chlamydia trachomatis*, it is endemic in parts of Africa and Asia. Repeated infections of the eye result in trichiasis, corneal inflammation, scarring, and ultimately blindness. Ocular herpes zoster is another cause of trichiasis that has serious sequelae.

CLINICAL FEATURES

- Trichiasis refers to abnormal eyelashes that are in contact with the globe (Fig. 5-5).
- Distichiasis refers to an extra row of eyelashes originating from the meibomian gland orifices on the posterior lid margin.
- With the eyelashes in contact with globe, patients may complain of epiphora and conjunctival irritation.
- Chronic irritation may present with keratitis and corneal ulceration.
- Most often, patients are asymptomatic.

DIAGNOSIS AND DIFFERENTIAL

- The diagnosis is most often a clinical one based on examination. However, if OCP or trachoma are suspected, a conjunctival biopsy is warranted.
- Entropion can present with or without trichiasis. Corneal abrasions and lesions separate from sequelae of trichiasis must also be distinguished. Systemic disease, including the aforementioned autoimmune and infectious diseases, must be diagnosed and treated.

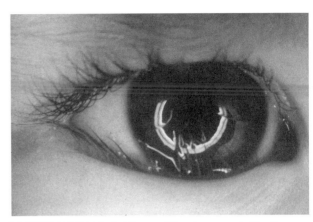

FIGURE 5-5 Trichiasis. The condition is aggravated by the presence of epiblepharon in this child.

TREATMENT

- Eye lubricants, as well as removal of the offending lashes, only provide temporary relief.
- The type of surgery is dependent on the nature of the lash abnormality. In cases of focal or segmental trichiasis, surgery may consist of radioablation, electrolysis, or cryotherapy of the lashes.
- Full correction of a malpositioned lid is warranted for entropion and posterior lamellar scarring.

INFLAMMATION

BLEPHARITIS

CASE 6

A 44-year-old man complained of a burning sensation in both eyes for several months. He often had crusting on his lids on awakening. Vision was normal. The lids showed erythema of the margins, with froth visible on slit-lamp examination.

PATHOPHYSIOLOGY

- Chronic eyelid inflammation is secondary to *meibomian gland dysfunction* (characteristic froth), related to chronic *bacterial* overgrowth (usually *Staphylococcus aureus*), *ocular rosacea* (telangectasia, pustules, papules), or *seborrheic dermatitis* (greasy scales observed).
- Other causes of inflammatory disease of the eyelid include infections such as herpes, varicella, and

molluscum contagiosum, as well as allergic, drug, and contact dermatitis.
- A distinction is often made between anterior (follicles and lashes) and posterior (meibomian gland) blepharitis, but this is not useful in management or classification with the degree of overlap.
- Histologically, seborrheic dermatitis is characterized by invasion of cell-mediated inflammatory cells in the superficial dermis and perivascular regions. Staphylococcus infections are characterized by neutrophil invasion in a chronic nongranulomatous immune reaction.

CLINICAL FEATURES

- Patients present with tired or sore eyes, worse in the morning.
- Five characteristic signs include (1) injection of lid margin, (2) blood vessel dilation, (3) cloudy meibomian gland plugging, secretion, and froth, (4) collarette formation around lashes, and (5) scales (Fig. 5-6).
- Additional symptoms include bacterial yellow crusting of the canthi, tearing, foreign body sensation, pain, photophobia, and even vision loss.
- Slit-lamp examination will reveal eyelash abnormalities such as trichiasis, meibomian plugging, and secondary corneal pathology and chalazia formation.
- If associated with seborrheic dermatitis, scaling, flaking, and greasy skin are observed.
- If associated with rosacea, an erythematous complexion with telangiectasia and pustules or papules can be observed.
- If associated with herpetic infection, vesicles and a dermatomal distribution can be observed.

DIAGNOSIS AND DIFFERENTIAL

- In general, an examination is sufficient for diagnostic purposes.
- Cultures of the eyelid are not necessary unless a rare pathogen is suspected.

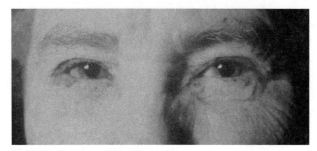

FIGURE 5-6 Seborrheic blepharitis.

- Other diagnoses to be considered in the differential include allergic and toxic conjunctivitis, preseptal cellulitis, chalazion, hordeolum, and lid tumors.

TREATMENT

- Hot compresses are necessary to free debris and open secretory glands. The eyelid margin should be thoroughly cleaned. A mixture of bicarbonate and diluted baby shampoo to remove debris is often used.
- Once the region is cleaned, erythromycin or sulfacetamide antibiotic ointment may be used. Fusidic acid gel has been used as well.
- In refractory cases where topical treatment is not efficacious, meibomian gland function is thought to be improved by oral tetracycline.
- Selenium shampoo should be used in cases of seborrheic dermatitis.
- Topical steroids should be avoided, as patients may become dependent on them (and susceptible individuals may develop glaucoma secondary to chronic steroid use). The exception is short-term use with blepharitis secondary to allergic dermatitis.
- Sequelae of trichiasis, chalazion, and structural eyelid disease should be monitored for and treated appropriately.

EXTERNAL AND INTERNAL HORDEOLUM

CASE 7

A 14-year-old girl noted pain and tearing of her right eye. The next day, her right upper lid was swollen. Her vision on examination was 20/15 OU. The involved lid was tender. When the lid was flipped, an area of erythema with purulent material at its center was found.

PATHOPHYSIOLOGY

- An internal hordeolum is an infection (abscess) which, unlike a chalazion, is painful. It may form within a meibomian gland.
- An external hordeolum is an acute infection (stye) of the glands of Moll or Zeis, at the base of an eyelash follicle. A cyst of Moll is a translucent cyst on the lid margin caused by obstruction of a sweat gland. A cyst of Zeis is caused by blockage of an accessory sebaceous gland.

CLINICAL FEATURES

- Patients present with pain and symptoms of infection in a localized region of the lid.
- Hordeola are differentiated as internal (abscess) or external (stye) with no clinical significance.
- The affected area is generally erythematous, and the patient complains of tearing and foreign body sensation. Vision is not affected. A history of blepharitis or meibomian cyst disease is often present. Symptoms of both internal and external hordeola include eyelid edema with erythema surrounding the cyst near the eyelid margin.
- On examination, evidence of localized inflammation can be found. Often, pus may be elicited. Cellulitis may have developed with infection of surrounding areas.

DIAGNOSIS AND DIFFERENTIAL

- Examination only. No laboratory tests are warranted. This is a clinical diagnosis.
- Again, to differentiate, a chalazion is not painful, whereas a hordeolum is.

TREATMENT

- Warm compresses, eyelid hygiene, and conservative management are the mainstays of treatment.
- Topical antibiotics may be warranted with secondary bacterial infection.
- Rarely is incision and drainage or steroid treatment warranted. The former is employed only if a large well-developed pocket of pus develops.
- Concomitant appropriate treatment of blepharitis and meibomian gland disease will prevent hordeolum formation.

CHALAZION

CASE 8

A 30-year-old man had a painless lump on his left upper lid for months. When he thought it was enlarging, he saw an ophthalmologist. His vision was 20/15 OU. A slightly rubbery, nontender mass was found. When the lid was flipped, slight erythema could be seen at the base of the lesion.

PATHOPHYSIOLOGY

- *Chalazion* derives from the Greek for "hailstone," which is not representative of its pathogenesis.
- A chronically obstructed meibomian gland causes a granuloma within the tarsal plate. The central portion of chalazia are often filled with inflammatory giant cells laden with cholesterol and lipid. There is thought to be an association of hypercholesteremic states with chalazia formation, although this is controversial.
- With chalazia, the obstruction is not painful in contrast to a hordeolum. A chalazion, if infected, may progress and present as a preseptal cellulitis (very rare).
- A chronic chalazion appears as a painless subcutaneous mass.

CLINICAL FEATURES

- Patients present with a nontender, painless lump on the eyelid (Fig. 5-7).
- Less common symptoms include erythema, lid discomfort, and edema.
- Other regions of sebaceous gland disease may be evident, such as acne and seborrhea.

DIAGNOSIS AND DIFFERENTIAL

- Examination only. No laboratory tests are warranted. A culture is rarely useful.
- The differential includes hordeolum (painful, and secondary to a pyogenic inflammatory process), cellulitis, blepharitis, and eyelid tumor.

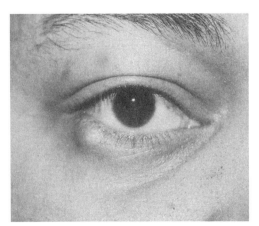

FIGURE 5-7 Chalazion, right lower eyelid.

TREATMENT

- Warm compresses are thought to aid in melting the lipid and promoting extrusion of the chalazion.
- Topical antibiotics can be employed if there is secondary infection, and surgical excision if conservative treatment fails.
- Steroid injection is sometimes used with chronic inflammation, but this is reserved for unremitting chalazia.

BENIGN TUMORS

FIBROUS POLYPS (FIG. 5-8A–D)

CASE 9

A 54-year-old man noted "skin tags" on his left lower lid. He showed them to his ophthalmologist when he went for a routine examination. Vision was 20/20 OU. Two benign small elongated papillomas were found.

PATHOPHYSIOLOGY

- These lesions are a benign upward proliferation of skin.
- Histologically, they show fingerlike projections of papillary dermis covered with epidermis. Although normal polarity is preserved, there is some degree of acanthosis, hyperkeratosis, variable parakeratosis, and elongation of rete pegs.

CLINICAL FEATURES

- This is one of the most common skin lesions, also known as fibroepithelial papilloma, acrochordon, soft fibroma, and fibroepithelial polyp.

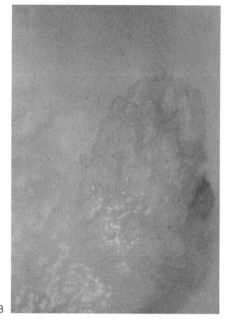

B

FIGURE 5-8B Close-up of a papilloma.

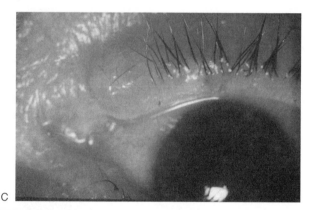

C

FIGURE 5-8C Inclusion cyst of gland of Moll.

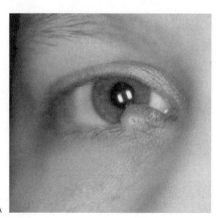

A

FIGURE 5-8A Lower lid papilloma.

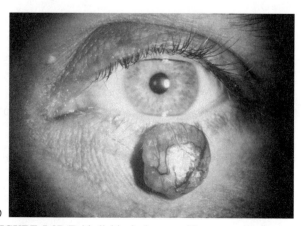

D

FIGURE 5-8D Epithelial inclusion cyst. Note normal lashes.

- These lesions are most commonly found in the neck and axillary areas in the middle-aged and the elderly.
- They tend to present as multiple lesions of varying sizes.
- They are polypoid, soft, skin-colored or slightly hyperpigmented lesions with a thin fibrovascular stalk.
- Occasionally, a lesion twists about its stalk, infarcts, and changes in color to black.

DIAGNOSIS AND DIFFERENTIAL

- The diagnosis is made clinically and is confirmed by histologic study.
- Differentials include other benign tumors such as warts, seborrheic keratosis, actinic keratosis, angiofibroma, and both pedunculated and intradermal nevi.

TREATMENT

- Simple surgical excision if symptomatic.

SEBORRHEIC KERATOSIS

CASE 10

A 69-year-old man presents with multiple raised brownish lesions over his left lower lid, both cheeks, and neck. They have been present for a few years and have not caused any ocular symptoms. These well-demarcated lesions have a greasy "stuck on" appearance. Results of his eye examination are otherwise within normal limits.

PATHOPHYSIOLOGY

- Chronic skin damage due to ultraviolet (UV) light is thought to play an important role in its pathogenesis.
- It is regarded by many as a delayed type of peridermal nevus.
- In most patients, these are incidental findings. However, a subset of patients develop seborrheic keratosis when afflicted by underlying malignancy.
- The sign of Leser-Trélat is a sudden eruption of seborrheic keratosis in persons with concomitant carcinoma, most commonly an adenocarcinoma of the gastrointestinal (GI) tract.
- Associations with leukemia, Sézary syndrome, and carcinoma of the prostate, breast, ovary, uterus, liver, or lung have also been reported.
- Seborrheic keratosis has been found in association with a variety of benign and malignant lesions, including basal cell carcinoma, squamous cell carcinoma,

malignant melanoma, keratoacanthoma, adenocarcinoma, Bowen's disease, and bowenoid transformation.

CLINICAL FEATURES

- These lesions are also known by many other names such as acanthosis verrucosa seborrhoica, acanthotic nevus, basal cell papilloma, keratosis pigmentosa, and verruca plana sinorum.
- They are among the most common human tumors, occurring in about 20% of the elderly with equal incidence in males and females.
- The trunk, neck, face, and arm are the most common sites.
- They generally appear as multiple well-demarcated brown or black raised lesions. Occasionally they may be pedunculated.
- Typically these lesions have a greasy, waxy, verrucous surface with friable scales and a "stuck on" appearance (Fig. 5-9).
- When traumatized, a lesion becomes crusted and pustular.
- A particular form, occurring mainly in blacks, is called dermatosis papulosa nigra. These are multiple small, soft, round keratoses on the face or torso of young adult black women. These lesions do not have greasy friable scales or a "stuck on" appearance.

DIAGNOSIS AND DIFFERENTIAL

- The diagnosis is made clinically and by biopsy.
- Most important, basal cell carcinoma and squamous cell carcinoma must be ruled out histologically.
- Other differentials include benign skin lesions such as verruca vulgaris (warts), hidroacanthoma, epidermal nevi, epidermal acantholysis, and intraepidermal epithelioma.

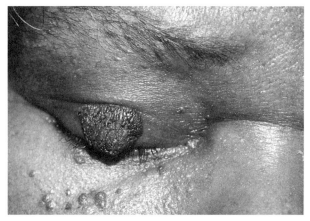

FIGURE 5-9 Seborrheic keratosis. This lesion has a "stuck on" appearance.

TREATMENT

- Shave removal or cryotherapy.
- It is important to keep in mind the association with malignancy of the rare eruptive form, and to make an appropriate referral if necessary.

ACTINIC (SOLAR) KERATOSIS

CASE 11

A 58-year-old woman presents with several lesions over her left lateral canthus, face, and neck. These fairly round, reddish lesions appear slightly raised, are well demarcated, and have greasy scales. The lesion in the lateral canthus itches occasionally. Results of her eye examination are otherwise within normal limits.

PATHOPHYSIOLOGY

- This is the result of skin damage from prolonged exposure to UV light.
- The lesion is precancerous. Many consider it to be equivalent to squamous cell carcinoma in situ.
- In 20–25% of patients with actinic keratosis, a squamous cell carcinoma will eventually develop.
- These lesions are also seen in patients who have received combined psoralen and long-wave UV ray treatment for psoriasis.

CLINICAL FEATURES

- These lesions are found in 11–25% of the elderly population, mainly those with fair complexion.
- Multiple lesions tend to appear in sun-exposed areas of aging skin: face, ears, alopecic scalp, and back of hands. They are rarely found on the eyelids.
- These lesions tend to be flat, rounded, or irregularly shaped, measuring less than 10 mm in diameter.
- The lesions are well demarcated and slightly red, with overlying white or gray or yellow scales. Some may show nodular or warty appearance, and occasionally they may resemble a cutaneous horn.
- Most lesions remain asymptomatic. Rarely, a lesion may be itchy or tender.
- Patients may also have other cutaneous premalignant or malignant lesions such as lentigo maligna, basal cell carcinoma, sebaceous carcinoma, adnexal carcinoma, and malignant melanoma.

DIAGNOSIS AND DIFFERENTIAL

- Diagnosis is made clinically and is confirmed by histopathologic study.
- Differentials include squamous cell carcinoma in situ, seborrheic keratosis, spongiotic dermatosis, and bowenoid papulosis.

TREATMENT

- Although cryotherapy or electrodessication may be used, surgical excision is preferred as it provides a specimen for histopathologic examination.

WARTS

CASE 12

A 32-year-old man presents with a lesion on his left lower lid. It does not cause any ocular symptoms and he desires surgical removal. His eye examination findings are essentially normal except for a papillomatous growth on the left lower lid.

PATHOPHYSIOLOGY

- Warts, or verrucae, are mucocutaneous intraepithelial tumors induced by human papillomaviruses (HPVs) which are DNA-containing viruses.
- Flat warts or verruca plana are caused by HPV 3 (Fig. 5-10).

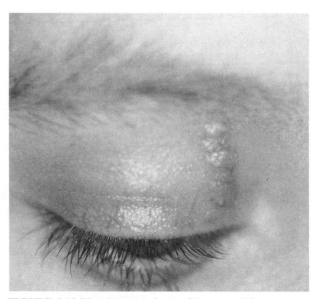

FIGURE 5-10 Wart (verruca plana) of the upper lid.

- The elevated papillomatous warts (verruca vulgaris) are caused by HPV 1, 2, 3, or 4.
- Most warts are benign, but a few of them are found to be associated with mucocutaneous malignancies (HPV 16, 18, 31, and 35 in anogenital cancers, and HPV 5 and 8 in patients with epidermodysplasia verruciformis).

CLINICAL FEATURES

- Four basic types of human warts are described: common wart (verruca vulgaris), flat wart (verruca plana), plantar wart (verruca plantaris), and genital wart (condyloma acuminatum).
- Common warts are small, circumscribed, elevated lesions with a papillomatous and hyperkeratotic surface. They may occur anywhere on the skin, but they have a predilection for the dorsal surfaces of hands and fingers.
- Flat warts tend to occur on the face and dorsal surfaces of hands. They are small, flat, flesh-colored to hypopigmented lesions.
- Plantar warts are on the soles of the feet, caused mainly by HPV 2.
- Genital or venereal warts are the most common venereal disease in the United States. These are cauliflower-like pedunculated nodules, caused by HPV 6, 8, 11, 16, and 18.
- Rarely, warts may appear on mucosal surface.

DIAGNOSIS AND DIFFERENTIAL

- The diagnosis is made clinically and is confirmed by histologic studies.
- The differentials include seborrheic keratosis, actinic keratosis, and skin tags.

TREATMENT

- Surgical excision and/or cryotherapy.

MOLLUSCUM CONTAGIOSUM

CASE 13

A 16-year-old male has been treated for a pink left eye over the past 4 weeks but shows no improvement. His visual acuity is 20/20 OD (right eye) and 20/30 OS (left eye) with pinhole to 20/20. There is mild conjunctival injection with follicular change in the left eye. The cornea is clear. There are two small pearly nodules near the left upper lid margin medially. They are dome-shaped and have an umbilicated center. There is no erythema or telangiectasis. All lashes are present.

PATHOPHYSIOLOGY

- This is a common viral skin and mucous membrane disease caused by a large DNA poxvirus.
- It appears to infect hair follicles, as evidenced by the presence of the virus in the wall of follicular cysts.

CLINICAL FEATURES

- When lesions are on the eyelids, patients frequently present with a chronic follicular conjunctivitis. Superficial punctate staining, superior pannus, or punctal occlusion may be seen.
- The distribution is worldwide and is spread by direct contact, autoinoculation, and fomites.
- The lesions are found anywhere on skin and rarely on mucosal surfaces in children, adolescents, and immunocompromised persons, such as those with AIDS.
- In children, the lesions are found in the face, limbs, and trunk. Outbreaks have been associated with swimming pools, hence they are known as water warts.
- Extensive eruption is usually seen in the immunocompromised.
- Sexual transmission results in multiple lesions in the genital and perineal area.
- Typically, the lesion is a small, flesh-colored, smooth, pearly papule a few millimeters in diameter. It progresses to develop a central depression. Many small ones may coalesce to form plaques (Fig. 5-11).

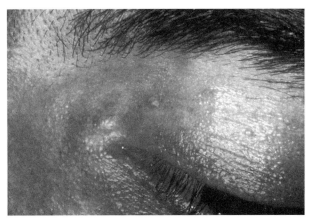

FIGURE 5-11 Molluscum contagiosum of the medial canthus.

- The lesions are asymptomatic unless they become irritated or inflamed.
- Incubation period ranges from 14 days to 6 months. In time, lesions become inflamed, suppurated, and crusted. In most cases infection is a self-limited course of 6 to 9 months.

DIAGNOSIS AND DIFFERENTIAL

- Intracytoplasmic inclusion bodies.
- The diagnosis is made clinically and is confirmed by histopathologic studies.
- Very large or giant lesions are usually found in AIDS patients.
- Large lesions may resemble keratoacanthoma.
- Differentials include basal cell carcinoma, squamous cell carcinoma, keratoacanthoma, sebaceous hyperplasia, syringoma, sebaceous adenoma, warts, papillomas, milia, lichen planus, varicella, and benign and malignant lymphocytic infiltrates.

TREATMENT

- Cryosurgery, curettage, electrodesiccation, alone or in combination, are effective.
- Topical application of various agents such as cantharidin, trichloroacetic acid, silver nitrate, phenol, podophyllin, carbolic acid, tincture of iodine, and Retin-A cream.
- Surgical excision or laser ablation is effective.
- Universal precaution and appropriate referral in the case of an AIDS patient is warranted.

KERATOACANTHOMA

CASE 14

A 49-year-old woman presents with a single, rapidly enlarging lesion on her right cheek. It first appeared 3 weeks ago. It now measures greater than 15 mm in diameter. The lesion has a crusty central depression with a dirty appearance. There was no history of trauma to the cheek or to the lesion. The lesion does not cause pain or ocular symptoms. The woman is otherwise healthy and results of her ocular examination are normal.

PATHOPHYSIOLOGY

- Keratoacanthoma (KA) is also known as invasive acanthosis, invasive acanthoma, molluscum sebaceum, or vegetating sebaceous cyst.

- The lesion is thought to arise from hair follicles in sun-exposed skin and is often associated with solar keratosis. Trauma and UV light are implicated in its pathogenesis.
- Exposure to HPV type 25, radiation, tar, pitch, and podophyllin has been reported in some patients.
- Although most of the lesions occur as a solitary tumor and are generally self-limiting, some experts view it as a low-grade squamous cell carcinoma.

CLINICAL FEATURES

- Peak incidence begins in the sixth decade, with males affected about three times as frequently as females.
- It is generally found on the face, hands, and forearms in men and on the face and legs of fair-skinned women.
- Characteristically, the lesion enlarges rapidly for 3 to 8 weeks to its maximal size and involutes spontaneously over 6 to 12 months, leaving a faint scar. Typically, it has an umbilicated, crater-like central keratin core.
- Some giant variety can reach a size of greater than 10 cm in diameter.
- Multiple KAs of Ferguson Smith is an autosomal dominant disorder that begins in childhood or early adulthood. The patient develops numerous lesions over the years.
- Multiple KAs may be seen in association with the Muir-Torre syndrome, an autosomal dominant inherited condition in which patients develop multiple sebaceous neoplasms and adenocarcinoma of the GI tract.
- Multiple persistent KA occurs sporadically and consists of slow-healing tumors.
- Multiple small KAs may involve the nonexposed skin and are often found in immunosuppressed patients.
- Patients with eruptive KAs of Grzybowski develop hundreds or thousands of small (2 to 3 mm in diameter) pruritic KAs. Familial inheritance is not found.
- Keratoacanthomas have been found in association with numerous benign and malignant lesions, herpes simplex infections, radiodermatitis, and drug eruptions.
- Conjunctival and vulvar keratoacanthoma have also been reported.

DIAGNOSIS AND DIFFERENTIAL

- The diagnosis is made by history, clinical findings, and biopsy.
- Well-differentiated squamous cell carcinoma and basal cell carcinoma must be ruled out when a patient presents with a locally aggressive tumor or a history of multiple recurrences.

• Other differentials include prurigo nodularis (pruritic nodules on extremities in middle-aged women), infundibular cyst (epidermoid cyst), and resolving inflamed wart.

TREATMENT

• Radiotherapy, topical 5-fluorouracil (5-FU), or retinoic acid are often effective.
• Intralesional 5-FU, bleomycin, interferon, triamcinolone, or methotrexate may be used.
• Cryotherapy and surgical excision are used if the lesion is not extensive or is not strategically located.
• Systemic retinoids, methotrexate, and etretinate are used for multiple KAs. Appropriate referral should be made.

XANTHELASMAS

CASE 15

A 54-year-old otherwise healthy man requests surgical removal of disfiguring lesions in the medial canthus bilaterally. There are several irregularly shaped, slightly raised yellowish plaques on all four eyelids medially. These lesions do not cause any ocular symptoms and results of his eye examination are otherwise normal.

PATHOPHYSIOLOGY

• These are lipid deposits in histiocytes in the dermis or tendon.
• One third of patients with xanthelasmas are found to have type IIa hypercholesterolemia [increased beta lipoprotein or low-density lipoprotein (LDL)] and type III dyslipoproteinemia (increased intermediate-density lipoprotein) with elevated cholesterol.
• Infiltrates of foamy or lipid-containing macrophages are seen histologically.

CLINICAL FEATURES

• Xanthelasmas are slightly raised yellowish plaques on the upper and lower eyelids, particularly, the inner canthi. Rarely do they affect other sites (Fig. 5-12).
• They are usually found in the middle-aged or elderly.
• Some patients may develop premature cardiovascular disease.

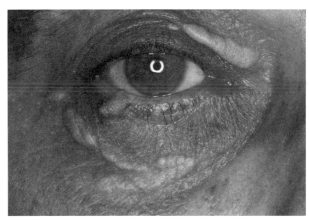

FIGURE 5-12 Xanthelasma. Typical appearance and location of the lesion.

DIAGNOSIS AND DIFFERENTIAL

• The diagnosis is made clinically and is confirmed by histopathologic studies.
• Differentials include xanthoma disseminaturum, necrobiotic xanthogranuloma, lipoid proteinosis, lichen sclerosus et atrophicus.

TREATMENT

• Surgical excision, laser, and 35% trichloroacetic acid may be used to remove large or multiple xanthelasmas.

EPIDERMAL NEVUS

CASE 16

A healthy 14-year-old boy comes in for a routine eye examination. Results of his eye examination are entirely within normal limits. There is a small pigmented nodule in the right upper eyelid laterally. The patient states that it has been there since birth, stayed about the same size, and never bothered him.

PATHOPHYSIOLOGY

• The patient's nodule is a benign collection of epidermal adnexal cells.
• There are several hypotheses. Some postulate it is secondary to an induction defect involving the mesoderm and ectoderm or the neuroectoderm and ectoderm. Others believe it is due to an insult in early development or an abnormal growth factor release or response. An error in cell migration has also been proposed.

CLINICAL FEATURES

- These are acanthomas of the skin or local overgrowth of keratinocytes.
- Lesions generally appear as pigmented papules, nodules, dome-shaped, papillomatous or pedunculated lesions. They rarely become malignant (Fig. 5-13).
- Lesions usually appear at birth or in infancy but may appear in childhood and occasionally in adult life.
- About 50% of the patients are younger than 20, and 33% of the lesions are in the head and neck region.
- Epidermal nevi comprise several clinical variants: nevus verrucosus, nevus unius lateris, systematized nevus, and ichthyosis hystrix. All present as solitary or grouped asymptomatic papules.
- Nevus verrucosus is a local collection of verrucous papules, referred to as squamous papillomas.
- Nevus unius lateris is a unilateral linear verrucous nevus.
- Ichthyosis hystrix is systematized in that it has a pattern of wide distribution.
- Lesions may be seen with multiorgan involvement in the epidermal nevus syndrome.

DIAGNOSIS AND DIFFERENTIAL

- The diagnosis is made clinically and is confirmed by biopsy.
- The differentials include verruca vulgaris, sebaceous keratosis, acanthosis nigricans, and yellow-brown verrucous papules.

TREATMENT

- Surgical excision, cryotherapy, laser, or topical retinoids or 5-FU.

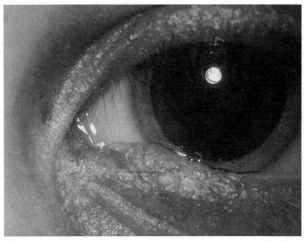

FIGURE 5-13 Lower lid nevus.

CAPILLARY HEMANGIOMA

CASE 17

A 5-month-old healthy female infant has a rapidly enlarging red mass on her left upper eyelid. Her conjunctiva and cornea are clear. Both fundi show good red reflex and clear media. There is a soft spongy mass on the left upper eyelid. It distorts the left upper eyelid and covers her pupil. The mass becomes larger when she cries.

PATHOPHYSIOLOGY

- This is a vascular hamartoma derived from endothelial cell rests.
- There is often positive family history for infantile hemangiomas.

CLINICAL FEATURES

- This is the most common benign periocular tumor of infancy.
- While an occasional capillary hemangioma appears at birth, the vast majority appear before 6 months of age. They go through a rapid growth phase during the first few months before spontaneous regression. By 7 years of age, 75% of the tumors have regressed.
- The mass is typically soft and spongy in consistency and it blanches with pressure. It enlarges when the patient is crying or is placed in a dependent position.
- Clinical appearance varies with the depth of the lesion. When close to skin surface, it tends to be bright red or purple in color. A deeper lesion assumes bluish color (Fig. 5-14A, B).
- Ultrasound, CT, or MRI studies are not necessary to make the diagnosis but are helpful to determine the extent of tumor.
- The tumor mass may cause refractive error or amblyopia, or may induce strabismus.
- The involved eye tends to be more myopic and astigmatic with the axis of (+) cylinder pointing toward the tumor.
- Rarely it is associated with the Kasabach-Merritt syndrome, in which entrapment of platelets within a large capillary hemangioma causes thrombocytopenia and bleeding diathesis.

DIAGNOSIS AND DIFFERENTIAL

- The diagnosis is made clinically and is confirmed by histological studies.

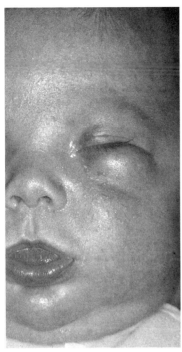

A

FIGURE 5-14A Capillary hemangioma of the lower lid. A superficial lesion involves the lid only. A deep lesion involves the orbit. A combined lesion involves both the lid and orbit. Note the bluish discoloration.

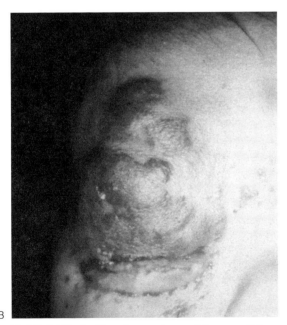

B

FIGURE 5-14B Capillary hemangioma of the upper lid.

- Congenital hydrops of the nasolacrimal sac is generally located in the lacrimal sac area and does not have the typical discoloration. It does not enlarge when the patient cries nor does it spontaneously regress.

- Port-wine stain (Sturge-Weber syndrome) is usually a flat noncompressible lesion.
- Histologically, the dermis shows a well-circumscribed collection of well-formed small, thin-walled capillaries with a flattened endothelial cell lining and occasional buds of endothelial cells with minimal inflammatory infiltrate.

TREATMENT

- If no active treatment is instituted, a child with an eyelid hemangioma must be followed closely and undergo frequent cycloplegic retinoscopy to prevent amblyopia.
- Slow, careful, and controlled intralesional steroid injection is the preferred modality.
- Systemic steroids are necessary if there is subglottic hemangioma causing airway obstruction or cardiac failure.
- Surgical excision or superficial radiotherapy may be used in selected cases.
- Sclerosing agents generally produce unpredictable results.

MALIGNANT TUMORS

SEBACEOUS CANCER OF THE LID

CASE 18

A 56-year-old woman presents with a history of constant ocular irritation and recurrent chalazion of the right upper eyelid. There is no history of weight loss, malaise, or fever. Her vision, motility, and funduscopic examination results are normal. Examination of the everted right upper eyelid shows an irregular conjunctival surface with pits and lines. Most of the eyelashes of the right upper eyelid are missing.

PATHOPHYSIOLOGY

- This is one of the most lethal eyelid tumors.
- Genetic factors may account for its higher incidence in Asians.
- A history of previous irradiation for ocular or orbital tumor is found in some.

CLINICAL FEATURES

- There is great variability in presentation and the diagnosis is frequently missed.

- It commonly presents as a painless enlarging mass.
- It may present as recurrent chalazion or chronic blepharo-conjunctivitis refractory to treatment (Fig. 5-15A).
- When lashes are missing spontaneously, malignancy is always possible.
- Look for enlarged preauricular, cervical, and submandibular lymph nodes. Lymph node metastasis ranges from 17 to 23% and orbital extension from 6 to 16%. With orbital extension, the mortality rate goes up to 76% (Fig. 5-15B).
- Poor prognostic indicators include involvement of both upper and lower lids, a tumor with >10 mm diameter, duration greater than 6 months, multicentricity, highly infiltrative pattern, poor differentiation, and vascular, lymphatic, and orbital extension.

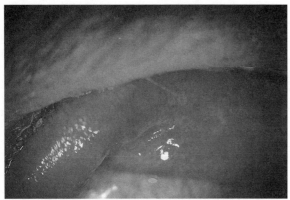

FIGURE 5-15A Sebaceous cell carcinoma of the lid. Note the white lines and pits in the tarsus surrounded by diffusely injected conjunctiva. This patient complains mainly of tearing with discharge. (See Color Plate.)

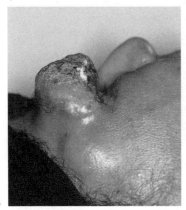

FIGURE 5-15B Sebaceous cell carcinoma of advanced stage. Note the large swollen regional lymph node.

DIAGNOSIS AND DIFFERENTIAL

- Properly prepared tissues and oil-red-O stain are keys to make the diagnosis. The tumor usually displays lobules, sheet, and cords of tumor cells with different degrees of sebaceous differentiation and infiltration into surrounding tissues. The well-differentiated cells contain foamy or vacuolated basophilic cytoplasm, whereas the less-differentiated cells contain more deeply basophilic cytoplasm and more mitotic figures.
- Some tumors demonstrate squamous features with foci of keratinization, which may be confused with squamous cell cancer.
- Differentials include squamous cell cancer, basal cell cancer, sebaceous adenoma, and sebaceous hyperplasia.

TREATMENT

- Systemic work-up and appropriate consultation.
- Wide surgical excision, radical neck dissection, and possible radiation therapy.

BASAL CELL CARCINOMA

CASE 19

A 62-year-old white man presents with a lesion in the right lower eyelid. It has been there for a year without causing any ocular symptoms. His vision is 20/20 OU. There is a well-circumscribed, raised, nontender lesion near the lid margin centrally. It has a waxy, pearly appearance with a crater-like depression in the center and telangiectatic changes at the base. Eyelashes next to the lesion are missing. Results of the eye examination are otherwise within normal limits.

PATHOPHYSIOLOGY

- This slow-growing neoplasm is often a result of skin damage secondary to UV light.

CLINICAL FEATURES

- Basal cell carcinoma is the most common malignancy of the eyelid.
- More than 60% are located on lower lids. The ratio of lower to upper lid involvement ranges from 3:1 to 5:1.
- In order of decreasing frequency, it is located in the medial canthus, upper lid, and lateral canthus.

- There are four different types: nodular, diffuse (morpheaform), ulcerative, or multicentric.
- Metastasis to lymph nodes, lung, and bones is extremely rare.

DIAGNOSIS AND DIFFERENTIAL

- Diagnosis is made clinically, confirmed by biopsy with frozen or permanent section (Fig. 5-16A–E).
- Rarely, this tumor may be pigmented.
- Tumor located in the medial canthus tends to be more extensive, often because of neglect.
- Involvement of deeper tissues may be determined clinically by assessing the mobility of the overlying skin.
- The differential includes other eyelid tumors such as actinic keratosis, senile keratosis, keratoacanthoma, pseudoepitheliomatous hyperplasia, adenoacanthoma, and squamous cell carcinoma.

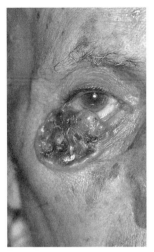

FIGURE 5-16C Basal cell carcinoma of the lid, advanced stage. (See Color Plate.)

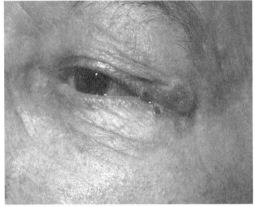

FIGURE 5-16A Basal cell carcinoma of the lid. This lesion involves both the upper and lower lids. (See Color Plate.)

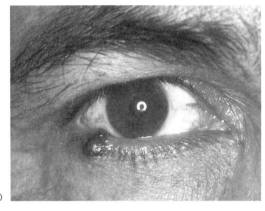

FIGURE 5-16D Pigmented basal cell carcinoma. (See Color Plate.)

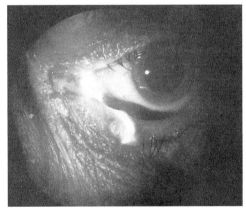

FIGURE 5-16B Basal cell carcinoma of the lid. Note the absence of lash and lack of pigmentation of the lesion. (See Color Plate.)

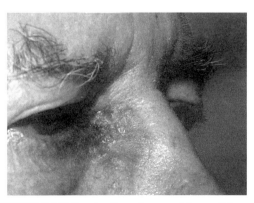

FIGURE 5-16E Basal cell carcinoma of the medial canthus. (See Color Plate.)

TREATMENT

• Tumor excision followed by lid reconstruction is the preferred modality although cryosurgery or radiotherapy is used occasionally.
• The clinical extent of a morpheaform basal cell carcinoma is ill defined, and deep invasion is frequent.
• Either Mohs' chemosurgery or fresh frozen section control technique may be used to delineate the extent of tumor involvement when dealing with a morpheaform tumor.
• Up to 4% of the cases are sufficiently advanced to require orbital exenteration.

SQUAMOUS CELL CARCINOMA

CASE 20

A 57-year-old white woman presents with a nonhealing lesion in the left lower lid. It first began 6 months ago and has gotten bigger. She does not have other medical problems. Her vision is 20/20 OS. There is an ulcerative lesion with all lashes missing at the left lower lid margin laterally. The lesion has irregular fissures and some crusting.

PATHOPHYSIOLOGY

• Squamous cell carcinoma may arise from precancerous dermatosis or de novo.
• Many factors have been implicated: exposure to hydrocarbon, UV light, arsenic, and tar; genetic factors (e.g., xeroderma pigmentosum), irradiation (treatment for retinoblastoma), Bowen's disease, and chronic skin damage.

CLINICAL FEATURES

• It tends to grow more rapidly than basal cell carcinoma.
• The ratio of basal cell carcinoma to squamous cell carcinoma ranges from 11.4:1 to 39:1. There are conflicting reports regarding the ratio of upper to lower eyelid involvement.
• There is no pathognomonic clinical presentation. Most commonly it presents as a red, scaly patch with induration and elevated border that shows ulceration, fissures, and crusting (Fig. 5-17A, B).
• Although it may frequently present in an ulcerative form, it can manifest itself as a papillomatous growth,

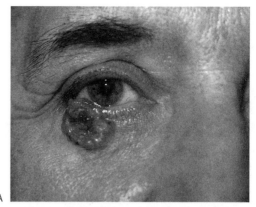

FIGURE 5-17A Squamous cell carcinoma of the lid. Lashes are absent. (See Color Plate.)

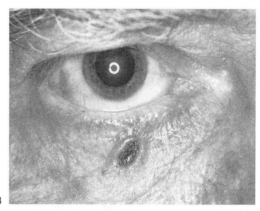

FIGURE 5-17B Squamous cell carcinoma presented as a non-healing ulcer. (See Color Plate.)

a rounded nodule, a cystlike lesion, or a cutaneous horn. Keratinization is the most consistent feature.
• It can spread to the orbit, sinuses, and lacrimal system by direct invasion. It may also spread along nerve sheaths, lymph channels, blood vessels, fascial planes, periosteum, and embryologic fusion planes.
• Patients with squamous cell carcinoma often have other skin tumors, such as basal cell carcinoma, Bowen's disease, and senile keratosis.

DIAGNOSIS AND DIFFERENTIAL

• It is difficult to make the diagnosis based on clinical findings alone. It takes an experienced dermatopathologist to make the correct diagnosis.
• Differentials include actinic keratosis, Bowen's disease, inverted follicular keratosis, senile keratosis, keratoacanthoma, pseudoepitheliomatous hyperplasia, and adenoacanthoma.

TREATMENT

- Surgical excision with frozen section control or Mohs' technique is the preferred modality.
- Radiation therapy, cryotherapy, topical chemotherapy (5-FU), photoradiation therapy, curettage, and electrodessication have been tried. Their effectiveness remains unproven.
- Exenteration is necessary when there is orbital invasion.
- Prognosis is correlated with the histologic grade of malignancy, the presence of predisposing condition such as radiation or xeroderma pigmentosum, and the site of the lesion.
- Reported mortality rates range from 0 to 30%. Patient selection bias and other factors may account for the difference.
- Higher mortality rates are noted when upper lid and medial canthus are involved and with tumors with a higher grade of malignancy.

MALIGNANT MELANOMA

CASE 21

A 66-year-old white man has noticed a dark-pigmented lesion in the left lower eyelid for about 18 months. It appears to have increased in size slightly. His vision is not affected and there is no history of eye irritation. A discrete pigmented mass is located near the left lower eyelid margin laterally, with most of the lashes missing.

PATHOPHYSIOLOGY

- It may arise de novo, from a preexisting nevus. Exposure to UV light is implicated.
- The role of histologic type in the behavior of eyelid melanoma is unclear.

CLINICAL FEATURES

- Malignant melanoma of the eyelid skin accounts for 1% of all lid tumors and mainly affects elderly whites. The incidence in males and females is about equal (Fig. 5-18A, B).
- Up to 40% of the melanomas found on the eyelids may be amelanotic.
- There are four clinicopathologic forms of cutaneous melanoma: lentigo maligna melanoma, superficial spreading melanoma, acral-lentiginous melanoma, and nodular melanoma.

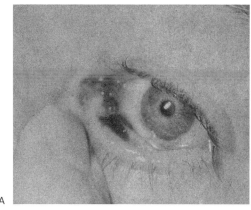

FIGURE 5-18A Malignant melanoma of the lid. This lesion infiltrates the full thickness of the lid and involves the conjunctiva.

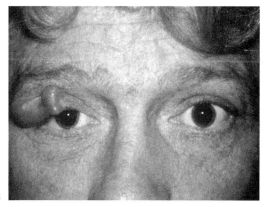

FIGURE 5-18B Malignant melanoma of the lid. Note the amelanotic appearance and absence of lashes.

- Lentigo maligna melanoma is the most common type found on the eyelids. These are flat lesions. They are found only on sun-exposed areas, more commonly involving the lower eyelid and the canthi. Superficial spreading melanoma, however, also affects skin that is not exposed to sun and affects a somewhat younger population than those with lentigo maligna melanoma.
- Lentigo maligna melanoma and superficial spreading melanoma have irregular feathery or notched borders with haphazard color arrangement. Nodular melanoma, by contrast, has discrete borders.
- Lentigo maligna melanoma and superficial spreading melanoma start with a radial growth phase. The development of a nodule in these lesions means a radical change in tumor behavior. It signals deeper invasion and the capability of spawning metastasis.
- In nodular form, there is no radial growth phase but a direct progression toward a biologic virulent disease. The vertical growth phase is the initial and only growth phase.

• Melanoma with the histologic features of acral-lentiginous melanoma has not been found in the eyelid skin.

DIAGNOSIS AND DIFFERENTIAL

• The diagnosis is made clinically and confirmed by histopathologic studies.
• The differential includes pigmented actinic keratosis, pigmented seborrhic keratosis, inverted follicular keratosis, pyogenic granuloma, pigmented squamous cell carcinoma, pigmented basal cell carcinoma, Spitz tumor, blue nevus, and cellular blue nevus.
• Evert the lid to exclude conjunctival involvement, check preauricular and submandibular nodes.

TREATMENT

• Pigmented lesions that are suspect should never be treated with destructive techniques such as cryosurgery, cautery, or electrodessication. The diagnosis should not be based on frozen section technique.
• Full-thickness incisional biopsy should be performed first to confirm the clinical impression. This also helps plan the extent of surgery (surgical margins and lymph nodes dissection or not). Tumor thickness is an important risk factor for recurrence and prognosis.
• Depth of invasion is determined by two different but complementary techniques: levels of invasion and tumor thickness. Level I: Tumor is confined to the epidermis. Level II: Tumor extends into the papillary dermis. Level III: Tumor fills and expands the papillary dermis to the margin of the reticular dermis. Level IV: Tumor cells permeate into the reticular dermis. Level V: Tumor extends into the subcutaneous fat.
• When the tumor is found to be no deeper than level II, it is designated as being in the radial growth phase and has no capacity to metastasize.
• In general, tumors less than 0.76 mm thick have an excellent prognosis. Tumors with thickness greater than 1.50 mm have a poor prognosis. Tumors with thickness between 0.76 and 1.50 mm have an indeterminate prognosis.
• Generally, for a tumor on the lid or face with thickness less than 0.85 mm, a surgical margin of 1–1.5 cm may be adequate. For a thicker tumor, the surgical margin may be 2–3 cm.
• Orbital exenteration or adjuvant radiotherapy is often used as palliative procedure.

LACRIMAL DISORDERS

NASOLACRIMAL DUCT OBSTRUCTION

CASE 22

A 7-month-old child was brought to the pediatrician because of constant tearing of the left eye. This had been present for some time. The child fixed and followed with either eye, and pupils were normal. There was no erythema or purulent discharge.

PATHOPHYSIOLOGY

• The most common congenital nasolacrimal system dysfunction is the failure of the nasolacrimal duct cord to canalize completely.
• Between 30 and 60% of term infants may exhibit some tearing at birth. Ultimately, however, about 5% remain symptomatic.

CLINICAL FEATURES

• Tearing with mattering (mucous accumulation) is typical (Fig. 5-19).

DIAGNOSIS AND DIFFERENTIAL

• History and examination. Occasionally, discharge may be expressed with pressure over the lacrimal sac area.
• Dye disappearance test is helpful in children.
• Dacryocystography or dacryoscintigraphy may be indicated in selected patients.
• The differential includes amniotocele (also known as mucocele, lacrimal sac cyst, or dacryocele), dacryocystitis, keratitis, and conjunctivitis.

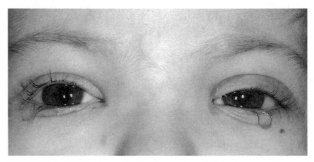

FIGURE 5-19 Tearing and discharge in a child with nasolacrimal duct obstruction and an upper respiratory infection.

TREATMENT

- In infants, the condition usually resolves spontaneously by age 1 year.
- Initially, topical antibiotics-steroids combination eye drops and massage may be helpful. If not resolved after a few weeks or months, probing may be considered.
- The timing of probing is somewhat controversial. It ranges from 3 months to 2 years of age.
- Probing may be performed under general anesthesia or without anesthesia in the office.

DACRYOCYSTITIS

CASE 23

A 60-year-old woman complained of tearing and pain in her right eye. She had no history of trauma or surgery of the eyelids, nose, or sinuses. She had had tearing and discharge for several months. Recently she had developed a painful red lump near the right inner canthus. Examination showed her vision to be 20/20 OU. There was an erythematous swelling over the right lacrimal sac. Purulent material was expressed when pressure was applied over the right lacrimal sac area.

PATHOPHYSIOLOGY

- In primary acquired nasolacrimal duct obstruction, the etiology remains obscure. Currently it is thought to be caused by involutional narrowing of the membranous nasolacrimal duct as a result of chronic inflammatory process within the duct.
- Secondary acquired lacrimal drainage obstruction may be categorized into five groups: *infectious, inflammatory, neoplastic, traumatic,* and *mechanical.*
- Infectious causes include various bacteria (*Staphylococcus aureus, Streptococcus pneumoniae, Actinomyces israelii, Mycobacterium* species, *Chlamydia trachomatis*), viruses (herpes simplex, herpes zoster, varicella), and fungi (*Aspergillus* species, and *Candida* species).
- Endogenous inflammatory causes include Wegener's granulomatosis, sarcoidosis, Stevens Johnson syndrome, cicatricial pemphigoid, sinus histiocytosis, and toxic epidermal necrolysis.
- Exogenous inflammatory causes include various antiviral and antiglaucoma eye drops, silver nitrate, thiotepa, radiation therapy, granulomas, chemical and thermal burns.

- Primary tumors of the lacrimal drainage system are uncommon. Papillomas and squamous cell carcinomas are the most frequent neoplasms that affect the lacrimal drainage system.
- Various secondary and metastatic tumors can cause lacrimal drainage system obstruction. These include adenoid cystic carcinoma, leukemia, lymphoma, capillary hemangioma, basal cell carcinoma, papilloma, squamous cell carcinoma, sebaceous gland carcinoma, and metastatic breast carcinoma, prostatic carcinoma, and melanoma.
- Trauma such as laceration of the lacrimal sac or canaliculus, or fractures involving the nasolacrimal duct can result in obstruction.
- Iatrogenic causes include surgical complications in sinus surgery, transantral orbital decompression, various nasal surgery, craniofacial surgery, and various procedures of nasolacrimal system repair.
- Mechanical causes include dacryolith, epinephrine cast, quinacrine deposits, migrated or retained punctal plug, Veirs rod, silicone tube fragment, and BB pellet.

CLINICAL FEATURES

- Tearing with discharge is the most common presentation. In more severe cases, there is a warm, tender, swollen pyocele (Fig. 5-20).
- Female to male ratio is about 3:1. The shape, length, and angle of the bony nasolacrimal duct may be responsible for the increased incidence in females.
- Patients with a narrow face, flat nose, and underdeveloped lacrimal bones and maxillae have a higher incidence of dacryocystitis.

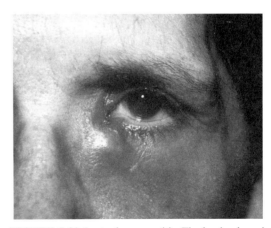

FIGURE 5-20 Acute dacryocystitis. The lacrimal sac is swollen, with overlying erythema and tenderness.

DIAGNOSIS AND DIFFERENTIAL

- History, examination, and Jones I and II tests are most helpful. A Jones I test assesses the patency of the nasolacrimal system using fluorescein dye. If the Jones I test fails, the duct can the irrigated (Jones II) to assess if a partial obstruction is present. If both tests fail, a complete obstruction is present.
- Many ophthalmologists avoid probing of the lacrimal system in acute cases.
- Nasal examination is essential to rule out nasal pathology such as polyps, mucosal mass or erosion, impacted turbinate, or rhinitis. This also helps assess the anatomy of the nasal septum and the distance between the middle turbinate and the lateral wall of the nose in preparation for an eventual dacryocystorhinostomy (DCR).
- CT scan is helpful to study the anatomy and condition of the paranasal sinuses and to rule out space-occupying lesions or a foreign body.
- Dacryocystography may be indicated in selected cases.
- The differential includes orbital cellulitis, lacrimal sac tumors, sinus mucocele, fronto-ethmoiditis, canaliculitis, and lacrimal diverticulitis.
- Other treatable causes of tearing such as eyelid or eyelash abnormalities, glaucoma, and refractive errors must be ruled out first.

TREATMENT

- Hot compress, topical and (when necessary) systemic antibiotics are used to quiet the infection.
- If a pyocele or abscess is present, a simple incision and drainage may be necessary.
- Definitive treatment is a dacryocystorhinostomy.

CANALICULITIS

CASE 24

A 43-year-old woman presents with constant tearing and discharge in the left eye over the past 2 years. She had been to several different ophthalmologists and had tried various antibiotic and steroids drops to no avail. Reportedly, her left lacrimal drainage system was patent by probing. Her left upper lid appeared chronically irritated. The skin was red, puffy, and scaly, particularly in the area over the punctum. The punctum was open and "pouted." When pressure was applied to the lacrimal sac, nothing was expressed. However, some yellowish cheesy material was expressed when pressure was applied directly over the punctum. Results of her eye examination were otherwise within normal limits.

PATHOPHYSIOLOGY

- The etiology of canaliculitis includes herpes simplex, herpes zoster, vaccinia, various bacteria, and fungi such as *Candida albicans* and *Aspergillus niger*, and *Actinomyces*, with the last being the most commonly found organism.
- Chronic canaliculitis is frequently due to a canalicular diverticulum in which organisms proliferate.

CLINICAL FEATURES

- Symptoms are similar to chronic dacryocystitis and there is papillary conjunctivitis with mucopurulent discharge.
- Redness is usually located medially and involves bulbar conjunctiva, caruncular area, and eyelid.
- The involved punctum is erythematous and enlarged and has a raised (or pouted) orifice (Fig. 5-21).
- Yellow cheesy material may be expressed from the canaliculus.

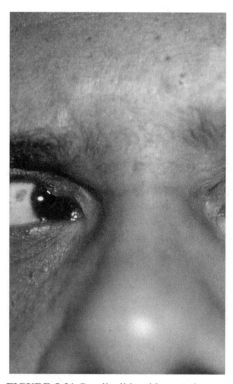

FIGURE 5-21 Canaliculitis with pouted punctum, right upper eyelid.

DIAGNOSIS AND DIFFERENTIAL

- The history of a unilateral medial conjunctival injection with discharge refractory to antibiotic eye drops and a supposedly patent lacrimal drainage system is typical.
- The differential includes chronic papillary conjunctivitis, toxicity to medications, keratoconjunctivitis sicca, blepharoconjunctivitis, superior limbic keratoconjunctivitis, floppy eyelid syndrome, retained foreign body, and a masquerade syndrome secondary to sebaceous cell carcinoma.

TREATMENT

- Using the flat end of two forceps, the involved lid may be squeezed to express the material. A Gram's stain and acid-fast stain should be obtained, and the patient's exudate cultured for anaerobic and aerobic bacteria and fungi.
- Curettage and irrigation with antibiotics is effective in most cases.
- Three-snip punctoplasty and/or canaliculotomy may be necessary in some cases.

CONJUNCTIVA AND SCLERA

Don Liu
Scott Lee

TRAUMA

SUBCONJUNCTIVAL HEMORRHAGE

CASE 1

A 45-year-old man with a history of hay fever had an episode of severe sneezing. He later noted his right eye was red. There was no pain, and vision was normal. Examination disclosed a localized, bright red patch in the right conjunctiva.

PATHOPHYSIOLOGY

- This is the result of a rupture of small conjunctival vessels with blood accumulated under the conjunctiva or Tenon's capsule (Fig. 6-1).
- It is often preceded by a bout of severe coughing, sneezing, or other Valsalva maneuver.
- Other common etiologies include minor trauma and hypertension. Rarely, anticoagulant therapy or blood dyscrasias can cause it.

CLINICAL FEATURES

- Although generally asymptomatic, the patient can be in distress, worrying about losing vision.

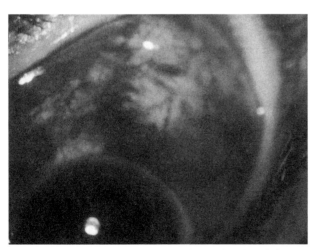

FIGURE 6-1 Subconjunctival hemorrhage. The globe is intact.

- Rarely, the subconjunctival hemorrhage may be large enough to cause a mild to moderate degree of conjunctival prolapse and mild ocular irritation.

DIAGNOSIS AND DIFFERENTIAL

- The diagnosis is made based on history and examination. Blood pressure is taken to rule out severe hypertension.
- A ruptured globe must be ruled out if there is any suspicion of it by patient history or examination.
- Differentials include conjunctival laceration, foreign body, tumor, and conjunctivitis.

TREATMENT

- A conservative approach with patient reassurance is adequate in most cases. The hemorrhage generally reabsorbs within 2 weeks.
- If the hemorrhage is bilateral or recurrent, a medical work-up is warranted.

CONJUNCTIVAL LACERATION

CASE 2

A 9-year-old boy was struck in the left eye with a pencil while wrestling with a classmate. He had pain and bloody tearing from the eye. He was brought to the emergency department, where his vision was found to be 20/25 OU (both eyes). The conjunctiva was injected with subconjunctival hemorrhage. There was a 5 mm laceration of the conjunctiva temporally, but the underlying sclera looked intact. The pupils were normal, and the anterior chambers deep and quiet. Intraocular pressure was 15 mm Hg OU. A dilated fundus examination showed both eyes to be normal.

PATHOPHYSIOLOGY

- The condition was caused by a tear in the conjunctiva, Tenon's capsule, or both.

CLINICAL FEATURES

- The initial presentation varies depending on the specific conditions. Some patients may show slight conjunctival injection while others may present with a large subconjunctival hemorrhage or hematoma (Fig. 6-2).
- A foreign body may or may not be present.

DIAGNOSIS AND DIFFERENTIAL

- The diagnosis is based on patient history and physical examination.
- Involvement of other structures, presence of foreign bodies, and ruptured globe must be ruled out.

TREATMENT

Small lacerations require only topical antibiotics or ointment. Larger ones require surgical closure.

CONJUNCTIVITIS

- Conjunctivitis may be caused by bacteria, viruses, allergens, or chemicals. It may be unilateral or bilateral. Patients may complain of redness, itching, and discharge. Pain, photophobia, or visual loss should not be attributed to conjunctivitis alone.
- Physical findings include conjunctival injection and discharge. Visual acuity should be normal. The cornea should be clear, the pupil normal (Fig. 6-3).
- It can be difficult to determine the cause of conjunctivitis from clinical examination.
- Usually conjunctivitis is benign and self-limited.
- Treatment with topical antibiotics may shorten the course of the condition.

Several types are described in more detail below.

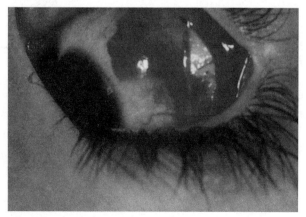

FIGURE 6-2 Conjunctival laceration. The globe is intact.

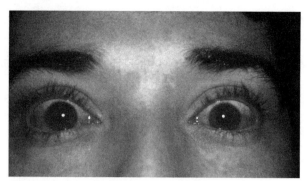

FIGURE 6-3 Bilateral viral conjunctivitis.

ALLERGIC CONJUNCTIVITIS

CASE 3

A 22-year-old healthy woman complains of itchy, watery red eyes for 6 months. She has been to different doctors and has used various antibiotics, decongestants, and other over-the-counter eye drops to no avail. Her vision is 20/20 OU. Her conjunctiva shows moderate injection and chemosis. Her eyelids are slightly swollen and erythematous. Results of her eye examination are otherwise normal.

PATHOPHYSIOLOGY

- Nonspecific inflammation of the conjunctiva may be caused by allergens.
- Indiscriminate use of topical medication is often the cause of contact allergy.

CLINICAL FEATURES

- The condition is usually bilateral and without photophobia or purulent discharge.

DIAGNOSIS AND DIFFERENTIAL

- The diagnosis is made clinically and is supported by patient history.
- The presence of eosinophils in the conjunctival scraping confirms the diagnosis but the absence of them does not exclude the diagnosis.
- History of having a new pet, using a new cosmetic, chemical exposure, and other environmental factors is helpful in identifying a possible cause.
- Seasonal allergic conjunctivitis presents essentially in the same manner but has a seasonal pattern. It is usually

associated with other symptoms or signs of allergic rhinitis such as sneezing and nasal discharge.

TREATMENT

- The patient should discontinue all topical eye drops in the case of contact-allergic conjunctivitis due to indiscriminate use of eye medication, and avoid contact with the specific allergen if identified.
- If the allergy is seasonal, topical mild steroids, antihistamine, mast cell stabilizer, and general symptomatic relief should be considered.

GIANT PAPILLARY CONJUNCTIVITIS

CASE 4

A 27-year-old woman complains of blurred vision and irritated eyes with discharge. Her visual acuity is 20/30 OU with soft contact lenses. There are deposits on the lenses. There is a small amount of mucoid material in both eyes. Her corneas show no staining. Bulbar conjunctiva appears slightly injected. The everted upper eyelids reveal numerous irregularly sized giant papillae.

PATHOPHYSIOLOGY

- It is likely the result of combined mechanical trauma and presence of antigens. Deposits on contact lenses predispose to the development or exacerbation of this condition. It is also seen in patients with a prosthetic eye, band keratopathy, filtering blebs, exposed sutures, or scleral buckle.
- There is histopathologic evidence of both an IgE-mediated type I immediate hypersensitivity reaction and a cell-mediated type IV delayed hypersensitivity reaction.
- The conjunctival epithelium is thickened, irregular, and often shows erosion. The substantia propia is infiltrated by lymphocytes, mast cells, plasma cells, eosinophils, and basophils. Degranulation is seen in many of the mast cells. An increased number of goblet cells accounts for the mucoid discharge.

CLINICAL FEATURES

- The appearance and location of papillae may vary. Giant papillae are those with a diameter greater than 1 mm (Fig. 6-4).
- In soft contact lens wearers, papillae usually start in the uppermost portion of the tarsoconjunctiva and

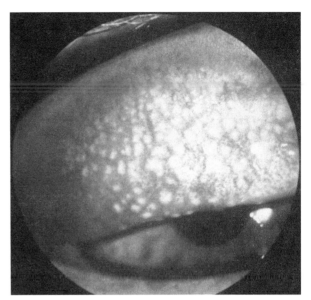

FIGURE 6-4 Giant papillary conjunctivitis. The upper lid is everted to show the giant papillae.

progress toward the lid margin. In hard contact lens wearers, the progress is reversed.
- Mucoid material or ropy discharge may be seen.

DIAGNOSIS AND DIFFERENTIAL

- The diagnosis is made clinically.
- Vernal keratoconjunctivitis usually affects children and resolves by the late teens or early twenties.
- Contact or seasonal allergic conjunctivitis may be diagnosed by patient history and lack of giant papillae.

TREATMENT

- Inciting factors such as suture material or polish or should be removed or an ocular prosthesis should be remade.
- Contact lens wearers should be informed about proper lens hygiene and disinfection technique, and advised to use a preservative-free disinfection solution. If necessary, they should change to a different type of lens.
- Steroidal or nonsteroidal antiinflammatory agents, antihistamine preparations, vasoconstrictors, or mast cell stabilizers may provide symptomatic relief.

EPIDEMIC KERATOCONJUNCTIVITIS

CASE 5

A 25-year-old woman complains of itchy, watery, red, painful eyes with photophobia. The symptoms began in the right eye 5 days ago and have gotten progressively worse. Now she feels the left eye is also involved. Her conjunctiva shows injection and chemosis, more on the right than the left. There is diffuse superficial punctate keratitis (SPK) on the right but none on the left eye. Although she has no fever or malaise, there is a tender preauricular node on the right side.

PATHOPHYSIOLOGY

- This disorder is most frequently caused by adenovirus 8, 19, and 37. It has a limited course with complete recovery.
- The subepithelial infiltrates indicate a delayed hypersensitivity response.

CLINICAL FEATURES

- The condition may be either unilateral or bilateral. It is transmitted by direct contact with the patient or contaminated instruments (Fig. 6-5).
- Clinical symptoms usually appear 8 days after initial exposure.
- An enlarged or tender preauricular node is often noted on the side of initial involvement.
- Early on, diffuse punctate epithelial erosions are seen on the cornea. Seven to 10 days later, larger, coarse epithelial infiltrates become evident. In another 7 to 10 days, these are replaced by focal subepithelial

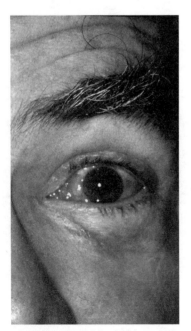

FIGURE 6-5 Epidemic keratoconjunctivitis.

infiltrates. Epithelial keratitis and round subepithelial opacities may be seen even grossly.
- Typically, there is a follicular reaction, mainly in the inferior fornix.
- Vision may be decreased for many weeks or months.

DIAGNOSIS AND DIFFERENTIAL

- The diagnosis is made clinically and is supported by a positive culture.
- Most patients are culture negative 7 to 10 days after the initial symptoms. However, positive cultures may not be obtained even 12 months following the initial exposure.

TREATMENT

- A cold compress on the eyelids, a topical vasoconstrictor, artificial tears, and analgesics will give symptomatic relief.
- Topical antibiotics should be considered to prevent or treat superinfection.
- Topical steroids are used to treat the immunologic response and the subepithelial infiltrates.
- Hands and instruments should be washed after examining patient and contaminated eye drops should be discarded.

CHLAMYDIAL INFECTION

CASE 6

A 55-year-old woman who recently came to this country from the Middle East complains of decreased vision and constant irritation in both eyes. Her past ocular history includes an old eye infection. Her visual acuity with best correction is 20/80 OD (right eye) and 20/200 OS (left eye). The conjunctiva shows no injection but appears very dry. There is a horizontal white line in the tarsoconjunctiva of both upper lids. Her cornea appears hazy and has neovascularization, more on the left side. In addition to a superior pannus in both eyes, there are several small dimples noted at the limbus. Entropion of both upper eyelids is noted. Her ocular motility is normal.

PATHOPHYSIOLOGY

- *Chlamydia trachomatis* species is an obligate intracellular parasite. It infects the mucosal cells and causes ocular, respiratory, and genital tract problems.

- Vision-threatening trachoma is caused by serovars A, B, Ba, and C, and is usually due to multiple reinfections.
- Cytokines are likely responsible for scarring. Limbal follicles, when necrosed, give rise to subsequent Herbert's pits. There is subepithelial infiltration of polymorphonuclear leukocytes and lymphocytes near Bowman's membrane. Corneal pannus, neovascularization, scarring, opacification, and entropion eventually become evident.

CLINICAL FEATURES

- Trachoma is perhaps the most significant cause of preventable visual loss in the world, particularly in North Africa, The Middle East, and South Asia.
- Initially patient presents with a red, sore eye with purulent discharge; often there is a palpable preauricular lymph node. Palpebral conjunctival follicles are noted early. Findings vary as the disease progresses.
- The disease process goes through various stages. There is formation of follicles, which later regress. There is prolonged papillary hypertrophy and subepithelial infiltration of lymphocytes and plasma cells, followed by subsequent conjunctival contraction and scarring.
- The MacCallan classification has four stages. *Stage 1*: immature follicles on the upper tarsal plate with minimal papillary conjunctivitis, diffuse SPK, faint subepithelial corneal opacities, fine superior pannus (Fig. 6-6A). *Stage 2a*: follicular hypertrophy, mature follicles, corneal haze, subepithelial infiltrates, and more pronounced pannus. *Stage 2b*: marked papillary hypertrophy and some necrosis of follicles. *Stage 3*: conjunctival subepithelial fibrosis and scarring (von Arlt's lines), necrosis of follicles (Herbert's pits), trichiasis, and entropion. *Stage 4*: Conjunctiva appears smooth, cornea has subepithelial scarring. Pannus,

trichiasis, entropion, and dry eyes are more pronounced (Fig. 6-6B).

DIAGNOSIS AND DIFFERENTIAL

- Clinical diagnosis is based on meeting at least two of the four criteria. (1) superior tarsal follicles, (2) limbal follicles or Herbert's pits, (3) subepithelial conjunctival scarring, and (4) superficial corneal neovascularization.
- Diagnosis may be confirmed by various laboratory tests: Giemsa stain (Diff-Quik) of conjunctival scrapings with identification of intracytoplasmic inclusions, fluorescein-labeled monoclonal antibody tests (MicroTrak Direct Specimen Test kit), and enzyme-linked immunoassay (Chlamydianyme) (Fig. 6-6C).
- Differentials include chronic follicular conjunctivitis, Axenfeld's chronic follicular conjunctivitis, oculoglandular syndrome (cat scratch fever), and adult inclusion disease (due to serovars D, E, F, G, H, I, J, and K).

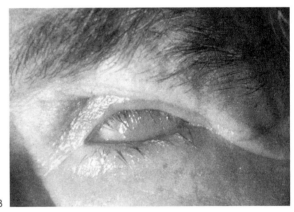
B

FIGURE 6-6B End-stage trachoma. The cornea is totally opacified.

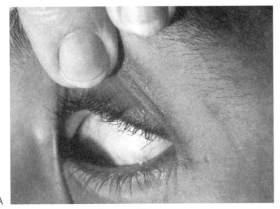
A

FIGURE 6-6A Trachoma. Note pannus on superotemporal cornea. (See Color Plate.)

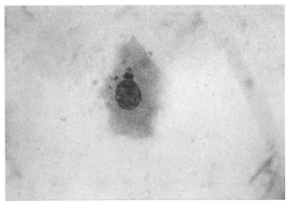
C

FIGURE 6-6C Cytoplasmic inclusion bodies in a case of trachoma.

TREATMENT

- Multiple organs and tissues may be involved in varying degrees. It is important to consult specialists in infectious disease and sexually transmitted diseases.
- Prevention is important and repeated treatment is necessary in endemic areas.
- A 2-week course of tetracycline 250 mg four times daily or doxycycline 100 mg twice daily is effective. Topical antibiotics and lubricants are helpful, and repair of trichiasis and entropion should be done when appropriate.

SUSPECTED CHILD ABUSE OR MUNCHHAUSEN BY PROXY

CASE 7

A 7-month-old otherwise healthy baby is brought in by the stepfather for the third time in 10 days. Bilateral corneal abrasion in both eyes that healed 2 days ago has now recurred. Although both eyes are injected, there is no foreign body or purulent discharge. There is no evidence of trauma to the eyes or the lids. There is no family history of unusual eye disease or genetic defect. Cultures taken by other physicians elsewhere 3 and 4 weeks ago were negative for organisms.

PATHOPHYSIOLOGY AND CLINICAL FEATURES

- This is an unusual problem with clinical findings difficult to explain (Fig. 6-7).

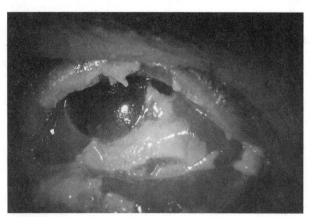

FIGURE 6-7 Munchhausen or self-inflicted injury. This patient gives an inconsistent history. There is no corneal involvement despite extensive conjunctival erosion and maceration. (See Color Plate.)

DIAGNOSIS AND DIFFERENTIAL

- Suspected child abuse or Munchhausen (feigned disease) by proxy. Look for clues in the inconsistencies in history and awkward chemistry between the parents or grandparents. Doctor-shopping also raises a red flag.

TREATMENT

- Antibiotics and supportive treatment may help.
- The case must be reported to the appropriate agency and involve social worker if child abuse is suspected.

PTERYGIUM

CASE 8

A 53-year-old man notices a "white spot" growing in his right eye and complains of nonspecific irritation. Findings of an eye examination are normal except for minimal astigmatism in that eye and a triangle-shaped, yellowish white lesion at the 3 o'clock position, covering 2 mm of cornea at the limbus.

PATHOPHYSIOLOGY

- Sun exposure, windy, sandy, dusty environment, or dry climate may contribute to its development.
- There are typically fibrovascular degenerative changes involving Bowman's membrane.

CLINICAL FEATURES

- The lesion is usually located medially. It can present bilaterally but is usually asymmetric (Fig. 6-8).
- A Stocker's line (iron deposit at the leading edge in the corneal epithelium) may be present.

DIAGNOSIS AND DIFFERENTIAL

- The diagnosis is made clinically.
- Differentials include pseudopterygium and pinguecula.

TREATMENT

- Surgical excision is warranted if the lesion is encroaching on a visual axis or posing a cosmetic problem.

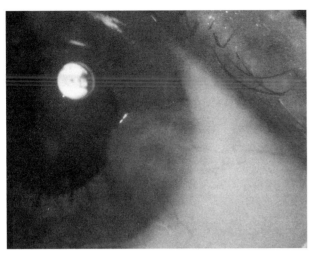

FIGURE 6-8 Pterygium.

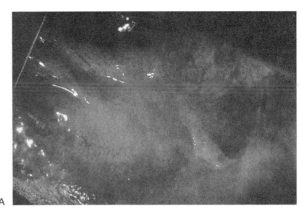

FIGURE 6-9A Acute case of Stevens-Johnson syndrome with severe conjunctival injection, chemosis, and pseudomembrane. (See Color Plate.) [Courtesy of Dr. C. Stephen Foster.]

- Adjunct therapy includes thiotepa or Mitomycin-C application, beta radiation, and topical steroids for frequent recurrence.
- Argon and excimer lasers have been used, but their effectiveness has not been proven.

STEVENS-JOHNSON SYNDROME

CASE 9

A few days ago in this 30-year-old male, a bacterial conjunctivitis was diagnosed and he was treated with a sulfa eye drop. He now presents with red, irritated eyes and mild fever. His visual acuity is 20/30 OU. Bilateral conjunctiva injection, erythema of the eyelids with crusting, and a few maculopapular skin lesions in both palms are noted.

PATHOPHYSIOLOGY

- This condition is also known as erythema multiforme major. It is a disease of the mucous membrane and skin from an acute hypersensitivity reaction in otherwise healthy individuals.
- Infections caused by *Mycoplasma pneumoniae* and herpes simplex are identified in some of the patients.

CLINICAL FEATURES

- Other symptoms include fever, rash, malaise, arthralgia, and respiratory symptoms. Development of target skin lesions in the palms and feet, and bullae with erosion and crusting in the oral mucosa are common.
- Pseudomembrane may be present (Fig. 6-9A).

DIAGNOSIS AND DIFFERENTIAL

- A history of allergy to medications is particularly important. These included sulfa, penicillin, barbiturates, isoniazid, phenytoin, and aspirin.
- Look for recent history of cough, sore throat, fever, and malaise.
- Examination should include mucous membrane surface and skin of extremities.
- Conjunctival cultures and stains are not helpful.
- Chemical burn, ocular cicatricial pemphigoid, pseudopemphigoid, and carcinomas should be considered and ruled out.

TREATMENT

- In mild cases, topical lubrication is prescribed for symptomatic relief. Topical antibiotics and/or steroids may be added when indicated.
- In severe cases with systemic involvement, the patient should be admitted and appropriate consultation obtained. Fluid management with systemic steroids is often the top priority in these patients. There may be devastating sequelae without treatment.
- In later stages, one may consider punctal occlusion, bandage contact lens, symblepharon ring, tarsorrhaphy, or another surgical procedure to protect the cornea (Fig. 6-9B, C).

DRY EYE SYNDROME

CASE 10

A 67-year-old woman complains of blurry vision, irritation, and constant tearing OU. Her vision is 20/30 OU.

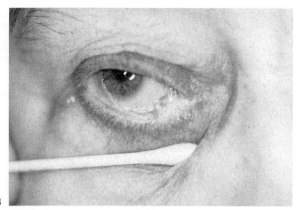

B

FIGURE 6-9B Late sequela of Stevens-Johnson syndrome. Symblepharon of the inferior fornix.

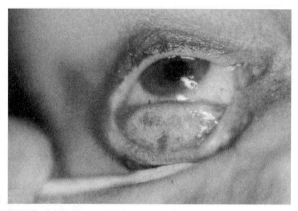

C

FIGURE 6-9C Stevens-Johnson syndrome. Conjunctival scarring, with secondary corneal changes.

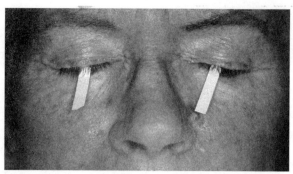

A

FIGURE 6-10A Dry eyes. Schirmer test. This is one of the many tests used to evaluate lacrimal function. Note absence of wetting on paper strips.

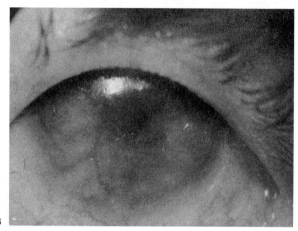

B

FIGURE 6-10B Severe dry eye (keratoconjunctivitis sicca) with corneal scarring and vascularization.

There is trace conjunctival injection with minimal superficial punctate keratitis (SPK). There is an increased tear lake with debris OU. Tear break-up time is 3 to 4 seconds OU. Lacrimal drainage systems are patent by probing. Schirmer I test shows wetting of more than 30 mm OU. Schirmer II test shows less than 3 mm of wetting OU. The Schirmer test is used to measure eye dryness. A strip of paper is placed in the lower fornix and the length of paper that absorbs moisture from the eye determines the degree of desiccation (Fig. 6-10A).

PATHOPHYSIOLOGY

• The condition is mainly caused by decreased tear production and/or deficient mucin or oil component in tears secondary to physiologic change or pathologic conditions. These include hormonal imbalance, aging, destruction of lacrimal tissues by injury, surgery, tumor, pseudotumor, sarcoidosis, tuberculosis, diabetes, chronic blepharitis, and dysthyroidism.

• It may be associated with rheumatoid arthritis, psoriatic arthritis, juvenile chronic arthritis, polymyositis, systemic lupus erythematosus, systemic sclerosis, Hashimoto thyroiditis, polymyositis, and primary biliary cirrhosis.

CLINICAL FEATURES

• Patients complain of dry eye.
• Secondary sequelae from lack of a tear film can include diplopia, decreased visual acuity, and conjunctival injection and erythema from irritation (Fig. 6-10B).

DIAGNOSIS AND DIFFERENTIAL

• Often it may not be possible to identify an underlying systemic cause.
• Other treatable etiology should be excluded first, such as refractive error, glaucoma, obstructed

lacrimal drainage system, lid and lashes abnormalities, foreign body, allergy, and other environmental factors.
• Schirmer tests and a Rose bengal dye are helpful. Patency of the lacrimal system should be verified by probing and/or irrigation.

TREATMENT

• Tear substitutes in the form of drops, ointment, and gel are available for symptomatic relief.
• Mucolytic agents, topical vitamin A, and control of room temperature and humidity are helpful.
• In more severe cases, punctal plugs, permanent occlusion of puncta, and lateral tarsorrhaphy (a procedure where the eyelids are partially sewn to provide greater coverage of the eye) should be considered.

CONGENITAL OCULODERMAL MELANOCYTOSIS

CASE 11

A 9-month-old baby girl of Asian origin has a bluish discoloration of the left eye and skin of the left periorbital area. Eye examination shows that the baby is able to fix and follow light. Eyes are straight and there is good red reflex OU. No lesion is palpable.

PATHOPHYSIOLOGY

• Congenital increase in the number, size, and pigmentation of melanocytes.

CLINICAL FEATURES

• Nevus of Ota is commonly seen in female Asians but it may affect any race.
• After instilling an anesthetic drop in the eye, use a cotton Q-tip applicator to determine if the discolored lesion moves with the conjunctiva. If immobile, it is in the episclera (Fig. 6-11A, B).
• Usually there is ipsilateral hyperpigmentation of the iris and deep facial skin. It tends to follow the distribution of the first and second divisions of the fifth cranial nerve.
• Tiny regularly spaced villiform iris lesions may be present.

DIAGNOSIS AND DIFFERENTIAL

• The diagnosis is made clinically.
• Secondary acquired melanosis attributable to racial, metabolic, or toxic factors should be considered and excluded.

TREATMENT

• Intraocular pressure should be checked regularly since ipsilateral glaucoma develops in about 10% of patients.
• Regular dilated examination should be performed since uveal melanoma can rarely develop in whites.

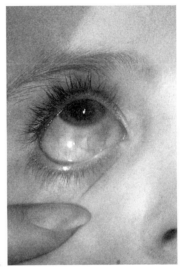
A
FIGURE 6-11A Melanosis bulbi. The pigmentation is in the episclera. (See Color Plate.)

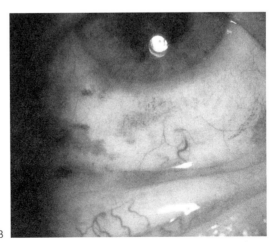
B
FIGURE 6-11B Melanosis of conjunctiva. This may be a primary or an acquired condition. (See Color Plate.)

CONJUNCTIVAL NEVUS

CASE 12

A 25-year-old man presents with a lesion in the right eye. It has been there for many years but it has been growing recently. A small, slightly elevated, nonpigmented lesion is noted at the right lower lid margin centrally. Eye examination results are otherwise completely normal.

PATHOPHYSIOLOGY

- It is a histologically benign condition. There are large spindle cell or epithelioid melanocytes and inflammatory cells.

CLINICAL FEATURES

- Conjunctival nevus is usually a unilateral condition.
- The nevus may be pigmented or nonpigmented (Fig. 6-12).
- It tends to be a solitary, well-demarcated lesion that moves with the conjunctiva.
- The lesion may enlarge or pigment may increase at about puberty.
- Most conjunctival nevi are compound or subepithelial and tend to be elevated. The intraepithelial or junctional nevi are found in the young and tend to be flat.

DIAGNOSIS AND DIFFERENTIAL

- The diagnosis is made clinically and is confirmed histologically.

- Frequently, cystic spaces within the lesion are observed.
- Sudden growth and/or increase in pigment may be a sign of a rare malignant transformation.
- Conjunctival melanoma must be considered and ruled out by biopsy.

TREATMENT

- Observe or surgically excise the lesion.

CONJUNCTIVAL PAPILLOMA

CASE 13

A 42-year-old male presents with a red spot over the right eye. It has been present for several years and appears to have slowly enlarged. There is no history of trauma or surgery of the eye. Eye examination shows a 6 × 4 × 1 mm sessile lesion on the bulbar conjunctiva in the inferonasal quadrant. It has numerous finger-like blood vessels arranged in groups. There is no conjunctival injection or involvement of the cornea.

PATHOPHYSIOLOGY

- Presence of koilocytotic cells with hyperchromatic nuclei surrounded by clear cytoplasm strongly suggests viral etiology.

CLINICAL FEATURES

- It may occur anywhere on the conjunctival surface (Fig. 6-13).
- Pigmentation may be present in persons of dark race.

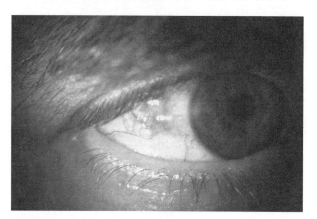

FIGURE 6-12 Conjunctival nevus. Note cysts within the lesion. (See Color Plate.)

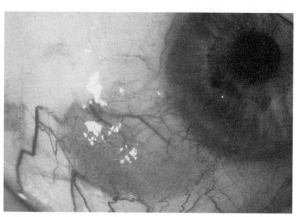

FIGURE 6-13 Large conjunctival papilloma.

- There is an association with high ultraviolet exposure.
- Signs of dysplasia include inflammation, keratinization, and symblepharon formation.
- Typically there is acanthotic nonkeratinizing squamous epithelium.

DIAGNOSIS AND DIFFERENTIAL

- The diagnosis is made clinically and supported by the patient's history.

TREATMENT

- Local excision is often effective.
- Adjunct therapy includes the use of cryotherapy and alpha interferon.

CONJUNCTIVAL PAPILLOMA (SQUAMOUS CELL)

CASE 14

A 27-year-old woman has noticed a growth in the corner of her right eye and desires surgical removal. There is a small pedunculated lesion inferior to the caruncle. Findings of her eye examination are otherwise normal.

PATHOPHYSIOLOGY

- Multiple lesions are highly suggestive of an infection with human papillomavirus (HPV) type 6 and 11.

CLINICAL FEATURES

- Pedunculated or exophytic papillomas of the conjunctiva are commonly found in children and young adults.
- They tend to be found in the fornices and near the caruncle. Occasionally they can be multilobular and bilateral (Fig. 6-14).

DIAGNOSIS AND DIFFERENTIAL

- The diagnosis is made by clinical findings and supported by the patient's history.

TREATMENT

- Surgical excision or cryosurgery and alpha interferon are recommended.

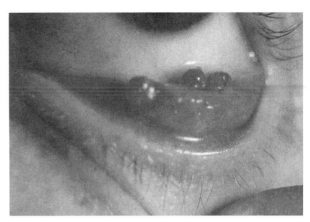

FIGURE 6-14 Pedunculated conjunctival papilloma.

CONJUNCTIVAL INTRAEPITHELIAL NEOPLASIA

CASE 15

A 57-year-old man presents with a growth over the right eye. It has been there for several years without causing any ocular symptoms. His vision and motility are normal. There is a slightly elevated mass that moves freely with the conjunctiva. It encroaches on the cornea medially, has a fleshy appearance, and has tufted blood vessels with hairpin configuration.

PATHOPHYSIOLOGY

- Sun exposure, heavy smoking, and infection with human immunodeficiency virus (HIV) or HPV (type 16, 18) have been implicated.
- There is partial to full thickness conjunctival epithelial dysplasia. Cells have a mild to marked increase of the nucleus to cytoplasm ratio. Mitotic figures may be present at all epithelial levels. Two cell types have been recognized: spindle cells and epidermoid cells.

CLINICAL FEATURES

- This is a slow-growing tumor with 95% of the lesions located at the limbus (Fig. 6-15).

DIAGNOSIS AND DIFFERENTIAL

- The diagnosis is made based on clinical findings and is confirmed by histopathological studies.
- Conjunctival squamous cell carcinoma and pseudo-epitheliomatous hyperplasia should be included in the differentials.

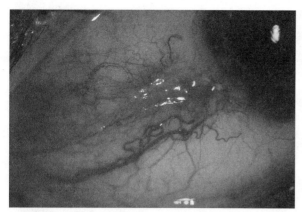

FIGURE 6-15 Conjunctival intraepithelial neoplasm (CIN) at the limbus. (See Color Plate.)

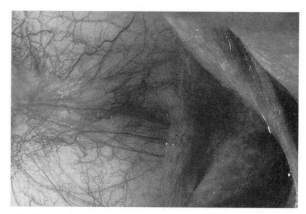

FIGURE 6-16 Squamous cell carcinoma of the conjunctiva. (See Color Plate.)

TREATMENT

• Surgical excision with either cryosurgery or application of Mitomycin-C is often effective.

CONJUNCTIVAL SQUAMOUS CELL CARCINOMA

CASE 16

A 63-year-old man complains of a constant red, irritated right eye. He has had the condition for more than a year and has had only temporary relief by using various antibiotic drops and artificial tears. The conjunctiva of his right eye appears slightly elevated with an irregular surface in the superotemporal quadrant. Conjunctival injection is more intense over that area and there are two larger blood vessels nearby.

PATHOPHYSIOLOGY

• Conjunctival intraepithelial neoplasia (CIN) is often the precursor. The histopathological findings are similar to those found in CIN except tumor cells penetrate the underlying basement membrane and into the subconjunctival space.
• HPV has been implicated in some cases.

CLINICAL FEATURES

• The lesion may appear gelatinous, leukoplakic, or papillaform (Fig. 6-16).
• If the lesion is fixed to the underlying sclera, this represents deep invasion.

DIAGNOSIS AND DIFFERENTIAL

• Diagnosis is made based on clinical findings and histopathological studies.
• Nonpigmented melanoma and mucoepidermoid carcinoma must be considered and ruled out.

TREATMENT

• Wide surgical excision with either cryosurgery or application of Mitomycin-C followed by conjunctival graft is the recommended treatment modality.
• Enucleation should be considered in advanced cases.

KAPOSI'S SARCOMA

CASE 17

A 28-year-old person with AIDS notices a painless, slowly enlarging, bright red mass in the left lower fornix. Eye examination results are otherwise normal.

PATHOPHYSIOLOGY

• This is a slow-growing vascular lesion frequently seen in patients with AIDS.
• Three histologic types have been described. Type 1 has dilated endothelial cell–lined vascular spaces without spindle cells. Type 2 consists of plump fusiform endothelial cells with patches of spindle cells. Type 3 shows densely packed spindle cells with many slitlike spaces.

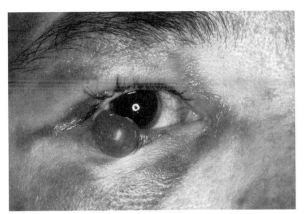

FIGURE 6-17 Kaposi's sarcoma. (See Color Plate.)

CLINICAL FEATURES

- The male to female ratio is about 4 : 1.
- The lesion is often elevated. It may be nodular or diffuse (Fig. 6-17).
- An association between Kaposi's sarcoma and other cancers exists.

DIAGNOSIS AND DIFFERENTIAL

- The diagnosis is made clinically and is confirmed by histopathological studies.
- Differentials include subconjunctival hemorrhage, foreign body, pyogenic granuloma, and cavernous hemangioma.

TREATMENT

- Procedures include local irradiation alone, or surgical excision with cryosurgery or radiotherapy.
- Apply universal precautions if diagnosed in a patient with known AIDS.

CONJUNCTIVAL LYMPHOMA

CASE 18

A 50-year-old man notices a constant red spot in his right eye. He is otherwise healthy and does not have any symptoms associated with the lesion. His vision, motility, and funduscopic examination results are normal. There is a smooth, mobile, slightly elevated, salmon-colored patch in the superonasal quadrant of the right conjunctiva. No feeder vessels are identified.

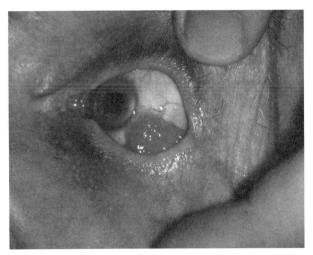

FIGURE 6-18 Conjunctival lymphoma.

PATHOPHYSIOLOGY

- Histologic description varies depending on the specific diagnosis: small or large cells, poorly or well differentiated, monoclonal or polyclonal.
- Fresh tissue is necessary to do many of the immunochemical studies or to identify receptors.

CLINICAL FEATURES

- This condition tends to affect adults and usually causes no symptoms (Fig. 6-18).
- It could be an early manifestation of a malignancy with systemic involvement.

DIAGNOSIS AND DIFFERENTIAL

- Biopsy and systemic work-up are necessary to determine the nature of the lesion.

TREATMENT

- Full systemic work-up and radiotherapy are recommended.
- The overall prognosis is good.
- It should be kept in mind that up to 20% of patients with initial "benign" polyclonal lymphoid lesions eventually develop systemic lymphoma.

CONJUNCTIVAL MELANOMA

CASE 19

A 63-year-old white man presents with a painless pigmented lesion in his left eye. He first noticed it 2 years ago, and the lesion seems bigger now. It is flat and well circumscribed. It has dark pigmentation and is located in the inferior fornix. There is no evidence of ulceration or bleeding. The lesion moves with the conjunctiva, and the underlying sclera appears normal. His ocular examination reveals no other abnormalities.

PATHOPHYSIOLOGY

- Malignant melanoma may arise de novo, from a pre-existing nevus, or from primary acquired melanosis.
- Atypical melanocytes, mitotic figures, spindle cells, and epithelioid cells are found, frequently in a desmoplastic stroma.

CLINICAL FEATURES

- There is a predilection for this in adult whites. Some may be amelanotic (Fig. 6-19A–C).
- Preauricular, intraparotid, submandibular, and cervical lymph nodes must be checked.
- Limbal lesions tend to have a better prognosis.
- Increased mitotic activity, enlarged regional lymph nodes, and involvement of eyelid skin margin, sclera, or orbit are poor prognostic indicators.

DIAGNOSIS AND DIFFERENTIAL

- Special silver stains should be used in suspected amelanotic lesions to identify fine melanin granules.
- Amelanotic conjunctival melanomas also show a positive immunohistochemical reactivity for HMB-45 and S-100.

- Most authorities believe a thickness of 1.8 mm separates the most lethal from nonlethal conjunctival melanomas. Others feel a tumor with a thickness of less than 0.8 mm could still metastisize.
- Differentials include nevus, pyogenic granuloma, extraocular extension of an intraocular melanoma, and melanocytoma.

TREATMENT

- For a well-circumscribed tumor, wide surgical excision with cryosurgery is recommended.
- For a diffuse tumor, local excision with application of cryosurgery or Mitomycin-C is necessary.
- All patients must be followed closely, i.e., every 4 to 6 months.
- If there is deep tissue invasion, orbital extension, or lymph node involvement, surgical excision with adjunct radiotherapy and chemotherapy is necessary. Orbital exenteration is necessary in advanced cases but does not appear to affect the survival rate.

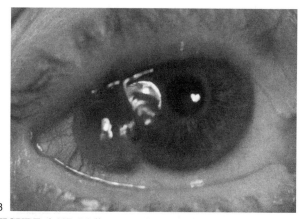

FIGURE 6-19B Malignant melanoma of the conjunctiva. (See Color Plate.)

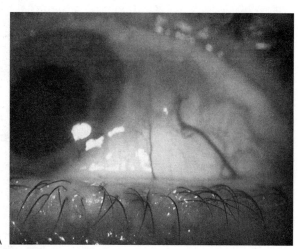

FIGURE 6-19A Malignant melanoma of the conjunctiva. Note the relative amelanotic appearance. (See Color Plate.)

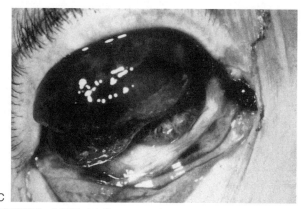

FIGURE 6-19C Malignant melanoma of the conjunctiva, advanced stage. (See Color Plate.)

CONJUNCTIVAL CHALASIS

CASE 20

A 66-year-old woman complains of constant tearing. She does not have glaucoma, refractive errors, or lid or lash abnormality. Dry eyes have been diagnosed and she has used artificial tears to no avail. Her Schirmer test shows wetting of 25 mm OD and 30 mm OS. Tear break-up time was 8 seconds OD and 6 seconds OS. Probing and irrigation shows a patent lacrimal system OU. At the slit lamp, there is a fold of redundant conjunctiva hanging over the lower lid margin when she moves her eyes from up- to downgaze.

PATHOPHYSIOLOGY

- Tearing and/or shooting pain are due to redundant conjunctiva incarcerated between the globe and the eyelid margin.

CLINICAL FEATURES

- This is usually a bilateral condition. The redundant conjunctiva may be located medially and cover the punctum. It may be located centrally or laterally and is incarcerated between the lower lid margin and the globe (Fig. 6-20).
- It is best observed when the patient's eyes move from up- to downgaze.
- Some patients may present with an occasional shooting pain in the eye.

DIAGNOSIS AND DIFFERENTIAL

- This is a rare condition and is often a diagnosis of exclusion. When many of the known and treatable causes of tearing have been ruled out, one needs to look diligently for redundant conjunctiva.

TREATMENT

- Either local excision or tagging down the redundant conjunctiva is effective treatment.

CONJUNCTIVA PROLAPSE

CASE 21

A 15-year-old male who had a left levator resection in one eye 2 days ago notices red swollen tissue in that eye. Examination reveals conjunctiva prolapse in the superior fornix. It is chemotic and covers the pupil.

PATHOPHYSIOLOGY

- A vicious cycle of irritation and fluid transudation causes conjunctival chemosis. When chemosis becomes severe, it disrupts the suspensory ligament of the superior fornix and causes prolapse of conjunctiva.

CLINICAL FEATURES

- Severe conjunctival chemosis with or without prolapse is also seen in patients following retina surgery, large levator resection, craniofacial procedure, repair of blow-out fractures, and in patients with inferior oblique myositis or chronic fistula (Fig. 6-21).

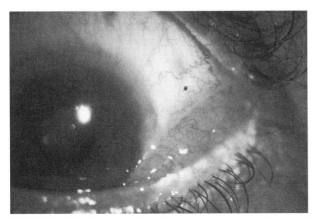

FIGURE 6-20 Conjunctival chalasis. It may be located centrally or medially, and the finding is not always so obvious.

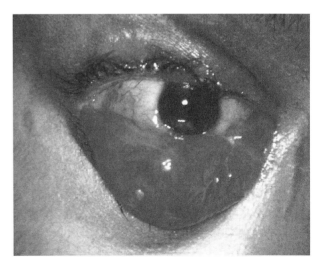

FIGURE 6-21 Conjunctival prolapse. Most frequently the inferior fornix is involved, as seen in this patient following orbital surgery.

- Severe conjunctival chemosis may be seen in patients with occult malignancy or in those who are undergoing chemotherapy for known malignancy.

DIAGNOSIS AND DIFFERENTIAL

- The diagnosis is made clinically.
- The differentials include chemosis secondary to seasonal or contact allergy.

TREATMENT

- In milder cases constant lubrication is useful.
- The prolapsed conjunctiva should be reattached with sutures.
- The prolapsed tissues should be deposited with a small strip of gauze saturated with antibiotics; pressure patching should be done.

EPISCLERITIS

CASE 22

A 40-year-old woman complained of having a red left eye for several weeks. There was no pain, photophobia, or discharge. On examination her vision was found to be normal. There was injection of the left conjunctiva and episclera temporally. Results of the remainder of the eye examination were normal.

PATHOPHYSIOLOGY

- In most cases this is an idiopathic, localized inflammation of the vascularized connective tissue overlying the sclera.
- In 30% of patients, an associated disease is found. Most commonly, it is rheumatoid arthritis, Crohn's disease, rosacea, gout, or herpes zoster.
- It is a relatively benign and self-limiting condition.

CLINICAL FEATURES

- It generally affects patients in the fourth or fifth decade age group.
- No gender predilection has been found in a large series in the United States of America. In contrast, a 3:1 female to male preponderance was found in a British series.

- Bilateral involvement was seen in up to one third of the patients in both series. In 26 to 32% of these patients, other associated diseases were found.
- Most patients present with an asymptomatic red eye(s).
- Occasionally, a patient may complain of a mild foreign body–like discomfort, a vague hot sensation in the eye, or photophobia.
- The condition may present in simple or nodular form (Fig. 6-22).
- In 67% of the simple form, only one sector of the globe is affected.
- Lid edema and conjunctival chemosis may be seen in severe cases.

DIAGNOSIS AND DIFFERENTIAL

- Diagnosis is made by patient history and examination.
- Conjunctival injection is typically found in the interpalpebral area.
- Red-free light should be used to delineate the vascular pattern. The superficial episcleral capillary plexus maintains a normal radial orientation despite engorgement.
- To blanch the conjunctival blood vessels so that the pattern of deeper vasculature can be seen, 2.5% phenylephrine should be used. This enables one to examine the episcleral and scleral vascular pattern and to distinguish conjunctivitis from episcleritis or scleritis.
- To blanch deep episcleral capillary plexi, 10% phenylephrine should be used. This helps distinguish episcleritis from scleritis, but hypertensive crisis must be monitored for.
- Differentials include scleritis and viral and phlyctenular conjunctivitis.

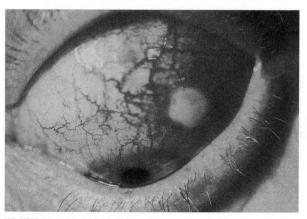

FIGURE 6-22 Episcleritis with nodular infiltration. Note the vascular patterns.

TREATMENT

- The condition usually resolves spontaneously. NSAIDs, artificial tears, and mild steroids may be prescribed for symptomatic relief.
- If there is an associated disease, therapy should be directed at the underlying cause.
- The nodular type of episcleritis is known to cause more discomfort, has a more prolonged course, and tends to recur.
- Recent reports have shown that, rarely, episcleritis can progress to scleritis. It is important to treat the nodular type of episcleritis, to prevent progression to scleritis.
- If recurrent and severe, investigation into collagen-vascular diseases with screening tests should be initiated and proper referral made.

SCLERITIS

CASE 23

A 38-year-old woman complained of redness and pain in the left eye for 2 weeks. She had mild photophobia. There was no discharge. On examination, her vision was found to be 20/20 OU. There was marked injection of the conjunctiva and episclera temporally OS, with slight elevation of the inflamed area. The remainder of the examination findings were normal.

PATHOPHYSIOLOGY

- This is a serious condition in which inflammation of the sclera, characterized by cellular infiltration, vascular changes, and collagen destruction, is seen and vision may be threatened.
- Inflammation may be (a) immunologically modulated (72–96%) or (2) initiated by infection. (4–18% of cases).
- Although the exact mechanism remains unknown, in immunologically modulated cases, an underlying systemic disease is found in more than 50% of the patients.
- Infectious agents include various bacteria, fungi, viruses, and parasites such as *Acanthamoeba, Toxoplasma gondii, Toxocara canis*, and insect larva.
- Exogenous infection is the most common type. This includes posttraumatic and postsurgical infections, and extension from adjacent infections. Infectious scleritis tends to be acute, suppurative, and destructive.
- Extension from other infected structures includes conjunctivitis, keratitis, choroiditis, chorioretinitis, endophthalmitis, panophthalmitis, orbital cellulitis, dacryocystitis, and sinusitis.

- Rarely, infectious scleritis may result from trauma with or without a foreign body.

CLINICAL FEATURES

- Scleritis affects persons in the fourth to sixth decade age group with no racial predilection. The female to male ratio is about 1.6:1.
- More than half of the cases are bilateral and more than half of these bilateral cases present with simultaneous involvement.
- Patients typically complain of vision loss, eye pain, photophobia, or diplopia.
- Depending on the type and severity of scleritis, examination may show conjunctival chemosis, scleral edema, inflamed scleral vessels, a deep violaceous discoloration of the globe, proptosis, lid edema, lid retraction, disc edema, exudative retinal detachment, macular edema, choroidal folds, or ophthalmoplegia.
- Clinical signs of infectious scleritis include conjunctival ulceration, conjunctival and episcleral hyperemia, mucopurulent discharge, subconjunctival nodule, hemorrhage or abscess, scleral necrosis, uveitis, uveal prolapse, and scleral perforation (Fig. 6-23A–C).

DIAGNOSIS AND DIFFERENTIAL

- Diagnosis is made by patient history and examination.
- When looking for an underlying disease, screening tests should include complete blood counts, ESR, circulating immune complexes, complements, ANA, RA factor, HLA typing, U/A, BUN, chest and joint x-rays.
- The natural history, disease course, clinical presentation, and ocular findings of a patient with infectious scleritis depend on the precipitating cause. In most cases, it is obvious.
- If there is no obvious infection, look for history or signs of surgery, trauma, collagen vascular diseases, tuberculosis, and syphilis.
- Corneal scraping for Gram's and Giemsa stains and cultures from the cornea or vitreous are helpful in suspected cases of infectious scleritis. Biopsy of sclera may be necessary in selected cases.
- Differentials include conjunctivitis, episcleritis, and Mooren ulcer if anterior. If posterior, orbital pseudotumor, choroiditis, endophthalmitis, and uveal effusion syndrome should be considered.

TREATMENT

- Oral NSAIDs are usually effective in the control of non-necrotizing types of scleritis. In some cases, a prolonged course of treatment is necessary.

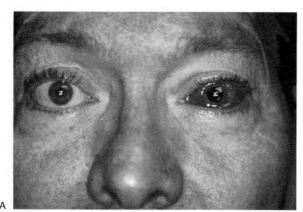

FIGURE 6-23A Scleritis.

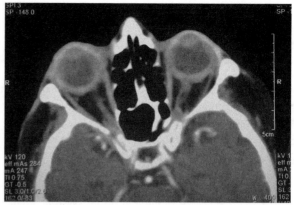

FIGURE 6-23B CT scan of posterior scleritis. Note thickened sclera.

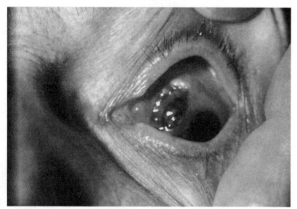

FIGURE 6-23C Scleromalacia perforans. (See Color Plate.)

• Systemic steroids are indicated in some cases of severe non-necrotizing scleritis unresponsive to oral NSAIDs and in necrotizing scleritis. The dose should be started at 1 mg/kg/day and slowly tapered according to response. Intraorbital steroid injection is used in selected cases although most ophthalmologists feel it is contraindicated in non-necrotizing scleritis.

• Systemic immunosuppressive agents such as methotrexate and cyclophosphamide may be required in severe necrotizing scleritis and in scleritis of any type in association with Wegener's granulomatosis or polyarteritis nodosa.

• In the case of infectious scleritis, therapy is also directed at the causative agent proven by culture or histopathological studies.

• A foreign body, if any, should be removed.

• Cryotherapy appears to be a useful adjunct to topical and parenteral antibiotics, especially against a *Pseudomonas* infection.

• Combining surgical debridement of infected tissue with cryotherapy improves the response to medical therapy.

• Lamellar or full thickness scleral and corneal grafting is reserved for special cases.

7 CORNEA

Kathryn Colby
Anh Nguyen

INFECTIOUS KERATITIS

CASE 1

A 30-year-old woman complains of a red left eye and a watery discharge. For the past 2 days, she has been having foreign body sensation and light sensitivity. Her son came from school with a pink eye a week ago. The involved eye appears diffusely injected with a follicular reaction and chemosis. Slit-lamp examination reveals scattered superficial punctate staining. Her anterior chamber is quiet. A preauricular node is also palpated on the same side. This patient presents with typical features of epidemic keratoconjunctivitis, most probably from contact with her infected son. This condition is self-limited. She is told to apply cold compresses to her eyes and to use cold artificial tears for symptomatic relief. She is also cautioned to limit spread of the disease by avoiding close contact and by frequent hand washing.

EPIDEMIC KERATOCONJUNCTIVITIS

PATHOPHYSIOLOGY

- Epidemic keratoconjunctivitis (EKC) is most commonly caused by adenoviruses, serotype 8 and 19. It usually follows an upper respiratory tract infection or occurs after close contact with an infected person. The disease is much more prevalent during the fall and winter months. It usually starts in one eye, but spread to the other eye can occur from autoinoculation.
- The conjunctivitis is generally self-limited and lasts about 2 weeks during which the patient is very contagious. Corneal involvement can occur, usually starting a week into the disease. Corneal subepithelial infiltrates can persist for many months after the first onset of symptoms and are thought to represent a delayed hypersensitivity reaction to viral antigens.

CLINICAL FEATURES

- The typical presentation is a red eye with watery discharge and tender preauricular nodes. Patients can be photophobic with a foreign body sensation.

- Examination shows conjunctival follicles, superficial punctate keratopathy and subepithelial infiltrates at a later stage (Fig. 7-1). Membrane or pseudomembrane formation can occur in severe cases (Fig. 7-2).

DIAGNOSIS AND DIFFERENTIAL

- Diagnosis can usually be made by history and typical clinical picture.
- An exhaustive work-up is usually not needed.

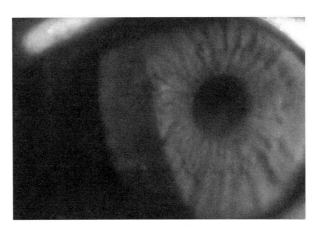

FIGURE 7-1 EKC. Subepithelial infiltrates.

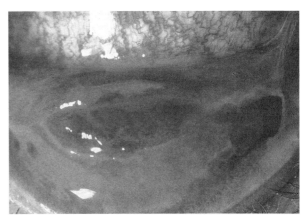

FIGURE 7-2 Pseudomembrane in EKC.

101

- Differential:
  - Bacterial conjunctivitis
  - Pharyngoconjunctival fever
  - Other viral infections such as Epstein-Barr virus in Parinaud's oculoglandular syndrome

TREATMENT

The treatment is mainly supportive as the disease is self-limited. The following are recommended:
- Cold compress
- Cold artificial tears
- Topical vasoconstrictor/antihistamine for redness and itching (VasoCon A or NaphCon A). Common ophthalmic drugs are listed in Table 7-1.
- Topical steroid reserved for severe cases with membrane or pseudomembrane formation and for subepithelial corneal infiltrates. However, steroid treatment may prolong viral shedding.
- Patients should be instructed to avoid close personal contact during the first 2 weeks, to wash their hands frequently, and to avoid rubbing their eyes.

CASE 2

A 5-year-old boy with a history of atopy was recently started on prednisone for a flare-up of his eczema. His mother brought him in because his right eye is red and painful. He had a similar episode during last summer's vacation on the beach with his family. The right eye is very sensitive to light and the conjunctiva is injected. Staining of the cornea with fluorescein shows a dendritic pattern. He also has some anterior chamber reaction. This case has key elements that point to a diagnosis of recurrent herpetic eye disease: the history of atopy, the immunosuppressive state (on prednisone), the history of previous episodes and the typical dendrite that stains with fluorescein. This boy is given liquid acyclovir 200 mg t.i.d. orally for 2 weeks and cyclopentolate 1% b.i.d. He should be reassessed in 1 week to document improvement of his ocular symptoms and resolution of the corneal dendrite.

HERPES SIMPLEX KERATITIS

PATHOPHYSIOLOGY

- Herpes simplex keratitis is typically caused by herpes simplex virus (HSV) type 1. Primary HSV infection most commonly has no symptoms, but may occasionally present as a vesicular, periocular dermatitis with or without corneal involvement. The virus then invades

TABLE 7-1 Common topical ophthalmic medications

CATEGORY	GENERIC	BRAND
Antibiotics	Bacitracin	AK-Bac
	Erythromycin	Ilotycin
	Polymyxin B/ bacitracin	Polysporin
	Polymyxin B/ Trimethoprim 0.1%	Polytrim
	Tobramycin 0.3%	Tobrex
	Ciprofloxacin 0.3%	Ciloxan
	Ofloxacin 0.3%	Ocuflox
	Levofloxacin	Quixin
Antihistamines	Levocabastine 0.05%	Livostin
Antivirals	Trifluridine 1%	Viroptic
	Vidarabine 3%	Vira-A
Mast-cell stabilizers	Cromolyn sodium 4%	Crolom
	Lodoxamide 0.1%	Alomide
Antihistamine-mast-cell stabilizer combinations	Nedocromyl sodium 2%	Alocril
	Olopatidine 0.1%	Patanol
Vasoconstrictor-antihistamines combinations	Naphazoline/pheiramine 0.025%/0.3%	Naphcon-A
	Naphazoline/antazoline 0.05%/0.5%	Vasocon-A
NSAIDs	Diclofenac 0.1%	Voltaren
	Ketorolac 0.5%	Acular
Corticosteroids	Prednisolone acetate 1%	Pred Forte
	Fluorometholone 0.1%	FML
Dilating agents	Cyclopentolate 0.5%, 1%, 2%	Cyclogyl
	Scopolamine 0.25%	Isopto Hyoscine
	Atropine 0.5%, 1%, 2%, 3%	Isopto Atropine

the trigeminal nerve in a retrograde manner and remains dormant in the ganglion until it is reactivated. Suspected triggers for reactivation include fever, ultra violet (UV) light, stress, trauma, immunosuppression, and menstruation.
- The most common manifestation of corneal HSV is dendritic keratitis, which is an acute infection of the corneal epithelium.
- HSV can affect all layers of the cornea, however. See below (Case 3).
- Bilateral disease is very rare and occurs in only about 2% of patients.
- With each reactivation, there is an increased risk of corneal scarring that can ultimately lead to loss of vision.

CLINICAL FEATURES

- The classic picture is that of a dendrite with terminal bulbs that stains brightly with fluorescein (Fig. 7-3).
- Other features include skin vesicles, preauricular nodes, unilateral red eye, pain, photophobia, tearing,

decreased vision, conjunctival follicles, superficial punctate keratopathy, and decreased corneal sensation. Keratic precipitates can be seen when there is concurrent intraocular inflammation (Fig. 7-4).

DIAGNOSIS AND DIFFERENTIAL

- Diagnosis is based on a history of previous episodes in the presence of a typical dendrite. Corneal sensation may be reduced, especially if there have been previous episodes.
- There is often a history of previous perioral cold sores, recent use of steroids or immunosuppressive agents, or immunodeficient states such as eczema, malignancy, or AIDS.
- In indeterminate cases, Giemsa staining of corneal scraping, viral culture or ELISA can be helpful.
- Differential
  - Herpes zoster keratitis (dendrite has different appearance—see Case 3)

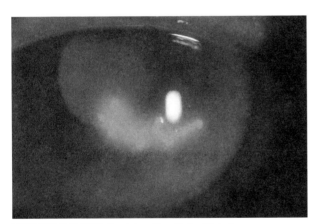

FIGURE 7-3 HSV dendrite. (See Color Plate.)

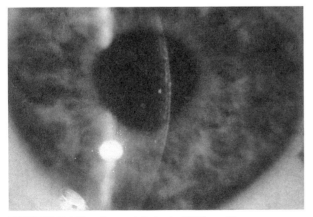

FIGURE 7-4 Keratic precipitates in HSV uveitis.

- Healing epithelial defects often have a dendritiform appearance and may be mistaken for HSV

TREATMENT

- Warm compresses are applied to the skin to dry out the vesicles.
- Viroptic drops (trifluridine 1%) 5–9 ×/day or
- Vira A (vidarabine) ointment 3 ×/day for 7–14 days or
- Acyclovir 400 mg by mouth 5×/day is sometimes given in primary disease and can be given t.i.d. for recurrent dendritic keratitis. The dosage for children is adjusted for their weight.
- Cycloplegics (homatropine, scopolamine b.i.d.) can be given if iritis is present
- Topical steroids are not given because they can prolong the healing of the dendrite.
- Patients should be seen weekly to monitor resolution of the dendrite and other signs of inflammation.
- In patients with more than 2 recurrences a year, oral acyclovir 400 mg b.i.d. significantly reduces the number of these episodes.

CASE 3

An 80-year-old woman was brought in from a nursing home with an excruciating headache. She also has a weeping vesicular rash covering her left forehead to the midline and also involving her left upper lid. Her vision is 20/40 OD (right eye) and 20/200 OS (left eye). Ocular examination is very difficult because of severe photophobia. Moderate conjunctival injection is noted. Corneal sensation tested with a cotton wisp is decreased in the left eye. The slit-lamp examination of the left eye reveals an ill-defined dendrite that stains poorly with fluorescein and dense superficial punctate keratopathy. There is a moderate anterior chamber inflammation, and intraocular pressures (IOP) are 14 and 25. This is herpes zoster ophthalmicus. The treatment consists of an oral antiviral for 7 days (famcyclovir 500 mg by mouth t.i.d.). Topical steroid drops (1% prednisolone acetate q.i.d.) and a cycloplegic (cyclopentolate b.i.d.) are given for the iritis; topical glaucoma medications (timolol or brimonidine) are given to control the inflammatory glaucoma. She is instructed to apply bacitracin ointment b.i.d. to the skin lesions and onto the ocular surface to prevent suprainfection and to keep the ocular surface lubricated. In addition, artificial tears q.i.d. are given to maximize lubrication of this numb cornea. She will need to be seen weekly.

HERPES ZOSTER OPHTHALMICUS KERATITIS

PATHOPHYSIOLOGY

- Herpes zoster virus (HZV) is a DNA virus in the same family as herpes simplex. It causes varicella (chicken pox) as the primary infection. Like the simplex virus, it stays latent in the sensory ganglia. Reactivation occurs when the homeostasis between the virus and the host immune system is disturbed. The virus then travels down the sensory nerve to infect the dermatome supplied by that nerve causing inflammation and necrosis, i.e., causing shingles. The disease is much more prevalent in the older population probably because of depressed cell-mediated immunity. When zoster is found in a patient younger than 50, an immunodeficient state should be considered.

CLINICAL FEATURES

- Patients present with a painful vesicular eruption in the distribution of the fifth cranial nerve (CNV) (Fig. 7-5). If the tip of the nose is involved, ocular involvement should be suspected since both of these areas are supplied by the nasociliary nerve. This is called Hutchinson's sign.
- Patients complain of headache, red eye, eye pain, and blurry vision.
- Slit-lamp findings include dendritic keratitis (can be differentiated from the HSV dendrite by the lack of terminal bulbs and poor staining with fluorescein) (Fig. 7-6), superficial punctate keratopathy, iritis, inflammatory glaucoma, and patchy iris atrophy. Retinitis and optic neuritis occur infrequently. Corneal sensation is typically markedly reduced following herpes zoster ophthalmicus (HZO) and this can complicate the long-term management of these patients.
- Postherpetic neuralgia can be severe and debilitating.

DIAGNOSIS AND DIFFERENTIAL

- The dermatomal rash is pathognomonic.
- A dilated fundus examination is required as both the retina and the optic nerve can be involved.
- A medical work-up is necessary to identify immunodeficiency in young patients.
- Differential:
  - HSV keratitis

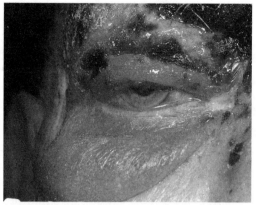

FIGURE 7-5 HZV dermatomal rash. (See Color Plate.)

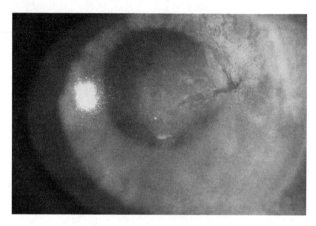

FIGURE 7-6 HZV dendrite. (See Color Plate.)

TREATMENT

- Oral antivirals (famcyclovir 500 mg t.i.d × 7 days, acyclovir 800 mg 5 ×/day for 10 days, or valcyclovir 1 g b.i.d. for 1 week) reduce the duration and severity of the infection and help reduce the incidence of postherpetic neuralgia. Ideally, oral antivirals should be started as soon as possible after the diagnosis is made.
- Immunodeficient patients may need to be admitted for intravenous (IV) antiviral treatment.
- Bacitracin or erythromycin ointment is applied to the skin lesions to avoid bacterial suprainfection.
- HZO dendrites are adequately treated by the oral antivirals. A bland ophthalmic antibiotic ointment, such as erythromycin, can be applied to the ocular surface to prevent bacterial infection and to soothe the eye.
- Topical cycloplegics with or without topical steroids are given when uveitis is present.
- Control of intraocular pressure is needed for inflammatory glaucoma.
- Post-herpetic neuralgia can be treated with a variety of medications including amytriptyline and gabapentin.

Capsaicin ointment applied to the skin can alleviate symptoms of post-herpetic neuralgia in some patients.

• The treatment of herpes zoster extends beyond the acute disease, especially in the setting of an anesthetic cornea.

CASE 4

A 26-year-old man comes into the emergency department with a red right eye and purulent discharge. He is a contact lens wearer but had to stop wearing them 2 days ago because of irritation. His vision with his glasses is 20/400 and 20/20. Slit-lamp examination of the right eye reveals a markedly injected and chemotic conjunctiva. A 3 × 3 mm white, central infiltrate extending deep into the stroma is seen with an adherent plaque of purulent exudate. There is an overlying epithelial defect that stains with fluorescein. A hypopyon is also seen with marked anterior chamber cells and flare. The first step in the management is to obtain microbiological studies of the infiltrate. Samples are obtained with a blade and transferred onto blood agar, chocolate agar, Sabouraud's dextrose agar, and thyoglycolate broth. Slides are also sent for Gram's and Giemsa stains. The patient is then admitted for aggressive fortified topical antibiotics with broad-spectrum coverage every hour around the clock. The usual empiric choices are fortified cefazolin 133 mg/cc and fortified tobramycin 14 mg/cc while waiting for culture results.

BACTERIAL KERATITIS

PATHOPHYSIOLOGY

• The corneal epithelium is a very effective barrier to infection. Bacterial keratitis usually occurs following a break in the corneal surface that allows entry of pathogens. The most common causative bacterial organisms are *Staphylococcus*, *Streptococcus*, and *Pseudomonas* (Table 7-2).

• Only a few organisms can penetrate an intact epithelium. These include *Neisseria gonorrhoeae*, *Corynebacterium diphtheriae*, *Listeria monocytogenes*, and *Haemophilus aegyptius*.

• Predisposing factors for corneal ulcers are contact lens wear, trauma, ocular surface diseases, blepharitis, use of topical steroids, and immunosuppression.

CLINICAL FEATURES

• Patients usually present with a red eye and pain, photophobia, and decreased vision.

TABLE 7-2 Common Corneal Pathogens

ORGANISMS	CELL WALL	DRUG OF CHOICE
Staphylococcus aureus	Gram + cocci	Cefazolin, vancomycin for MRSA*
Staphylococcus epidermitis	Gram + cocci	Cefazolin
Streptococcus pneumoniae	Gram + cocci	Cefazolin
Enterobacteriaceae (*Klebsiella, Serratia, Proteus*)	Gram − rods	Fluoroquinolones, aminoglycosides
Pseudomonas aeruginosa	Gram − rods	Fluoroquinolones, aminoglycosides

*Methicillin-resistant *Staphylococcus aureus*.

• The hallmark is an infiltration of the stroma with an overlying epithelial defect and an adherent mucopurulent exudate.

• A hypopyon, layered white blood cells within the anterior chamber, may be present in severe cases (Fig. 7-7). It is typically sterile.

DIAGNOSIS AND DIFFERENTIAL

• Definitive diagnosis is made with cultures and stains (Table 7-3).
• Differential:
  ○ Fungal infection
  ○ *Acanthamoeba* infection
  ○ Staphyloccocal hypersensitivity reaction (immune reaction—see Case 11)
  ○ Sterile ulcers (neurotrophic)
  ○ Geographic HSV ulcers
• Fungal ulcers most typically present as multiple fluffy white infiltrates with feathery borders and satellite lesions. Risk factors include history of outdoor trauma, chronic use of topical steroids, and ocular surface diseases.

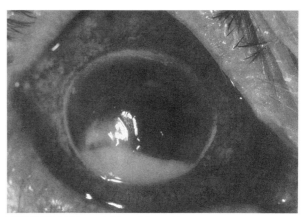

FIGURE 7-7 Bacterial keratitis and hypopyon.

TABLE 7-3 Common Plates and Stains Used

Blood agar	Aerobic organisms
Chocolate agar	Aerobic organisms
Sabouraud's agar	Fungi
Thioglycolate broth	Anaerobic organisms
Gram's stain	Bacteria
Giemsa	Bacteria, fungi, *Chlamydia, Acanthamoeba*
Calcofluor white	*Acanthamoeba*, fungi
Page's saline	*Acanthamoeba*

- *Acanthamoeba* infections are usually linked to contact lens wearers using homemade saline solution to clean their lenses or swimming or using a hot tub while wearing contact lenses. Features that make *Acanthameoba* more likely include (1) pain out of proportion to the clinical findings; (2) radial keratoneuritis (infiltration of corneal nerves)—this is a pathognomonic finding but is only present in 2% of cases; and (3) ring infiltrate (Fig. 7-8). Definitive diagnosis requires cultures for identification of the pathogen.

TREATMENT

- Patients with corneal ulcers should be promptly referred to an ophthalmologist for treatment since some ulcers can progress very rapidly, causing thinning and corneal perforation.
- General guidelines for treatment are:
  - An attempt to identify the most likely causative pathogen in view of the risk factors is important to guide empiric treatment. Adjustment should be made after the organism has been identified through cultures and the susceptibility established.
  - Contact lens wear is associated with *Pseudomonas* and *Acanthamoeba* ulcers. Immunosuppressed patients and those with a history of trauma with a vegetable material are at higher risk for fungal

infections. Patients on ventilators have a well-established association with *Pseudomonas* ulcers. Patients with sexually transmitted diseases are at risk for chlamydial and gonococcal ulcers.
  - Small ulcers can be started on a broad-spectrum topical antibiotic drop such as a fluoroquinolone given hourly. Treatment should be modified according to culture results and clinical response.
  - The more severe ulcers are started on broad-spectrum fortified antibiotics on an hourly basis. These patients may need hospital admission.
  - Topical steroids to minimize the devastating effect of inflammation may be considered once the ulcer has shown response to treatment.
  - Topical steroid use is contraindicated in fungal keratitis and controversial in *Acanthameoba* infection.
  - Cycloplegics are used as needed for patient comfort.

TRAUMA

CASE 5

A 40-year-old man comes in with a painful eye that is tearing profusely. He just cannot keep his eye open for you to examine him. He was playing with his 6-year-old daughter, who scratched his left eye with her fingernail. His vision is 20/20 and 20/60. Slit-lamp examination of the left eye shows perilimbal injection. Fluorescein is instilled and the patient feels immediate relief. There is a linear staining centrally. There is also a very mild anterior chamber reaction. This patient has a corneal abrasion. An antibiotic ointment such as bacitracin is given q.i.d. A small defect should close in 3 days.

CORNEAL ABRASION

PATHOPHYSIOLOGY

- Abrasions are very common corneal injuries (Fig. 7-9). They result from traumatic breaks in the corneal surface. The usual sources of trauma are fingernails, plants, and contact lens wear.

CLINICAL FEATURES

- Patients present with an acute pain, foreign body sensation, photophobia, and tearing following the injury.

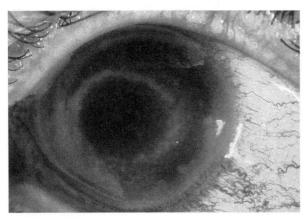
FIGURE 7-8 Ring infiltrate.

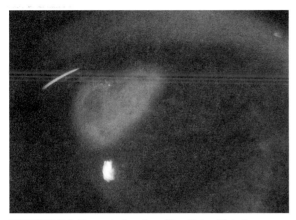

FIGURE 7-9 Corneal abrasion. (See Color Plate.)

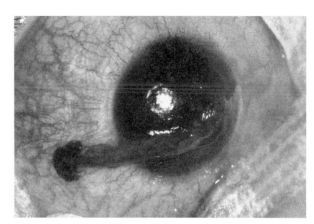

FIGURE 7-10 Open globe. (See Color Plate.)

DIAGNOSIS AND DIFFERENTIAL

- The physician should look for an epithelial defect that stains with fluorescein. It is important to identify any infiltrate that might indicate an infection.
- One should evert the lids to search for foreign bodies. Foreign bodies in the upper lid usually cause vertical lines of abrasion.

TREATMENT

The main goal is to provide comfort and to prevent infection.
- The small defects (less than $10\,\text{mm}^2$) can be treated with either a broad-spectrum topical drop or ointment.
- Topical antibiotic choices include: ciprofloxacin hypochloride 0.3%, ofloxacin 0.3% and polymyxin B/trimethoprim (Polytrim). Start q.i.d.
- Ointment choices are: erythromycin 0.5%, bacitracin, polymyxin B/ bacitracin (Polysporin).
- Pressure patching can be done for larger defects. The patch should be removed every day to verify the absence of an infection and the healing of the defect. Patching should not be done when the risk of infection is significant, as in trauma from a contact lens, from a fingernail, and from vegetable material.
- Topical cycloplegics may be given for pain relief. Corneal abrasions can be very painful and may require oral narcotics.

CORNEAL LACERATION

CASE 6

A young man is brought in by the police after being assaulted with a knife. He is screaming in pain and is

holding his hand over his left eye. He is also bleeding profusely from a laceration on his left forehead. He has bare light perception in the left eye. The lids are gently pried open for examination. His cornea is edematous with uveal tissue extruding through an opened corneal wound (Fig. 7-10). His anterior chamber is flat. This patient has a corneal laceration from the assault with the knife. A Fox shield should be placed on the eye while the patient is prepared for surgery.

PATHOPHYSIOLOGY

- Laceration of the cornea is usually from an injury with a sharp object.

CLINICAL FEATURES

- Patients usually present with decrease vision and eye pain following the injury. The anterior chamber may be flat, with iris prolapsing through the wound.
- The intraocular pressure is usually low from aqueous leak.

DIAGNOSIS AND DIFFERENTIAL

- A Seidel test is positive (fluorescein-stained aqueous seen streaming from the wound).

TREATMENT

- These patients should be immediately referred to an ophthalmologist and given nothing by mouth in anticipation of surgery.
- A shield should be placed over the eye.

- Putting any pressure on the globe is to be avoided.
- Imaging studies, typically thin-cut computed tomography (CT), should be performed before surgery if there is any suspicion of an intraocular foreign body.
- Lacerations are typically repaired in the operating room. The prognosis varies depending on the severity of the injury.

CASE 7

A 30-year-old construction worker comes in with right-eye pain. He was hammering a nail without protective goggles 2 days ago. His vision is 20/30 and 20/20. Slit-lamp examination of the right eye shows mild perilimbal injection. There is a small metallic foreign body lodged in the superficial stroma with an overlying epithelial defect. A rust ring is formed around the piece of metal. A very mild anterior chamber inflammation is seen. His IOP is 15 in that eye. His upper lid is everted and the fornix checked for any remaining particles. A drop of proparacaine is instilled in his right eye and the tip of a 25-gauge needle is used to dislodge the foreign body. Finally, a burr is applied to the surface to remove the rust ring. The patient is sent home with Polysporin ointment q.i.d. until he is seen again in 4–5 days. He is encouraged to wear safety glasses.

FOREIGN BODIES, RUST RINGS

PATHOPHYSIOLOGY

- Superficial foreign bodies lodge in the cornea following injury.
- Iron-containing foreign bodies will oxidize to form rust, which deposits in the cornea around the foreign body.

CLINICAL FEATURES

- Patients usually present with a history of trauma and foreign body sensation, pain, tearing, decreased vision, photophobia.
- The foreign body can be seen on the cornea. If the foreign body contains iron, a rust ring can be found on examination after 12–24 hours.

DIAGNOSIS AND DIFFERENTIAL

- Finding of a foreign body is diagnostic.

- The lids should be everted and fornices should be inspected for any remaining particles.
- A careful dilated fundus examination should be done to rule out intraocular penetration. Imaging studies such as CT or x-ray may be needed as well. Magnetic resonance imaging (MRI) is contraindicated if an intraocular metallic foreign body is suspected.

TREATMENT

- The physician should remove the foreign body and the rust ring after instilling a drop of topical anesthetic.
- The foreign body can be removed with a special instrument called a "golfstick" or with the tip of a 25-gauge needle. The rust ring can be removed with a burr.
- The resulting corneal abrasion can be treated as described above with a topical antibiotic to help prevent infection.
- Prevention is the best treatment—safety glass use should be encouraged.

CASE 8

A hairdresser comes in after she inadvertently splashed her face with the hair dye she was using on her client. She complains of extreme photophobia and foreign body sensation in both eyes. After a drop of proparacaine is instilled, her eyes are immediately irrigated in the emergency department with 2 liters of normal saline solution. The lids are everted and all fornices are thoroughly irrigated with an IV tubing. A pH paper in the fornices shows a pH of 7. Her vision is then checked and is 20/50 OU. She has marked conjunctival chemosis and injection but no perilimbal blanching. Her corneas are slightly edematous with dense punctate staining. The anterior chamber structures are well visualized. A moderate anterior chamber reaction is seen. Her IOP is 16 OD and 18 OS. She is started on bacitracin ointment, Pred Forte q.i.d. and Cyclogyl 1% b.i.d. She is instructed to come back in 1 day.

CHEMICAL BURNS

PATHOPHYSIOLOGY

- Chemical burns are true ocular emergencies. Alkali burns carry the worst prognosis because alkali penetrates the cornea and can cause damage to intraocular structures. Common alkali substances include ammonia, lye, wet plaster, and cement. Acid chemicals include sulfuric acid and hydrofluoric acid.

CLINICAL FEATURES

- Patients present with acute pain and a history of injury. Depending on the extent of the injury and the toxicity of the chemical, corneal findings can range from a mild superficial punctate keratitis to sloughing of the entire corneal epithelium. Vision can be markedly reduced following severe burns.
- Other features are chemosis, perilimbal blanching (Fig. 7-11), corneal edema, anterior chamber inflammation and elevated IOP from trabecular meshwork damage. A white eye following a severe burn signifies ischemia of the ocular surface. This is a poor prognostic sign.

DIAGNOSIS AND DIFFERENTIAL

- Patients can usually give a history of the burn. An attempt should be made to identify the noxious agent and the time of injury. This can be done by reviewing the material safety data sheet for the offending chemical.

TREATMENT

Immediate irrigation of the eye at the time of injury is key to limiting ocular damage. This can be done with any clean liquid, making sure to hold the eyelids open.
   To irrigate in the hospital:
- A lid speculum should be placed to maximize exposure. Topical anesthetic is instilled to provide comfort.
- The involved eye should be copiously irrigated with saline until the pH is 7.0. One should use the limited

range pH paper (6–8) and not the expanded range pH paper (5–11).
- Irrigation can be done with IV tubing.
- All particulate matters should be removed as they may trap chemicals. Do not forget to evert the lids and sweep the fornices.
- The treatment after irrigation depends on the severity of the burn and is best handled by an ophthalmologist.
- The main goals are:
  ○ To promote epithelial healing with either patching or placing a bandage contact lens.
  ○ To prevent infection with antibiotic ointment.
  ○ To control inflammation with topical steroid. However, prolonged steroid use can delay wound healing.
  ○ To control IOP as needed.
  ○ Prevention is the best treatment.

CASE 9

A 65-year-old woman complains of constant burning and watery eyes. She likes to read but her vision gets blurry after a long period of reading. Her vision is 20/30 OU. Slit-lamp examination reveals inspissated secretions along the lash margin. Her corneas show punctate staining mostly in the interpalpebral area. A 5-minute Schirmer test is done after a drop of proparacaine is placed in her eyes. The strips show wetting of 6 mm bilaterally. The diagnosis is a dry eye condition, exacerbated by the meibomian gland dysfunction. She is instructed to apply a warm compress to her closed eyes at bedtime and to apply bacitracin ointment along the lash margin after the soak. She should also use artificial tears at least q.i.d. If the above measures fail to improve her dry eye condition, punctual plugs can be inserted.

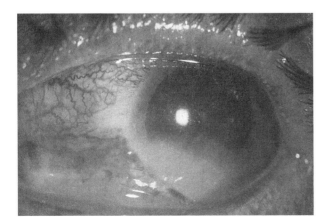

FIGURE 7-11 Chemical burn and perilimbal blanching.

DRY EYE

PATHOPHYSIOLOGY

- Keratoconjunctivitis sicca (dry eye syndrome) results from tear film abnormalities, either a decrease in tear production or an increase in tear evaporation.
- The tear film consists of three components: the outer lipid layer secreted by the meibomian glands along the lid margin, the middle aqueous layer secreted by the lacrimal glands, and the inner mucous layer produced by goblet cells in the conjunctiva. Abnormalities in any of these layers can give rise to a dry eye condition.

- Most cases are idiopathic and are more prevalent in older women. Dry eye is probably related to hormonal changes.
- Dry eyes can also occur as a result of eyelid inflammation (Fig. 7-12) (staphylococcal or seborrheic blepharitis or rosacea) and impaired eyelid gland function.
- Dry eye syndrome can be associated with collagen vascular diseases and Sjögren's syndrome, but most of the time it is idiopathic.

CLINICAL FEATURES

- The symptoms are chronic. Patients complain of burning, as well as foreign body sensation because of decreased surface lubrication. They may have excess tearing from a reflex mechanism in response to the dry eyes. Symptoms are more prominent in the evening and are exacerbated in dry conditions.
- One should look for superficial punctate staining of the cornea after fluorescein instillation. Mucous strands adherent to the corneal surface can appear at a later stage (filamentary keratopathy).

DIAGNOSIS AND DIFFERENTIAL

A number of tests can suggest the diagnosis.
- Low tear meniscus <1 mm
- A decreased tear breakup time (< than 10 seconds) reflects the instability of the tear film. A drop of fluorescein dye is placed on the corneal surface. As the dye disperses, it assumes a uniform dark blue-green appearance. If the film breaks up easily, diagnosis of tear film instability is diagnosed. This is typically due to eyelid gland dysfunction and a poor quality of oil coating the tear film (evaporative dry eye).

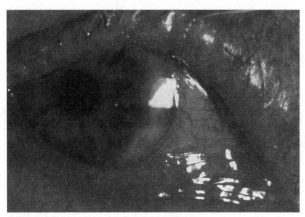

FIGURE 7-12 Blepharitis.

- Rose bengal and fluorescein are dyes that will stain the cornea and conjunctiva in the dry eye condition. The staining is typically more prominent in the exposed interpalpebral area.
- A Schirmer test can be done with or without anesthesia. The irritation from the strip placed without anesthesia causes a reflex tear production. When a drop of anesthetic is given, this reflex tearing is eliminated and only the basic tear secretion is measured. The Schirmer test with anesthesia is more commonly performed. Strip wetting <10 mm in 5 minutes is usually an indication of aqueous tear deficiency.
- The physician should identify other conditions mimicking or exacerbating dry eyes:
  ○ Exposure keratopathy: Graves' ophthalmopathy and eyelid retraction disorders
  ○ Cicatricial diseases (Stevens-Johnson, ocular cicatricial pemphigoid, chemical burns, radiation, graft versus host diseases in bone marrow transplantation)
  ○ Collagen vascular diseases (rheumatoid arthritis, systemic lupus erythematosus, Wegener's granulomatosis, scleroderma, systemic sclerosis, primary biliary cirrhosis)
- Systemic medications can also be a culprit (oral contraceptives, antihistamines, β-blockers, phenothiazine, atropine, morphine).
- Infiltration of lacrimal glands from sarcoid or a tumor can lead to an aqueous tear deficiency state.
- Vitamin A deficiency, although not very common in the industrialized world, may also cause dry eye syndrome because of poor mucin production.

TREATMENT

Treatment of dry eyes is symptomatic, the goal being control of symptoms rather than cure of disease. It is important to identify other conditions associated with dry eyes and treat them. The eyes should be kept well lubricated with the use of artificial tears and ointment. Frequency is dependent on the patient's symptoms, as frequently as every hour as needed. Many brands are currently available.
- When frequent use is needed, preservative-free tears are preferred to avoid toxic effects of preservatives on the corneal epithelium.
- Punctal occlusion with either punctal plugs or cautery can be of benefit when frequent lubrication is not enough.
- One should treat the eyelid problems contributing to the dry eye condition.
- A tarsorrhaphy to reduce exposure can be of benefit in some patients with decreased blink, as in seventh nerve (CN VII) palsy or in Graves' ophthalmopathy.

- The care of patients with collagen vascular diseases should be coordinated with a rheumatologist.

IMMUNE-MEDIATED DISEASES OF THE CORNEA

CASE 10

A 7-year-old boy with a history of asthma and eczema is brought in by his mother with swollen, itchy, and watery eyes. According to his mother, he can't stop rubbing his eyes. She says that this has been a chronic problem, usually worse during spring. Slit-lamp examination shows conjunctival chemosis and a papillary reaction. Giant papillae are seen in the upper tarsus on lid eversion. Both corneas show punctate staining. This is a typical picture of chronic vernal keratoconjunctivitis. This patient is given topical olopatadine (Patanol, a combination of an antihistamine and a mast cell stabilizer) t.i.d. OU. Cold compresses to the eyes can be of help to relieve symptoms. The patient should avoid rubbing his eyes. Treatment of systemic allergies and allergen avoidance should be coordinated with the child's allergist and pediatrician.

VERNAL KERATOCONJUNCTIVITIS AND ATOPIC KERATOCONJUNCTIVITIS

PATHOPHYSIOLOGY

- Both vernal and atopic keratoconjunctivitis are believed to be combined type 1 (IgE-mediated) and type 4 (delayed hypersensitivity reaction) immune responses, with activation of mast cells, eosinophils, and lymphocytes causing damage to the corneal surface. Patients with an atopic disposition (history of asthma, eczema, allergic rhinitis) are more prone to these disorders.
- Vernal keratoconjunctivitis typically affects young men. The symptoms show seasonal variation, and are often worse during spring and summer. This disease will often "burn out" after a few years.
- Atopic keratoconjunctivitis typically has no seasonal variation and has a more chronic course without spontaneous remission.

CLINICAL FEATURES

- The hallmark of vernal disease is intense itching and giant "cobblestone" papillae on the upper tarsus.

Patients also have photophobia, tearing, foreign body sensation, sticky mucoid discharge, shield ulcers (ulcers caused by mechanical irritation of the corneal surface by the giant papillae and by their release of toxic inflammatory mediators), and limbal papillae (limbal eosinophilic infiltrates called Horner-Trantas dots). Corneal vascularization and scarring can eventually result from prolonged inflammation.
- All the above features can also be found in atopic disease. In addition, the eyelids of these patients are usually thickened and scaly, a manifestation of their atopy.
- Both conditions affect atopic individuals. Vernal is seasonal and atopic keratoconjunctivitis is year-round in general.

DIAGNOSIS AND DIFFERENTIAL

- Diagnosis is made by the history of chronic eczema, asthma, or allergies in association with characteristic eye findings.
- Differential:
  - Atopic keratoconjunctivitis
  - Vernal keratoconjunctivitis
  - Allergic conjunctivitis. Associated with seasonal allergic rhinitis, this condition is a type 1 IgE-mediated acute response to an allergen such as ragweed. It is typically self-limited and without associated ocular signs. The diagnosis is made on history in the absence of specific eye findings.
  - Giant papillary conjunctivitis (see Case 20)

TREATMENT

- First, avoidance of allergen and inhibition of mast cell degranulation.
- Second, symptomatic relief:
  - Rubbing the eyes should be avoided.
  - Cold compresses and cold artificial tears can be helpful.
  - Topical mast cell stabilizers (cromolyn, lodoxamide, olopatadine) should be given chronically. Topical antihistamines can be useful for relief of acute itching.
- Systemic antihistamines can be helpful in addressing the underlying systemic disease.
- Other topical medications, including steroids or immunomodulators such as cyclosporin A, may be needed for corneal manifestations such as shield ulcers.

CASE 11

A 50-year-old man with chronic crusty lids in the morning comes in with an acutely red right eye. He complains of a foreign body sensation and photophobia. His vision is decreased in the right eye. Slit-lamp examination of the involved eye reveals dandruff-like flakes along the lashes. Three small infiltrates are seen near the inferior limbus that do not stain with fluorescein. There is also a moderate anterior chamber reaction. This is a typical picture of marginal infiltrates in the context of seborrheic blepharitis. The patient is given a mild topical steroid in addition to warm compresses, scrubbing of the lashes with a mild soap, and bacitracin ointment at bedtime. He should be reevaluated in 1 week to monitor response.

MARGINAL INFILTRATE

PATHOPHYSIOLOGY

- Marginal infiltrates are believed to be an immunologic reaction to staphylococcal antigens released from the organisms colonizing the lids. This condition is also appropriately termed staphylococcal hypersensitivity reaction.

CLINICAL FEATURES

- Characteristically, the epithelium overlying these infiltrates is intact (unlike infectious corneal ulcers—see Case 4). Marginal infiltrates are usually multiple, superficial, and located near the limbus but separated from it by a clear zone. They are often found where the eyelids touch the cornea.
- Patients present with pain, photophobia, and signs of blepharitis (collarettes, meibomian gland dysfunction).

DIAGNOSIS AND DIFFERENTIAL

- The appearance of the infiltrates associated with blepharitis is highly suggestive.
- Both infectious infiltrates and peripheral ulcerative keratitis (see Case 12) must be ruled out with appropriate cultures and laboratory work-up.
- The general rule is that infectious ulcers develop more centrally, hidden from the host immune surveillance, whereas immune ulcers arise near the limbus where limbal vasculature brings in inflammatory cells.

TREATMENT

- Immune infiltrates are typically treated with topical steroids, often with concomitant topical antibiotics to prevent infection.

- The blepharitis and meibomitis must be addressed to prevent recurrences, including treatment with warm compress, lid scrubs with a mild soap, oral doxycycline, and antibiotic ointment in the eyes at bedtime.

CASE 12

A 45-year-old woman with rheumatoid arthritis complains that her left eye is extremely irritated and sensitive to light. On examination, an injected eye is seen with a white infiltrate associated with some thinning near the limbus. She also has anterior chamber inflammation. In the context of rheumatoid arthritis, this infiltrate most likely represents a peripheral ulcerative keratitis. A set of cultures still needs to be sent to rule out an infectious process. The patient is cautiously started on topical steroid with antibiotic coverage until the culture results are obtained. An immunologic work-up is also started. Systemic anti-inflammatory treatment is often needed to control this condition.

PERIPHERAL ULCERATIVE KERATITIS

PATHOPHYSIOLOGY

- Peripheral ulcerative keratitis (PUK) results from a vasculitic process with immune complex deposition in the peripheral cornea. This attracts inflammatory cells that release enzymes, causing necrosis and melting of the tissue. Most of these patients will have systemic inflammatory diseases, most commonly collagen vascular diseases (rheumatoid arthritis, systemic lupus erythematosus, relapsing polychondritis, Wegener's granulomatosis, polyarteritis nodosa, inflammatory bowel diseases).

CLINICAL FEATURES

- Patients present with pain and photophobia.
- Examination of the cornea reveals a sterile ulcer with thinning.
- These lesions can ultimately perforate if underlying vasculitis is not controlled by systemic treatment.

DIAGNOSIS AND DIFFERENTIAL

- One needs to rule out infectious process with corneal culture and smears.

- Work-up for collagen vascular diseases is necessary. This includes an ANA, RF, ESR, CBC, ANCA.
- Differential:
  - Terrien's marginal degeneration
  - Mooren's ulcer
  - Dellen—an area of corneal thinning adjacent to a corneal or conjunctival elevation. This irregular surface causes abnormal drying and subsequent corneal thinning. The epithelium remains intact in the area of a dellen. This condition can be easily reversed with adequate surface hydration with artificial tears and bandage contact lens wear.
  - Staphyloccocal marginal infiltrates (see Case 11).
  - The marginal thinning in both Terrien's degeneration and Mooren's ulcers shares similarities with PUK. Terrien's degeneration is uncommon. The thinning is usually superior with bridging vessels. The epithelium remains intact and a lipid line at the edge of the thinned area is usually observed. The condition is typically bilateral, but may be asymmetric. Terrien's degeneration is not usually painful. Mooren's ulcers, on the other hand, are very painful with more inflammation. The corneal melting and thinning can be extensive, with overhanging edge of anterior cornea hiding much of the thinning. Mooren's ulcer is a diagnosis of exclusion when other disorders causing PUK have been ruled out.

TREATMENT

Treatment is directed at preventing further corneal melting and subsequent perforation. The underlying disease must be addressed with systemic immunosuppressive therapy.

CASE 13

An 8-year-old boy comes in for an evaluation of poor vision. His saddle nose and dental abnormalities are noted as he is examined. The slit-lamp examination reveals bilateral corneal haze associated with deep ghost vessels. These lesions are called interstitial keratitis. Syphilis is the most likely diagnosis for this constellation of findings. These corneal lesions are congenital and usually do not require treatment.

INTERSTITIAL KERATITIS

PATHOPHYSIOLOGY

- Interstitial keratitis (IK) is an inflammatory reaction in the corneal stroma (Fig. 7-13). It represents a reaction

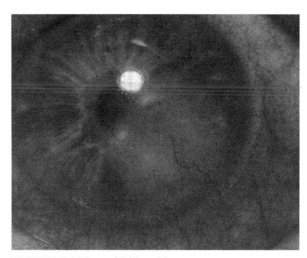

FIGURE 7-13 Interstitial keratitis.

to infectious organisms or their toxins entering the stroma from the limbal vasculature.
- It is classically associated with congenital syphilis but also found with herpes, sarcoidosis, tuberculosis, and Lyme disease.

CLINICAL FEATURES

- The hallmark of active disease is an area of stromal infiltrate associated with deep vessels. Patients present with decreased vision and pain. Corneal scars and ghost vessels are signs of old disease.

DIAGNOSIS AND DIFFERENTIAL

- Diagnosis of IK can be made by history and clinical presentation.
- Systemic disease needs to be ruled out.
- Work-up includes VDRL, FTA-ABS, PPD with anergy panel, chest x-ray, ESR, ANA, RF, Lyme titer.

TREATMENT

- The corneal inflammation can be controlled with topical steroid.
- A cycloplegic (such as cyclopentolate) is added to prevent synechiae.
- The underlying disease should be treated.

CASE 14

A 36-year-old female complains of pain in her left eye and extreme light sensitivity. She had an episode of herpes simplex keratitis 2 years ago, but has had no history of recurrence. Her vision is 20/20 OD and 20/100 OS. An examination reveals an area of edematous cornea but no dendrite. A few keratitic precipitates are seen on the endothelium. There is some anterior chamber inflammation. This patient probably has herpetic disciform keratitis. She is started on a topical steroid such as 1% prednisolone acetate q.i.d. and a cycloplegic such as cyclopentolate 1% q.i.d. to her left eye. Topical (e.g., trifluridine 5 × per day) or oral (acyclovir 400 mg b.i.d.) are also prescribed to prevent the recurrence of epithelial herpetic dendrite (see Case 2). She needs to be reevaluated in 1 week.

DISCIFORM KERATITIS

PATHOPHYSIOLOGY

- Disciform keratitis is most commonly associated with herpetic disease. It is believed to be an immune response to herpes antigens found in the stroma. The host inflammatory response causes stromal edema by causing dysfunction of the corneal endothelium.

CLINICAL FEATURES

- The lesion presents as a disk-shaped area of stromal edema with an intact epithelium associated with other signs of inflammation including keratic precipitates and anterior chamber cells. Patients complain of pain, photophobia, and decreased vision. The IOP may be increased.

DIAGNOSIS AND DIFFERENTIAL

- The classic disciform appearance with a prior history of dendritic HSV keratitis or anterior stromal scarring consistent with prior episodes of HSV infection is highly suggestive.
- Infectious process needs to be ruled out. For example, *Acanthameoba* keratitis can present as a disciform keratitis.
- *Acanthamoeba* is usually associated with a history of contact lens wear, and pain is more prominent because of the perineural infiltration, whereas herpetic lesions are associated with decreased corneal sensation and prior history of HSV.

TREATMENT

- Prednisolone acetate 1% q.i.d. to control stromal inflammation.

- Antiviral to prevent dendritic disease (topical trifluridine at least 5 ×/d or oral acyclovir 400 mg b.i.d.).
- Cycloplegics (scopolamine 0.5% t.i.d.).
- Slow taper of steroid drops is important in preventing recrudescence of the corneal inflammation. Patients need to continue antiviral prophylaxis until steroid dose is less than 1 drop of 1% prednisolone per day.

CASE 15

A 42-year-old woman is very anxious about the irritation and the decreased vision in her right eye. She had a corneal transplant 2 years ago for a corneal scar from herpetic disease. Her vision is decreased in the involved eye. Slit-lamp examination of her right eye reveals a sectoral area of corneal edema and fine keratic precipitates on the endothelium. No infiltrate is identified. There is a mild anterior chamber reaction. This is an episode of corneal transplant rejection that needs to be aborted with aggressive topical steroid every hour. However, an infectious process should also be kept in mind.

CORNEAL TRANSPLANT REJECTION

PATHOPHYSIOLOGY

- Although the cornea is considered to be an immune privileged site, rejection can occur after corneal transplantations (Fig. 7-14). Up to 30% of transplant patients experience a rejection episode during the life of their transplant. Early diagnosis and treatment can prevent most of these episodes from having long-term sequelae.

CLINICAL FEATURES

- The typical features are decreased vision, foreign body sensation, pain, redness, photophobia, corneal edema, anterior chamber inflammation, keratic precipitates on the endothelium, and a rejection line.

DIAGNOSIS AND DIFFERENTIAL

- A high index of suspicion should be maintained. It is very important to recognize early signs of rejection because prompt treatment can abort the acute episode and save the graft.
- Need to rule out:
  ○ Infection
  ○ Recurrent disease in the graft

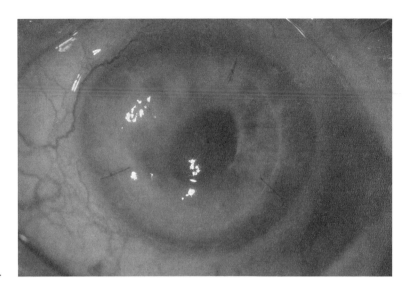

FIGURE 7-14 Acute corneal graft rejection.

○ Uveitis
○ Elevated IOP. High pressure can cause corneal edema.

TREATMENT

- The mainstay of treatment is frequent topical steroid (every hour) once infection has been ruled out. Occasionally injections of steroid into the orbit or underneath the conjunctiva are given.
- Cycloplegics as needed.
- Early diagnosis is key. Corneal transplant patients must remain vigilant for symptoms of rejection (decreased vision, redness of the eye, persistent foreign body sensation) throughout the rest of their lives.

DYSTROPHIES

CASE 16

A 50-year-old woman awoke with a severe pain in her right eye, redness, and profuse tearing. She states that she had a hard time opening her lids this morning and the pain appeared right after she opened them. She has had similar less severe episodes prior to this. Her vision is decreased in the right eye. On slit-lamp examination of the involved eye, an area of irregular epithelium is seen. This area also picks up fluorescein stain. Examination of the other eye shows a map, dot, and fingerprint pattern on the superficial surface of the cornea but no area of staining. This patient presents with a typical episode of recurrent erosion syndrome, and examination

of the other eye reveals the diagnosis of an anterior basement membrane dystrophy as the underlying cause of her recurrent erosions. Her dystrophy cannot be cured but her symptoms can be alleviated, and future episodes of erosions can be suppressed. The management is a step-ladder approach starting with artificial tears, ointment, and hypertonic drops. If these measures fail to improve her symptoms, a bandage contact lens or surgery may be needed.

MAP-DOT-FINGERPRINT DYSTROPHY

PATHOPHYSIOLOGY

- This is a bilateral progressive dystrophy of the anterior basement membrane leading to poor epithelial adherence and breakdown, which is manifested as recurrent corneal erosions (Table 7-4). This usually occurs in the adult without any definite pattern of inheritance.

CLINICAL FEATURES

- The typical appearance on the cornea is described as map, dot, and fingerprint lines in the epithelium. Histopathologically, the dots are intraepithelial cysts filled with nuclear debris. The fingerprints and maps are fibrillogranular material with thickened Descemet's folds projecting into the epithelial layer. The map, dot, and fingerprint changes are especially well visualized using retroillumination through a dilated pupil.
- Map-dot-fingerprint dystrophy typically presents as painful recurrent erosions from breakdown of poorly adherent epithelium. Occasionally it is asymptomatic

TABLE 7-4   Characteristics of Common Corneal Dystrophies

CORNEAL DYSTROPHIES	LAYER INVOLVED	INHERITANCE	EROSIONS
Map-dot-fingerprint	Anterior basement membrane	?	Common
Granular	Stromal	AD	Uncommon
Macular	Stromal	AR	Common
Lattice	Stromal	AD	Common
Fuchs'	Endothelial	?	Uncommon

and diagnosed by characteristic findings during slit-lamp examination.
• Vision can be decreased from surface irregularity.

DIAGNOSIS AND DIFFERENTIAL

• The appearance of the cornea and episodes of recurrent erosion are diagnostic.

TREATMENT

• Treatment is directed at promoting epithelial adhesion:
  ○ Lubrication
  ○ Debridement of the loose epithelium
  ○ Patching or bandage contact lens
  ○ Optimizing the quality of tear film by treating any eyelid disease that is present.
  ○ Surgery (mechanical or laser superficial keratectomy) may be required for patients who do not respond to medical management.

STROMAL DYSTROPHIES

PATHOPHYSIOLOGY

• Stromal dystrophies result from abnormal deposits of material in the stromal layer causing either decreased vision or pain when the corneal surface breaks down. Well-characterized variants include granular, macular, and lattice dystrophies. They are commonly bilateral, progressive and with an autosomal dominant inheritance, except for macular dystrophy, which is autosomal recessive. The material deposited and the clinical appearances are specific to each dystrophy.

CLINICAL FEATURES

• The stromal deposits can cause decreased vision, photophobia, glare, and recurrent erosions.
• Of the stromal dystrophies, macular dystrophy is the most visually debilitating.

DIAGNOSIS AND DIFFERENTIAL

• The stromal dystrophies can be differentiated by their clinical appearance and by the composition of the deposits. The material deposited can be examined histologically using different stains.
• Granular dystrophy has bread crumb–like deposits with clear intervening zones (Fig. 7-15). These deposits are hyaline and stain with Masson trichome.
• Macular dystrophy lesions are less well defined, with cloudy spaces in between. The material is mucopolysaccharide that stains with Alcian blue.
• Lattice dystrophy presents with branching lesions that are amyloid and demonstrate Congo red birefringence (Fig. 7-16).

TREATMENT

• Treatment is symptomatic with lubrication and bandage contact lens for recurrent erosions.
• Phototherapeutic keratectomy is also useful for removing visually significant opacities located in the anterior cornea.
• Corneal transplant is considered when the vision is markedly reduced.

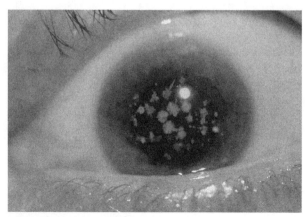

FIGURE 7-15 Granular dystrophy.

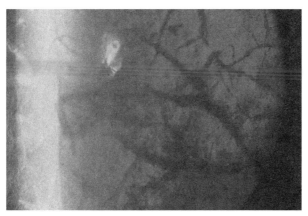

FIGURE 7-16 Lattice dystrophy.

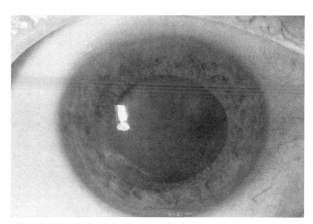

FIGURE 7-17 Epithelial edema Fuchs' dystrophy.

CASE 17

A 65-year-old woman comes in for new glasses because her vision is getting worse. Upon questioning, she states that her vision is fluctuating and usually worse in the morning. She also has disabling glare at night. Her vision is 20/30 OU. On slit-lamp examination, the corneal endothelium in both eyes has a beaten metal appearance. Stromal edema is present but there is no epithelial edema. Her IOP is 16 OU and her pachymetry values are 610 and 650. This patient has Fuchs' dystrophy with early corneal edema explaining her symptoms. Management is mostly expectant at this stage.

FUCHS' ENDOTHELIAL DYSTROPHY

PATHOPHYSIOLOGY

- Fuchs' dystrophy is characterized by dysfunction of the endothelium, the inner layer of the cornea. The number of endothelial cells is decreased with loss of their normal pumping function, resulting in progressive corneal edema (Fig. 7-17).
- This condition has a heritable component, although it is likely that both genetics and environmental factors contribute to its expression.

CLINICAL FEATURES

- Patients commonly complain that their vision is worse in the morning because of decreased evaporation of fluid from the cornea during sleep, when the eyelids are closed. As the disease progresses, they can also have pain from microcystic edema and ruptured bullae.
- Other symptoms are glare and halos from corneal edema.

- The typical findings are guttae on the endothelium that are described as having a beaten metal appearance.
- Other features are stromal edema, folds in Descemet's membrane, and pigment on the endothelium.

DIAGNOSIS AND DIFFERENTIAL

- The clinical appearance is diagnostic.
- Pachymetry is used to document progressive corneal edema.
- Specular microscopy is used to assess the size and the morphology of endothelial cells.

DIFFERENTIAL

- Elevated IOP causing corneal edema
- Aphakic or pseudophakic bullous keratopathy
- Congenital hereditary endothelial dystrophy—a rare bilateral and symmetric dystrophy of the endothelium present at birth and causing progressive corneal edema.
- Posterior polymorphous dystrophy—a bilateral, dominantly inherited disorder of the corneal endothelium, which is characterized by vesicles and areas of opacification. Corneal edema occurs infrequently. Iris irregularities may be seen as well. Often identified as an incidental finding.

TREATMENT

- Hypertonic drops are given to reduce epithelial edema (5% NaCl upon awakening).
- A hair dryer can be helpful to accelerate evaporation of the corneal fluid in the morning, reducing symptoms.

- Corneal transplant is recommended when the vision is poor or when the pain is debilitating.

DEGENERATIONS

CASE 18

A 19-year-old patient with Down's syndrome is having an acute episode of severe pain in his eye and profuse tearing. Slit-lamp examination of the right eye reveals a steep conic cornea with an iron line at the base of the cone. A focal area of corneal edema is located inferiorly, a little off the center. The cone in the left cornea is less prominent, but vertical stress lines can be seen. This patient has keratoconus. His symptoms and examinations are diagnostic of a typical episode of acute hydrops, a focal corneal edema resulting from a tear in Descemet's membrane. The other eye has less prominent keratoconus. An acute episode of hydrops is treated with hypertonic saline (NaCl 5%) to help resolve the corneal edema and Cyclogyl 1% b.i.d. for comfort.

KERATOCONUS

PATHOPHYSIOLOGY

- Keratoconus is a bilateral, progressive inferior thinning and steepening of the cornea causing reduced vision (Table 7-5).
- It is usually sporadic, but up to 10% of patients have a positive family history.
- It is often seen with eye rubbing and eye rubbing–associated diseases (atopy and Down's syndrome). Keratoconus can also be seen with connective tissue disorders (Ehler-Danlos and Marfan's syndromes, osteogenesis imperfecta).

CLINICAL FEATURES

- Irregular astigmatism, which is best seen on corneal topography.
- Vogt's striae can be seen (vertical stress lines in the posterior stroma that disappear with light pressure on the cornea).
- Munson's sign (convex deformation of the lower lid by the cone as the patient looks down).
- A Fleischer ring (iron line at the base of the cone) is an early finding.
- Hydrops (acute tears in Descemet's membrane, with fluid accumulation in the stroma causing corneal edema and pain) is relatively uncommon and can result in apical scarring when the acute edema resolves.

DIAGNOSIS AND DIFFERENTIAL

- Diagnosis is made by the typical clinical features.
- The topography shows steepening and irregularity with high keratometric value (K > 47D).
- Scissoring of the light reflex on retinoscopy.
- Differential (see Table 7-5)
  ○ Pellucid marginal degeneration.
  ○ Keratoglobus.

TREATMENT

- A rigid contact lens can neutralize the high astigmatism and provide good vision in most patients with keratoconus.

TABLE 7-5   Comparison between Major Ectatic Corneal Disorders

	KERATOCONUS	KERATOGLOBUS	PELLUCID MARGINAL DEGENERATION
Inheritance	Occasional	Not inherited	Not inherited
Age of onset	Puberty	At birth	20–40
Thinning	The apex of the cone is thinned	Diffusely thinned cornea with the periphery being the thinnest	Arcuate band of inferior thinning. The protrusion is above the band of thinning
Treatment	Contact lenses in the early stages and corneal transplant in the later stages	-Options limited -Contact lens not recommended because of risk of perforation -Corneal transplant is challenging because of the thinned sclera	-Hard contact lens fitting is difficult. -Lamellar keratoplasty (partial thickness transplant)
Prognosis	Good after corneal transplant	Not as good as keratoconus	Not as good as keratoconus

- Penetrating keratoplasty is considered when the vision deteriorates or when the patient is unable to wear contact lenses.
- Treatment for acute hydrops includes use of hypertonic saline to promote deturgescence of the corneal edema and cycloplegics for comfort.

CASE 19

During a routine ophthalmic examination on a 35-year-old woman with myopia, a whitish-gray circumferential opacification in the peripheral cornea of both eyes is noted. The patient has no complaints. The patient has arcus senilis in both of her eyes. These usually do not have any clinical significance unless unilateral or seen in the younger patient such as in this woman. This patient's lipid profile needs to be evaluated to identify hypercholesterolemia, hyperlipidemia, or hyperlipoproteinemia.

ARCUS SENILIS

PATHOPHYSIOLOGY

- This condition results from deposition of lipid and collagenous material in the stroma of the peripheral cornea. It is usually associated with aging. However, an arcus in a patient younger than age 40 can be associated with hyperlipidemia, hyperlipoproteinemia, or hypercholesterolemia. An asymmetrical arcus should prompt an evaluation of carotid disease on the side where the arcus is absent.

CLINICAL FEATURES

- Clinically it appears as a peripheral circumferential opacity along the limbus but separated from it by a clear zone. Patients are typically asymptomatic.

DIAGNOSIS AND DIFFERENTIAL

- Diagnosis is made by clinical observation.

TREATMENT

- These lesions are usually not symptomatic and do not require intervention unless they are associated with underlying diseases.

CASE 20

An African American woman with a history of chronic uveitis from sarcoidosis complains of a chronic foreign body sensation. When she looks in the mirror she sees a white opacity on her right cornea. Her vision is 20/200 OD and 20/30 OS. Slit-lamp examination of the right eye shows a white deposit extending across the interpapebral area. Details of the anterior chamber are obscured by this band. This is a band keratopathy in the context of chronic uveitis. Initial steps are lubrication with artificial tears and ointment. If the calcific band is thick enough as to cause decreased vision and pain, it should be removed surgically by chelation with EDTA.

BAND KERATOPATHY

PATHOPHYSIOLOGY

- Band keratopathy (Fig. 7-18) is a calcium precipitation in the cornea as a result of chronic ocular inflammation or systemic diseases such as hypercalcemia, hyperphosphatemia, chronic mercurial exposure, abnormal vitamin D metabolism, or increased uric acid. Deposition is most prominent in the interpalpebral area.

CLINICAL FEATURES

- Patients present with decreased vision, foreign body sensation, and pain.

DIAGNOSIS AND DIFFERENTIAL

- The appearance of band keratopathy is quite characteristic. It typically involves the interpalpebral area and is separated from the limbus by a clear zone. The

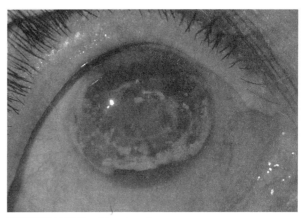

FIGURE 7-18 Band keratopathy.

calcific deposits are gray-white or brownish. Small holes in the calcium deposits can be seen giving a Swiss cheese pattern.

TREATMENT

- The goal is to provide symptomatic relief with lubrication. Occasionally, patients may require a bandage contact lens for relief of foreign body sensation.
- Surgical removal of symptomatic band keratopathy can be done using topical EDTA to chelate the calcium, in association with corneal scraping.

CONTACT LENS–RELATED COMPLICATIONS

CASE 21

A 28-year-old woman who has been wearing soft contact lenses for 10 years complains of increasing irritation and mucus production for the past 2 weeks. She is unable to wear her contact lens for more than 2 hours. Even when she takes them out, she still has a persistent foreign body sensation. Her vision with her glasses is 20/20 OU. Slit-lamp examination of both corneas show nothing remarkable except for scattered superficial punctate keratopathy. Upon lid eversion, giant papillae are seen in the upper tarsus bilaterally. This patient has giant papillary conjunctivitis from contact lens use. Lens wear should be deferred until symptoms resolve. The patient is started on lodoxamide (Alomide, a mast cell stabilizer) q.i.d. and seen in 1 month.

PATHOPHYSIOLOGY

- The most common problems associated with contact lens wear are infectious keratitis, sterile corneal infiltrates, giant papillary conjunctivitis, and corneal neovascularization.
- Extended-wear soft contact lenses, overnight wear, and careless lens cleaning are the greatest risk factors for infectious keratitis. Decreased oxygen supply, interference with nutrient supply by reduced tear flux underneath the lens, and microtrauma on the corneal surface created by the contact lenses, compounded with dirty lenses, all play a role in facilitating invasion and growth of pathogens. *Pseudomonas* is the most common bacterial pathogen associated with contact

lens–related corneal ulcers (see Case 4). *Pseudomonas* ulcers can be particularly aggressive, with devastating sequelae, including corneal perforation. Contact lens wear, especially in concert with use of homemade saline for lens cleaning, is a well-established risk factor for *Acanthameoba* keratitis.
- Sterile corneal infiltrates associated with contact lens represent a delayed hypersensitivity immune reaction to materials trapped by the lens. Agents known to stimulate delayed hypersensitivity include thimerosal, microbial byproducts, and proteins coating the lens. Differentiating sterile immune infiltrates from infectious ulcers is difficult. This condition is similar in etiology and management to the staphylococcal hypersensitivity described in Case 11.
- Giant papillary conjunctivitis (GPC) (Fig. 7-19) is a clinical syndrome most commonly associated with contact lens wear, but which can also be found with retained foreign bodies causing irritation to the ocular surface, such as exposed sutures or poorly fitting ocular prostheses. GPC is an inflammatory response to the extended mechanical irritation of a foreign body in a host with an allergic tendency. The response is similar to that of vernal keratoconjunctivitis (see Case 10) with activation of mast cells, lymphocytes, eosinophils, and fibroblasts causing increased collagen deposition and hyperplastic papillae in the upper palpebral conjunctiva. Protein deposits that coat the surface of the lens as the lens is worn and the preservatives used in certain cleaning systems, in particular thimerosal, may also be sensitizing agents.
- Corneal neovascularization is also most commonly found in patients who use extended-wear contact lenses, in response to a chronic low-grade hypoxia. The corneal neovascularization usually does not extend more than several millimeters onto the cornea. Progressive neovascularization is of concern, as vessels

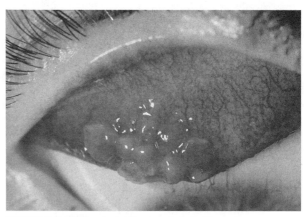

FIGURE 7-19 Giant papillary conjunctivitis.

can occasionally progress into the visual axis, causing reduced vision.

CLINICAL FEATURES

- All of these contact lens–related complications can present with similar symptoms ranging from irritation to pain, photophobia, and contact lens intolerance.
- Infectious keratitis presents as a corneal infiltrate with an overlying epithelial defect.
- Sterile infiltrates resemble staphylococcal marginal infiltrates with similar clinical presentation (Case 11). Patients have intolerance to contact lenses and photophobia. The infiltrates are usually multiple and located along the limbus in the superficial cornea. There is usually no overlying epithelial defect.
- Giant papillary conjunctivitis presents with tearing, itching, and excess mucus production. Giant papillae (> 0.3 mm) can be seen when the upper eyelid is everted. Contact lens tearing time is usually reduced.
- Corneal vascularization is seen on slit-lamp examination as fine blood vessels along the limbus progressing toward the central cornea.

DIAGNOSIS AND DIFFERENTIAL

- Diagnosis of each of these conditions can be made by clinical examination.
- Infectious keratitis needs to be confirmed by cultures and smears.
- When sterile infiltrates cannot be differentiated from infectious infiltrates on history and examination, they should also be cultured.
- Diagnosis of GPC is made by everting the upper lids and noting the giant papillae in the upper tarsus.

TREATMENT

- Infectious keratitis – see Case 4 for management
- Sterile infiltrates
  - Sterile infiltrates should be managed as infectious keratitis when there is any doubt about the diagnosis. Otherwise, contact lenses should be discontinued and a trial of topical steroids may be considered as described for marginal infiltrates (Case 11).
- GPC
  - When symptoms are mild, new soft lenses should be used, or even rigid gas-permeable contact lenses
  - Wearing time should be reduced
  - Patients should be instructed to perform more thorough cleaning of protein deposits with enzymes. A preservative-free cleaning solution might be helpful

in decreasing toxicity. Daily disposable lenses eliminate the issue of protein buildup and toxicity from cleaning solutions.
  - Topical mast cell stabilizers may be of benefit. Symptoms will abate before clinical signs.
- When symptoms are severe, contact lens use should be discontinued for an extended period in addition to the measures mentioned above.
  - Associated eyelid disease or dry eye should be treated.
- Progressive corneal neovascularization
  - Contact lens wear should be doscontinued.
  - Topical steroid q.i.d. for extensive neovascularization should be considered.
  - Refitting with lenses allowing higher transmission of oxygen should be considered.

CORNEAL MANIFESTATION OF SYSTEMIC DISEASES

CASE 22

A diabetic patient had a scratch on his cornea 4 weeks ago and he still has a red eye. His vision is poor in the involved eye. Corneal sensation is reduced. Slit-lamp examination shows an epithelial defect that stains with fluorescein. The edges of the defect are heaped up. This patient has a persistent defect from delayed epithelial closure. His diabetes predisposes him to poor healing. He needs a bandage contact lens and frequent preservative-free artificial tears to promote healing.

NEUROTROPHIC KERATITIS

PATHOPHYSIOLOGY

- Neurotrophic ulcers are noninfectious epithelial defects that result from loss of normal corneal innervation. Corneal nerves are thought to release trophic factors to the epithelium. The lack of these factors results in epithelium dysfunction with poor wound healing and persistent epithelial defects.
- Neurotrophic keratitis most commonly results from herpes simplex or zoster keratitis, prolonged contact lens wear, or diabetes mellitus.

CLINICAL FEATURES

- The cornea has a dull, irregular surface with punctate epitheliopathy. Persistent areas of epithelial breakdown with heaped up margins are present. Bacterial suprainfection and occasionally corneal perforation are well-recognized sequelae of persistent epithelial defects. Corneal sensation is decreased.

DIAGNOSIS AND DIFFERENTIAL

- One needs to rule out infectious ulcers by cultures and smears.
- The physician also needs to treat any exposure keratopathy (for example, from eyelid malpositioning or poor blink from seventh nerve palsy) that would exacerbate the neurotrophic keratopathy.

TREATMENT

- Frequent use of preservative-free tears and ointments are used to promote epithelial healing.
- Toxicity from preserved medication drops should be avoided.
- Lids should be taped at night if there is a history of nocturnal lagophthalmos.
- Associated eyelid disease (blepharitis, ectropion, entropion, trichiasis) should be treated.
- Bandage contact lens and tarsorrhaphy can be used if the defect is persistent despite the above maneuvers.
- An amniotic membrane graft may be useful for recalcitrant neurotrophic keratitis.

CASE 23

A female patient taking amiodarone for atrial fibrillation is sent for evaluation. She has no visual complaints. Her vision is 20/20 OU. Slit-lamp examination of both corneas shows a superficial haze in a vortex pattern. The rest of the ocular examination is otherwise unremarkable. This patient has vortex keratopathy from amiodarone toxicity. Vision is usually not affected. Her cardiologist should be informed.

VERTICILLATA

PATHOPHYSIOLOGY

- Verticillata results from accumulation of material in the epithelium in a whorl-like pattern. This pattern reflects the growth and centripetal migration of epithelial cells from the limbus toward the center of the cornea.

CLINICAL FEATURES

- Vortex keratopathy is usually asymptomatic.

DIAGNOSIS AND DIFFERENTIAL

- The appearance of the verticillata is pathognomonic and usually sufficient to make the diagnosis.
- The most common associations are use of amiodarone, chloroquine, or related compounds, chlorpromazine, indomethacin, or tamoxifen. Similar findings can occur in patients with or carriers of Fabry's disease.

TREATMENT

- Verticillata are usually asymptomatic. The decision whether to stop the causative medication should be made conjointly by the ophthalmologist and the internist.

CASE 24

A patient with Wilson's disease is referred for evaluation. His vision is 20/40 and 20/20. His corneas are clear. Gonioscopy shows a pigmented band at the border of Descemet's membrane. There is also a cataract forming in the right lens in a sunflower pattern.

WILSON'S DISEASE

PATHOPHYSIOLOGY

- Abnormal excretion of copper into bile can result in accumulation of copper in almost all body tissues.
- The condition is autosomal recessive.

CLINICAL FEATURES

- Kayser-Fleischer ring is a peripheral band of copper deposition in Descemet's membrane (Fig. 7-20). It is usually a late sign when neurologic impairment has already developed. It is found in 95% of patients with Wilson's disease.
- Early Kayser-Fleischer rings are best seen with gonioscopy.
- A "sunflower cataract" may also be present.

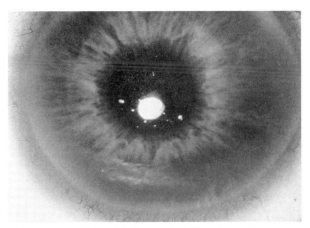

FIGURE 7-20 Kayser-Fleischer ring. (See Color Plate.)

DIAGNOSIS AND DIFFERENTIAL

Diagnosis is confirmed by laboratory values:
- High serum and urine copper level are present.
- Low serum ceruloplasmin is noted.
- Differential:
  - Any other causes of copper deposition
  - Primary biliary cirrhosis
  - Arcus senilis (see Case 19)

TREATMENT

- Systemic D-penicillamine can be given.
- Kayser-Fleischer ring will regress with treatment. It is a good indicator of response to treatment.
- Regression of the ring is also seen after liver transplant.

CASE 25

A 9-year-old boy with cystinosis is admitted for renal failure. An ophthalmology consultation has been requested. His vision is good. Slit-lamp examination of both eyes reveals fine needle-shaped, refractile, polychromatic crystals in the anterior stroma. Results of his retinal examination are unremarkable. This patient has the typical corneal crystals associated with cystinosis. If these cause recurrent erosions or photophobia, then topical cysteamine can be given.

THE CLOUDY CORNEA—METABOLIC DISORDERS

PATHOPHYSIOLOGY

- Of the metabolic disorders causing corneal clouding, the most important ones to recognize are the mucopolysaccharidoses and cystinosis. All mucopolysaccharidoses are autosomal recessive, except for Hunter's which is X-linked recessive. Corneal clouding is a feature of the following named mucopolysaccharidoses: Hurler, Scheie, Morquio, Maroteaux-Lamy, and Sly syndromes. Corneal clouding results from vacuolization of the cytoplasm of corneal epithelium, endothelium, and keratocytes (Table 7-6).
- Cystinosis is an autosomal recessive disorder with impaired efflux of cystine out of lysosomes that leads to accumulation of this material in tissues. There are three forms: infantile, adolescent, and adult. The infantile form is more aggressive, with renal failure and early death. Patients with the adult form have only the ocular manifestation.

CLINICAL FEATURES

- In the mucopolysaccharidoses, diffuse corneal opacification is associated with other systemic findings consistent with the disease process. Vision is reduced.
- Fine crystals are deposited in the cornea in cystinosis (Fig. 7-21). These deposits become denser with age. Typical symptoms are photophobia, recurrent erosions, and band keratopathy.

TABLE 7-6 Characteristics of Mucopolysaccharidosis

SYNDROMES	INHERITANCE	CORNEAL OPACIFICATIONS	RETINAL DEGENERATIONS	OPTIC NERVE ATROPHY
Hurler	Recessive	+	+	+
Scheie	Recessive	+	+	+
Hunter	X-linked recessive	−	+	+
Sanfilippo	Recessive	−	+	+
Morquio	Recessive	+	−	+
Maroteaux-Lamy	Recessive	+	−	−
Sly	Recessive	+	?	?

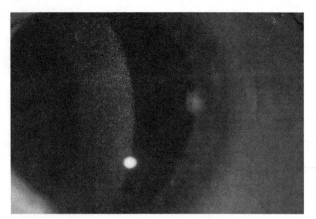

FIGURE 7-21 Corneal crystals in cystinosis.

DIAGNOSIS AND DIFFERENTIAL

• Mucopolysaccharidoses are diagnosed with the help of a geneticist.

• In cystinosis, high levels of cystine and cysteine can be demonstrated in leukocytes, cultured fibroblasts, or in biopsies of rectal mucosa.

TREATMENT

• Corneal treatment options for these patients with mucopolysaccharidoses are not well established. Many patients die at an early age as a result of systemic complications of their disease. Concomitant retinal and optic nerve disease often limits the visual potential of these patients.
• Cysteamine can be used to reduce the corneal crystal content in patients with cystinosis. It reacts with intracellular cystine and helps in the transport of cystine out of lysosomes.

8 ANTERIOR CHAMBER, IRIS, AND LENS

Sandra Lora Cremers

TRAUMA

HYPHEMA/MICROHYPHEMA

CASE 1

A 34-year-old athlete presents with pain and blurry vision in his right eye 6 hours after he was hit in that eye by a baseball. His vision is 20/100 OD and 20/20 OS. Examination shows a poorly reactive pupil OD with no afferent pupillary defect. He has red blood cells in his anterior chamber with a layered hyphema (Fig. 8-1A). His posterior chamber is normal. His left eye is normal.

PATHOPHYSIOLOGY

- Hyphema is defined as layering or clotting of blood in the anterior chamber.
- Microhyphema is defined as red blood cells suspended in the anterior chamber without significant layering.
- Traumatic hyphemas are postulated to result from the following: direct, contusive forces that cause mechanical tearing of the fragile blood vessels of the iris and/or angle, or concussive trauma causing a rapid rise in the intravascular pressure within these blood vessels, resulting in rupture.

  Spontaneous hyphemas are not as common as traumatic cases. They usually occur secondary to neovascularization of the iris.
- Red blood cells may obstruct the trabecular meshwork and outflow of aqueous humor, which may result in glaucoma. Cases with high pressure may also result in blood pigments staining the cornea (Fig. 8-1B). A few red blood cells in the anterior chamber are not always harmful, as can be seen after laser iridotomy.
- Hemolytic glaucoma results from direct obstruction of the trabecular meshwork by fresh blood.
- Hemosiderotic glaucoma results from the obstruction of the trabecular meshwork by degrading hemoglobin.
- Ghost cell glaucoma results from trabecular meshwork obstruction by the cell membranes of disintegrating red blood cells.

- Direct damage to the trabecular meshwork may result in a delayed reduction in aqueous drainage and late onset glaucoma.
- Hyphema patients with sickle cell disease or trait are at risk for abnormally high intraocular pressures (IOPs), rebleeding, and early optic nerve head damage because the environment of the anterior chamber promotes sickle hemoglobin polymerization, which can result in elevated IOP due to blockage of the trabecular meshwork.

CLINICAL FEATURES

- Patients may present with blurred vision, pain, photophobia, and tearing following blunt injury to the eye or orbit.
- Spontaneous hyphemas may present with pain or just a red area over the iris.
- Hyphemas may be visible without a slit lamp.
- The IOP may be normal or low initially.
- There may be significant associated ocular or adnexal injury in traumatic cases.
- Most hyphemas can be seen with a penlight examination.
- Microhyphemas require a slit-lamp microscope for diagnosis.
- Ocular examination should include an evaluation of the external adnexa. If necessary, order an X-ray or computed tomography (CT) scan to rule out an orbital fracture or extraocular muscle entrapment. Additionally, be sure to examine the cornea to assess for perforation, the sclera to assess for ruptured globe, the lens for phacodynesis or dislocation, the vitreous for blood or pigment, and the retina for any holes, tears, or a retinal detachment. If a clear view of the fundus is obstructed by the hyphema or vitreous hemorrhage, perform a B-scan ultrasound.
- The term *eight-ball hyphema*, or black hyphema, is reserved for a completely filled anterior chamber with black clots.
- Gonioscopy increases the risk of rebleeding and therefore is performed after the hyphema has resolved. Approximately 50% of patients with hyphema have angle recession (see next clinical case) and are thus at

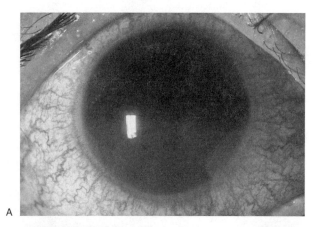

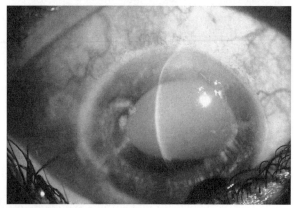

FIGURE 8-1 A. Hyphema. (See Color Plate.) B. Corneal staining after a resolving hyphema. (See Color Plate.)

risk of developing secondary glaucoma in the future. Optic nerve damage can occur between ages 12 months and 50 years after the initial hyphema in patients with angle recession. It is therefore important to follow the IOP in patients with angle recession at least once per year, depending on the degree of recession.

DIAGNOSIS AND DIFFERENTIAL

- The diagnosis is made by physical examination.
- Hyphemas may be due to following:
  - Trauma
  - Iris neovascularization (usually secondary to retinal vascular disease)
  - Blood dyscrasia, clotting disorders, hemophilia
  - Intraocular tumor: juvenile xanthogranuloma, retinoblastoma, leukemia
  - Postsurgical: bleeding from iris or corneal wounds
- Red color is characteristic of a hyphema, but the differential diagnosis of material layered in the anterior chamber includes the following:
  - Hypopyon: white blood cells layered in the anterior chamber
  - Iritis: white blood cells floating in the anterior chamber as a result of, for example, an infection such as from herpes simplex or zoster iritis
  - Metastasis to the anterior chamber: leukemia, breast cancer

TREATMENT

- It is necessary to obtain a complete history of the trauma, as well as a past medical history including any history of sickle cell anemia, clotting disorders, a past ocular history, and a list of current medications.
- If the patient is a poor historian, order systemic tests for sickle cell anemia (sickle prep or sickle dex) and bleeding disorders i.e., prothrombin time (PT) and partial thromboplastic time (PTT).
- A hyphema in patients with sickle cell disease is a medical emergency.
- Since patients with sickle cell disease are prone to central retinal artery occlusion and optic atrophy, even with mildly elevated IOP, they should be closely monitored as inpatients for IOP changes. It should not be allowed to exceed 25 mm Hg for longer than 24 hours.
- Hospitalization of non–sickle cell patients with hyphemas is controversial.
- Most ophthalmologists manage compliant patients with uncomplicated hyphemas on an outpatient basis.
- Medical treatment includes the following:
  - Cycloplegia with atropine 1% q.i.d.
  - Steroids, e.g., prednisolone acetate (Pred Forte 1%) or rimexolone (Vexol) q.2h to q.i.d.
  - High IOP (above 27 mm Hg in an otherwise healthy eye) should be treated with topical beta-blockers (Timolol 0.5% b.i.d.), alpha 2 adrenoreceptor agonists (brimonidine tartrate [Alphagan P b.i.d.], apraclonidine [Iopidine b.i.d.]), or carbonic anhydrase inhibitors such as dorzolamide [Trusopt b.i.d.] if there are no contraindications. When IOP requires acute attention (i.e., over 35 mm Hg) prescribe acetazolamide 500 mg by mouth b.i.d. if there are no contraindications (such as sickle cell anemia), until the pressure is adequately controlled. Do not use pilocarpine.
  - If there are corneal epithelial defects, use a topical antibiotic prophylactically.
  - Aminocaproic acid (Amicar 50 mg/kg), an antifibrinolytic, may reduce the risk of rebleeding. It appears to function best in children but is not universally accepted and remains controversial. It may cause postural hypotension during the first 24 hours and is contraindicated in patients who are pregnant, have coagulopathies, or renal, hepatic, cardiovascular or cerebrovascular disease.

- The patient should be instructed to:
  - Limit activity to the bathroom and bed rest.
  - Keep head of bed elevated at an angle of 30°.
  - Apply a Fox eye shield for additional protection.
  - Avoid aspirin and ibuprofen to prevent rebleeding.
- An anterior chamber washout should be considered for the following: corneal blood staining; IOP greater than 60 mm Hg; an eight-ball hemorrhage; IOP above 35 mm Hg for 7 days; high uncontrolled IOP despite medical management in a sickle cell patient. An anterior chamber washout involves the injection of balanced salt solution into the anterior chamber with subsequent aspiration of the anterior chamber to wash out the hemorrhage.
- Patients should be followed with checks of visual acuity, slit-lamp examinations, IOP, and dilated fundus examinations for 4 consecutive days, then as necessary.
- Spontaneous hyphema: treatment will depend on the underlying cause.
- A microhyphema is treated as a traumatic hyphema. Because by definition the hemorrhage is smaller, rises in IOP are generally not as severe. However, these patients should still have their pressures monitored and be examined for angle recession as noted above.

SUGGESTED READINGS

Albert DM, Jakobiec FA, eds: *Principles and Practice of Ophthalmology*, 2nd ed. Philadelphia: Saunders, 1994.

Basic and Clinical Science Course: American Academy of Ophthalmology, 2001.

Nasrullah A, Kerr NC: Sickle cell trait as a risk factor for secondary hemorrhage in children with traumatic hyphema. *Am J Ophthalmol* 1997;123:783–790P.

IRITIS

CASE 2

A 35-year-old police woman presents with a red painful left eye that began 2 days ago after she was hit in the eye by a suspect. She has been very sensitive to light since the pain began. Her examination is significant for a visual acuity of 20/20 OD and 20/100 OS. Her left eye has diffuse conjunctival injection. She has 1+ cells and flare in the anterior chamber and keratic precipitates on the corneal endothelium OS. Results of the rest of her examination, including a careful examination of her retina, are normal. Her diagnosis is traumatic iritis. For further information, refer to the section on INFLAMMATION.

ANGLE RECESSION

CASE 3

A 24-year-old athlete presents for follow-up for a resolving hyphema one month after she was hit in her right eye with a racquetball. Her vision is 20/25 OD and 20/20 OS and results of her examination are significant for a resolved hyphema and a pressure of 11 mm Hg. Her gonioscopy examination reveals angle recession from approximately the 5 o'clock to 8 o'clock positions (Fig. 8-2). The rest of her examination findings were within healthy limits.

PATHOPHYSIOLOGY

- Angle recession results from blunt trauma to the eye that tears the ciliary body between the longitudinal and circular muscles.
- A microhyphema or hyphema often occurs at the time of the trauma.
- The IOP may increase months to years after the initial injury.
- Approximately 15–20% of patients with angle recession develop secondary glaucoma, depending on the extent of angle recession. Typically, two-thirds of the angle must be compromised in order for glaucoma to develop.

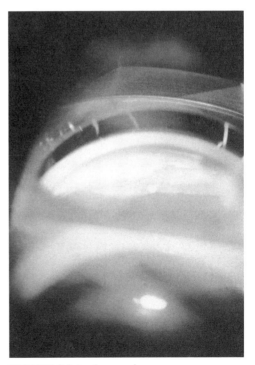

FIGURE 8-2 Angle recession.

- The etiology of IOP rise in traumatic angle recession is not completely understood. The following theories are postulated:
  - Direct traumatic damage to the trabecular meshwork.
  - Particulate matter such as pigment and hemosiderin released at the initial trauma damages the trabecular meshwork, causing scarring and poor filtration.
  - Endothelial cells migrate and proliferate over the trabecular meshwork in response to trauma, forming a Descemet's-like membrane that blocks filtration.
- There is a higher than expected incidence of primary open-angle glaucoma in the nontraumatized fellow eye, leading some to speculate that angle recession eyes that go on to develop glaucoma have a predisposition to IOP elevation.

CLINICAL FEATURES

- Because angle recession is diagnosed weeks to years after the initial injury, patients usually have no symptoms (except for symptoms associated with the trauma).
- Angle recession glaucoma may affect patients of any age.
- An associated traumatic cataract and/or an iridodialysis (which is a separation of the iris root from the ciliary body) in severe cases may also be present.
- A substantial rise in IOP may occur. An unexplained IOP rise in the fellow eye often occurs in unilateral cases.
- In cases of unilateral glaucoma, ask about a history of trauma and inspect the angle carefully for angle recession.

DIAGNOSIS

- Gonioscopy will reveal a deepening of the angle recession and an apparent widening of the ciliary body band, or the appearance of excessive gray tissue (ciliary body) posterior to the scleral spur.
- In some cases of angle recession glaucoma, the angle appears relatively normal, except that it reveals more of the posterior angle structures than is typical. The suspect eye should always be compared with the normal fellow eye to reveal asymmetry between the angles.
- A cyclodialysis cleft, which is a disinsertion of the ciliary body from the sclera at the scleral spur, must be ruled out. A cleft can cause future spikes of IOP if the cleft suddenly closes.

DIFFERENTIAL

- Cyclodialysis cleft
- Iridodialysis

TREATMENT

- Treatment of angle recession consists of monitoring the IOP and an optic nerve examination. Since 15% of patients with angle recession eventually develop changes in their optic nerve function, visual field, and thus glaucoma, it is imperative that these patients be followed every 6 months to 1 year to rule out early changes in their optic nerve and/or visual field.
- Miotics, prostaglandin analogs, and argon laser trabeculoplasty are rather ineffective in managing angle recession glaucoma since the outflow structures have likely been compromised. More appropriate topical medications include aqueous suppressants such as beta-blockers, carbonic anhydrase inhibitors, and alpha-adrenergic agonists.
- If medical therapy fails to control IOP, filtering surgery is an option.

SUGGESTED READINGS

Albert DM, Jakobiec FA, eds. *Principles and Practice of Ophthalmology*, 2nd ed. Philadelphia: Saunders, 1994.

Rich R, Shields B, Krupin T. *Glaucomas*, 2nd ed. New York: Mosby, 1996.

CYCLODIALYSIS

CASE 4

A 54-year-old construction worker presents after he fell and hit his left eye on the corner of a metal beam. He notes slight pain and mildly decreased vision. His examination is significant for 20/20 OD and 20/30 OS. He has 1+ cell and flare OS and an IOP of 11. Gonioscopy reveals a cyclodialysis cleft in the inferotemporal angle (Fig. 8-3). Results of the rest of his examination are within healthy limits.

PATHOPHYSIOLOGY

- Cyclodialysis is a disinsertion of the ciliary body from the sclera at the scleral spur. This results in a cleft, which is visible on gonioscopy examination (Fig. 8-4). The sclera may be visible through the disrupted tissue.
- Blunt or surgical trauma is the etiology.

CLINICAL FEATURES

- Patients may present with chronically low IOPs or hypotony following trauma or surgery.

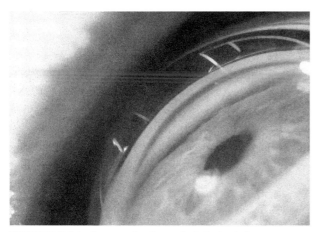

FIGURE 8-3 A photograph of a cyclodialysis cleft.

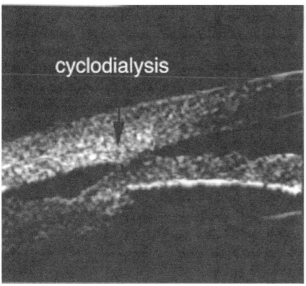

FIGURE 8-4 Ultrasonic biomicroscopy of a cyclodialysis shows a complete disinsertion of the ciliary body from the scleral spur accompanied by a 360° supraciliary effusion.

- A cleft is visible on gonioscopy examination.
- Macular edema or hypotony maculopathy may result from chronically low pressures.

DIAGNOSIS AND DIFFERENTIAL

- The diagnosis is made by inspection with gonioscopy.
- The differential diagnosis includes:
  ○ Iridodialysis
  ○ Angle recession

TREATMENT

- Cycloplegic agents such as Cyclogel 1% q.i.d. may help close the cleft.

- Persistent hypotony despite medical management is an indication for surgical repair.
- The ciliary body may be reattached to the sclera by using argon laser photocoagulation, diathermy, or cryotherapy, or by direct suturing with a McCannel suture.

SUGGESTED READINGS

Albert DM, Jakobiec FA, eds: *Principles and Practice of Ophthalmology*, 2nd ed. Philadelphia: Saunders, 1994.
Rich R, Shields B, Krupin T: *Glaucomas*, 2nd ed. New York: Mosby, 1996.

IRIDODIALYSIS

CASE 5

A 26-year-old stunt man presents 3 months after a bungee cord injury to his right eye. He had sustained a traumatic hyphema that cleared within 2 weeks. His vision is now 20/40 OD and 20/20 OS. The patient has an enlarged and irregular pupil due to traumatic iridoplegia, as well as an early traumatic cataract. An iridodialysis is noted temporally, and the iris is thinned and adherent to the underlying lens capsule, also in the temporal region (Fig. 8-5). Ophthalmoscopy findings are unremarkable. The left eye is normal. There is no other significant medical or ocular history.

PATHOPHYSIOLOGY

- Iridodialysis is a separation of the iris root from the ciliary body.

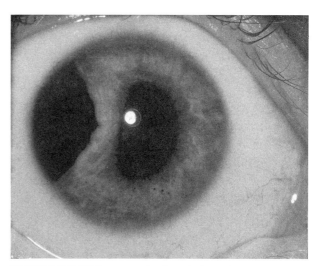

FIGURE 8-5 Slit-lamp examination photograph.

• An iridodialysis may occur in association with a hyphema resulting from blunt trauma. However, the iridodialysis may not be diagnosed until the hyphema has cleared.

CLINICAL FEATURES

• An iridodialysis is usually visible as a dark area at the base of the iris (where the iris meets the sclera). The pupil is usually irregular. As the iris is pulled away from its base, a second pupil may form.
• Patients may complain of monocular double vision or glare due to the formation of a second pupil. Symptoms may be mild if the upper eyelid of the patient masks the iridodialysis.

DIAGNOSIS AND DIFFERENTIAL

• Diagnosis is made by slit-lamp examination, gonioscopy, or ultrasound biomicroscopy (Fig. 8-6).

TREATMENT

• Repair is not necessary in all cases. If the patient has mild complaints of glare, halos, or diplopia, a cosmetic contact lens that blocks peripheral light rays from the area of the iridodialysis may be an option. If the iridodialysis is large or the patient has significant visual complaints uncorrected with a cosmetic contact lens, surgical correction is an option.
• Reattaching the iris to the sclera with a McCannel suture of 10-0 prolene on a special CIF-4 needle will repair an iridodialysis.

SUGGESTED READINGS

Albert DM, Jakobiec FA, eds: *Principles and Practice of Ophthalmology*, 2nd ed. Philadelphia: Saunders, 1994.
Hersh P, Zagelbaum B, Lora Cremers S: *Ophthalmic Surgical Procedures*, 2nd ed. New York: Thieme, 2003.
Rich R, Shields B, Krupin T: *Glaucomas*, 2nd ed. New York: Mosby, 1996.

IRIDOPLEGIA

CASE 6

A 26-year-old man presents 3 months after a baseball injury to his right eye. He had sustained a traumatic hyphema that cleared within 2 weeks. His vision is 20/20 OU. The patient has an enlarged and irregular pupil due to traumatic iridoplegia (Fig. 8-7). A small iridodialysis is noted inferotemporally. The lens is slightly dislocated superotemporally. Findings of ophthalmoscopy are unremarkable. Gonioscopy reveals multiple abnormalities including a superior angle recession and areas of peripheral anterior synechias. The left eye is normal. There is no other significant medical or ocular history.

PATHOPHYSIOLOGY

• Iridoplegia is defined as an altered pupillary reaction to light.
• Iridoplegia may result from the following:
  ○ Trauma may injure or tear the iris sphincter, which results in segmental contraction of the iris to light.
  ○ Ischemia with resulting neuronal injury to the iris sphincter may occur in herpes zoster infections and diabetes mellitus.

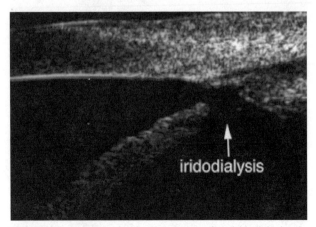

FIGURE 8-6 Ultrasonic biomicroscopy of an iridodialysis: the iris is disinserted at the scleral spur.

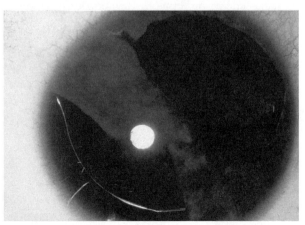

FIGURE 8-7 Traumatic iridoplegia.

- The following may cause iridoplegia:
  - Ocular trauma, the most common cause
  - Herpes zoster infection: Herpes zoster may result in an atrophic sphincter as well as transillumination defects secondary to ischemic injury
  - Diabetes mellitus
  - Autonomic neuropathies (e.g., Riley-Day syndrome)
  - Guillain-Barre syndrome
  - Adie's pupil
  - Syphilis
  - Idiopathic

CLINICAL FEATURES

- Patients with iridoplegia often complain of photophobia. They may also complain of anisocoria (asymmetric pupil size), glare, and blurred vision.
- Examination with a penlight will reveal an enlarged and often irregular pupil. The pupil will sluggishly or asymmetrically constrict to direct light.

DIAGNOSIS

- A diagnosis of iridoplegia is made by pupillary examination with direct illumination.
- A slit-lamp examination may reveal sphincter tears or segmental atony.

TREATMENT

- If there is no obvious history of trauma, a work-up for an underlying systemic disorder is indicated.
- The underlying cause should be treated if possible.
- If the patient has mild complaints of glare, halos, or light sensitivity, a cosmetic contact lens that limits central light rays may be an option. If the patient has significant visual complaints that cannot be corrected with a contact lens or if the patient is intolerant to contact lenses, surgical correction is an option.
- An irregular or enlarged pupil can be surgically corrected with a modified McCannel suture technique that allows for a "purse string" closure with prolene suture.

SUGGESTED READINGS

Albert DM, Jakobiec FA, eds: *Principles and Practice of Ophthalmology*, 2nd ed. Philadelphia: Saunders, 1994.
Hersh P, Zagelbaum B, Lora Cremers S: *Ophthalmic Surgical Procedures*, 2nd ed. New York: Thieme, 2003.

PIGMENTARY DISPERSION: SEE CHAPTER 9

INFLAMMATION

IRITIS

CASE 7

A 35-year-old woman presents with a red painful left eye she has had for 3 days. She has been very sensitive to light since the pain began. She denies any trauma. Her review of systems is significant only for a recent work-up by her doctor for difficulty breathing. Her examination is significant for a visual acuity of 20/20 OD and 20/100 OS. Her left eye has 1+ conjunctival injection. She has 3+ cells and flare in the anterior chamber and large "mutton fat" keratic precipitates on the corneal endothelium OS. Numerous cells are present in the vitreous and the view of her retina is hazy. Her ACE level is elevated. A PPD is negative. Her chest x-ray shows bilateral hilar adenopathy.

PATHOPHYSIOLOGY

- Uveitis is defined as inflammation of the uveal tract.
- The uveal tract consists of the pigmented structures of the eye, which include the iris, the ciliary body, and the choroid.
- Uveitis is thought to be due in part to an immune reaction against foreign antigens, which cause damage to the uveal tract and its blood vessels via immune complex deposition.
- Uveitis is associated with infections, neoplasms, and autoimmune diseases.
- Uveitis may be the initial presentation of an underlying systemic disease.
- Iritis is the inflammation specifically of the iris, ciliary body, or both, and includes anterior uveitis, iridocyclitis, and cyclitis.
- Iritis may occur after trauma to the eye.
- The pain associated with iritis is due to ciliary spasm and may cause referred pain over a larger area innervated by the trigeminal nerve (cranial nerve V).
- Inflammation of the iris, cornea, or ciliary body causes epiphora, photophobia, and blurry vision.

CLINICAL FEATURES

- **History:** In acute anterior uveitis, patients will complain of a painful red eye with blurred vision, light sensitivity, and tearing. In chronic anterior uveitis, patients may have few symptoms. In posterior uveitis, patients may have minimal pain. More often they complain of blurred vision, floaters, and mild light sensitivity.

- **Physical Exam:** Visual acuity may be decreased. Conjunctiva/ episclera reveals a ciliary flush. This is diffuse perilimbal injection that increases in intensity around the limbus. This is in contrast to conjunctivitis, where there is a relative clear zone around the limbus. Slit-lamp examination reveals white blood cells and flare (protein) in the anterior chamber. (White blood cells can be seen floating in the anterior chamber. A simulation of flare is a flashlight's beam in a dark smoky room.) Cells in the anterior chamber are graded on a scale of 1+ to 4+:
    - Zero = No cells
    - 1+ = Faint (barely detectable)
    - 2+ = Moderate cells present but the iris and lens are clearly visible
    - 3+ = Moderate cells but with a hazy view of the iris and lens
    - 4+ = Intense inflammation often with fibrin deposition
- Uveitis is classified as nongranulomatous and granulomatous.
- In nongranulomatous iritis, fine keratic precipitates (KPs) may be seen on the corneal endothelium. KPs are composed of white blood cells.
- In granulomatous iritis, large mutton-fat KPs are seen on the corneal endothelium. Clusters of white cells on the pupillary border are called Koeppe nodules and white cells on the anterior iris surface are called Busacca nodules.
- Other findings may include fibrin, a hypopyon, pupillary miosis, and anterior and posterior synechiae.
- The IOP may be normal or slightly decreased because of decreased aqueous humor production. High pressures may occur if significant inflammation is causing obstruction of the trabecular meshwork.

DIAGNOSIS AND DIFFERENTIAL

- A comprehensive history is critical to evaluate underlying systemic causes of iritis. A thorough examination of the fundus is necessary to rule out posterior uveitis, as is an evaluation for complications such as cataract and secondary glaucoma.
- In recurrent unilateral or in a bilateral case of uveitis, a systemic work-up is recommended. Baseline blood work includes the following: complete blood count (CBC) with a manual differential, ESR, FTA-ABS, RPR, ACE, ANA, RF, CXR, PPD, and anergy panel,

HLA-B27, Lyme titer (if in an endemic area). More extensive work-ups may be indicated in certain cases.
- A majority of patients have idiopathic uveitis, which is not associated with an underlying disease.
- Acute nongranulomatous uveitis is associated with ankylosing spondylitis, Reiter's syndrome, psoriatic arthritis, Behçet's disease, and inflammatory bowel diseases. Infectious causes include Lyme disease, mumps, influenza, adenovirus, measles, and *Chlamydia*. Trauma is the most common cause of acute nongranulomatous uveitis. Other causes include the following: postoperative iritis, glaucomatocyclitic crisis, lens-induced uveitis, medications (prostaglandin analogs, cidofovir, systemic sulfonamides, rifabutin), and tight contact lens.
- Chronic nongranulomatous uveitis (Fig. 8-8) is most commonly associated with juvenile rheumatoid arthritis in children and Fuchs' heterochromic iridocyclitis in adults.
- Acute and chronic granulomatous uveitis include infectious causes, such as, herpes simplex, herpes zoster, varicella, syphilis, and tuberculosis. Noninfectious causes include sarcoidosis (Fig. 8-9).

TREATMENT

- Topical steroid drops (e.g., Pred Forte 1% every hour to every six depending on the extent of inflammation).
- Topical cycloplegic drops (e.g., Cyclogyl 1% q.i.d. or atropine 1% b.i.d.) will break and prevent the formation of posterior synechiae and relieve photophobia secondary to ciliary spasm.
- Topical nonsteroidal drops q.i.d. may help relieve some of the discomfort.
- Close follow-up depending on the extent of the inflammation.

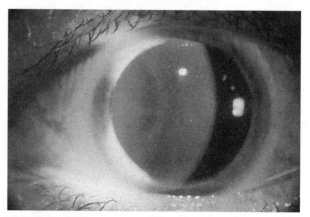

FIGURE 8-8 Nongranulomatous uveitis. [Courtesy of Dr. Stephen Foster.]

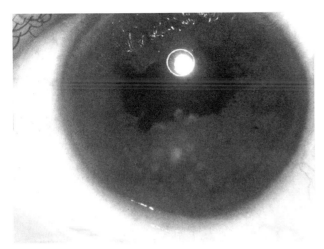

FIGURE 8-9 Granulomatous uveitis.

- Treat underlying etiology.
- Systemic steroids may be indicated in certain patients depending on the underlying etiology and the extent of the inflammation.

SUGGESTED READINGS

Albert DM, Jakobiec FA, eds: *Principles and Practice of Ophthalmology*, 2nd ed. Philadelphia: Saunders, 1994.

Foster S, Vitale M: *Diagnosis and Treatment of Uveitis.* Philadelphia: Saunders, 2002.

Nussenblatt RB, Whitcup SM, Palestine AG: *Uveitis: Fundamentals and Clinical Practice*, 2nd ed. St Louis: Mosby, 1996.

HYPOPYON

CASE 8

A 26-year-old man presents complaining of redness, pain, sensitivity to light, and decreasing vision in his right eye for the last 2 days. He has no significant past medical history but notes a history of oral aphthous ulcers. On examination, his vision is found to be 20/80 OD and 20/20 OS. His right eye shows severe diffuse conjunctival injection with 3+ white blood cells and a 1 mm layered hypopyon in the anterior chamber (Fig. 8-10). His IOP is 10 mm Hg. His posterior segment is within healthy limits with no evidence of retinal vasculitis.

PATHOPHYSIOLOGY

- Hypopyon is defined as a layering of white blood cells in the anterior chamber.

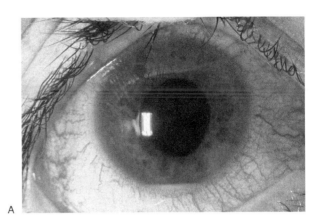

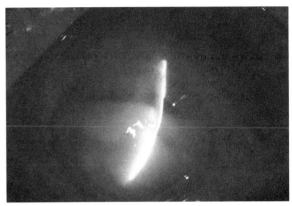

FIGURE 8-10 A and B. Small hypopyon in a patient with Behçet's disease. [Courtesy of Dr. Stephen Foster.]

- The etiologies for hypopyon include the following:
  - Infections: associated with corneal ulcers, endophthalmitis
  - Inflammation: uveitis, iritis, iridocyclitis
  - Drugs: rifabutin
  - Traumatic: retained intraocular foreign body, toxic lens syndrome, status post surgery (e.g., refractive surgery, pars plana vitrectomy with silicone oil injection)
  - Intraocular tumors or tumor necrosis: leukemia, non-Hodgkins lymphoma, retinoblastoma

CLINICAL FEATURES

- **History:** Patients may have a history of contact lens use (Figure 8-10B) or previous corneal ulcer due to other predisposing factors such as dry eyes, rosacea, diabetes mellitus, Bell's palsy, or cranial nerve V palsy.
- **Examination:** A hypopyon can be seen on slit-lamp examination. There may be other symptoms such as pain, injection of the conjunctiva. A white, quiet eye suggests an underlying tumor, drug-induced hypopyon, or pseudohypopyon.

DIAGNOSIS

- Hypopyon is diagnosed on slit-lamp examination.
- Obtaining a thorough history of contact lens use, prior trauma, medication use, and the medical and surgical history will aid in determining the underlying etiology.

DIFFERENTIAL

- The differential diagnosis includes the following:
  - Pseudohypopyon: retinoblastoma, accidental steroid injection, ghost cell glaucoma, and tight contact lens.
  - Metastasis to the anterior chamber: breast cancer, leukemia

TREATMENT

- Treat the underlying cause. See sections on endophthalmitis, uveitis, and corneal ulcers.

SUGGESTED READINGS

Albert DM, Jakobiec FA, eds: *Principles and Practice of Ophthalmology*, 2nd ed. Philadelphia: Saunders, 1994.
Foster S, Vitale M: *Diagnosis and Treatment of Uveitis.* Philadelphia: Saunders, 2002.

CONGENITAL AND DEVELOPMENTAL ANOMALIES OF THE IRIS

ANIRIDIA

CASE 9

The mother of a 6-month-old girl is concerned about her daughter's "funny-looking eyes." The mother notices that her baby avoids opening her eyes in lighted areas and has unusual eye movements. The baby's examination shows that she has significant inability to fixate on a target in both eyes has searching nystagmus of both eyes, and initially appears to have dilated, unresponsive pupils. Examining her is difficult because of her sensitivity to light. Further examination under sedation with a portable slit lamp shows essentially total absence of her iris, and a small central anterior polar cataract in

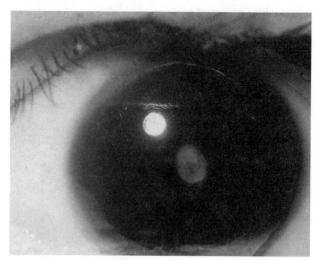

FIGURE 8-11 Aniridia.

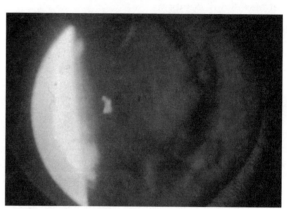

FIGURE 8-12 Aniridia.

both eyes (Figs. 8-11 and 8-12). Her IOPs are within healthy limits. Her dilated examination reveals optic nerve hypoplasia and foveal hypoplasia.

PATHOPHYSIOLOGY

- Aniridia is defined as an absence of the iris. The term *aniridia* is, however, a misnomer as rudimentary iris stumps are always present at the iris base circumferentially.
- Aniridia is a panocular, bilateral disorder.
- There are two forms of aniridia: familial and nonfamilial (sporadic).
- The familial form is inherited as an autosomal dominant or autosomal recessive trait.
- Almost all cases of aniridia occur from a defect of a developmental gene PAX6 that encodes a transcription factor responsible for eye development. The PAX6 gene is located on the short arm of chromosome 11 at 11p13.

- Rarely aniridia is inherited as an autosomal recessive trait. Gillespie's syndrome is the syndrome of autosomal recessive aniridia, cerebellar ataxia, metal retardation, and congenital cataracts.
- Nonfamilial or sporadic aniridia is associated with Wilms' tumor (sporadic cases, not autosomal dominant cases), ambiguous genitalia, genitourinary anomalies, and mental retardation known as the WAGR (**W**ilms', **a**niridia, **g**enitourinary abnormalities, **r**etardation) syndrome. Approximately 30% of sporadic aniridia cases are associated with Wilms' tumor.
- WAGR syndrome is associated with a small but variable interstitial deletion of the short arm of chromosome 11 (11p-). There is no association between autosomal dominant Wilms' tumor and aniridia.

CLINICAL FEATURES

- **History:** There may be a family history of aniridia. Aniridia is usually diagnosed at birth. Children with aniridia avoid light and rub their eyes due to light sensitivity and poor vision.
- **Examination:** Patients often have a decreased visual acuity, usually 20/100 or worse. Aniridia may present with a spectrum of almost total absence of the iris to relative mild hypoplasia. Patients may present at birth with the following symptoms and signs:
  - Congenital sensory nystagmus
  - Strabismus
  - Corneal pannus
  - Corneal opacities
  - Microcornea
  - Sclerocornea
  - Limbal dermoids
  - Ectopia lentis (lens subluxation)
  - Congenital absence of the lens
  - Persistent pupillary membrane
  - Glaucoma
  - Optic nerve hypoplasia
  - Foveal or macular hypoplasia
  - Choroidal colobomas
- Gonioscopy reveals the presence of some iris remnants even in severe cases. Peripheral synechiae from the contraction of rudimentary iris remnants bridging the angle may cause early angle closure.
- Glaucoma develops in about 50% of patients during late childhood or early adolescence.

DIAGNOSIS AND DIFFERENTIAL

- The diagnosis is most often based on family history and slit-lamp examination.

- In some cases a high-resolution banded chromosomal analysis will assist in the diagnosis.
- The differential includes the following:
  - Albinism
  - Iris coloboma
  - Iridocorneal endothelial syndrome

TREATMENT

- All children with sporadic aniridia should have chromosomal analysis for the Wilms' tumor gene defect. If this is positive, an oncologist should be consulted for a baseline intravenous pyelogram, periodic urinalysis for microscopic hematuria and/or repeated abdominal ultrasonographic and clinical examinations. Wilms' tumor is diagnosed before age 5 in 80% of cases. Familial aniridia patients are rarely at risk for Wilms' tumor.
- The patient's parents should be examined in efforts to detect variable expression of autosomal dominant aniridia.
- Female infants with isolated aniridia should have a high-resolution banded chromosomal analysis to rule out subtle genital anomalies associated with the deletion of 11p.
- Associated glaucoma should be managed with IOP control.
- Provide protective polycarbonate sunglasses and maximize vision with a low-vision specialist evaluation.

SUGGESTED READINGS

Albert DM, Jakobiec FA, eds: *Principles and Practice of Ophthalmology*, 2nd ed. Philadelphia: Saunders, 1994.
Yanoff M, Duker J: *Ophthalmology.* New York: Mosby, 1999.

IRIS COLOBOMA

CASE 10

The mother of a 6-month-old infant is concerned about an irregular black hole in her son's right eye. His examination, which shows that he can fix and follow in with both eyes, is significant for a keyhole-shaped defect in the inferior iris of the right eye (Fig. 8-13). His dilated fundus examination reveals an inferotemporal coloboma of the retina and choroid of his right eye.

PATHOPHYSIOLOGY

- Coloboma is defined as the absence of part of an eye structure.

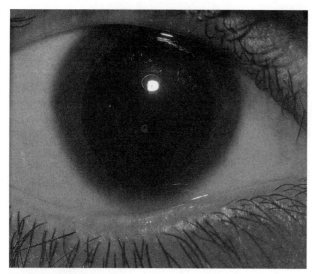

FIGURE 8-13 Iris colomoma.

- Colobomas may result from developmental aberrations, surgery, or injury.
- Congenital iris colobomas are classified as typical or atypical.
  - Iris colobomas are typical if they occur in the inferonasal quadrant. This occurs because the embryonic fissure fails to close in the 5th week of gestation. These colobomas are on a continuum that extends to microphthalmos and anophthalmos.
  - Atypical iris colobomas occur in areas other than the inferonasal quadrant and thus outside the region of the embryonic fissure. They are not associated with more posterior uveal colobomas. These colobomas likely result from fibrovascular remnants of the anterior hyaloid system and pupillary membrane.
- Uveal colobomas can be inherited as an autosomal dominant trait with incomplete penetrance and expressivity or as an autosomal recessive trait.
- More than half of typical colobomas are bilateral though they are often asymmetric.
- Areas of normal fusion of the embryonic fissure may alternate with areas of defective closure and thus, for instance, an optic disc coloboma may not be associated with an iris coloboma and vice versa.
- Lens colobomas result from hypoplasia of the corresponding ciliary body and zonular fibers causing a lack of zonular pull in that region. This causes peripheral flattening or indentation of the lens, usually inferiorly, and can be seen in patients with uveal colobomas.
- Iris colobomas can be associated with any chromosomal defect. The most common include the following:
  - Trisomy 13
  - Triploidy
  - Cat's-eye syndrome
  - 4p- Wolf-Hirschhorn syndrome
  - Trisomy 18
  - Klinefelter's syndrome
  - Turner syndrome (rare)
  - Other chromosomal defects including: 11q-, 18r (ring), 13r
- Uveal colobomas are associated with the following syndromes:
  - CHARGE syndrome occurs in 15% of cases. CHARGE stands for ocular **c**oloboma, **h**eart defects, choanal **a**tresia, mental **r**etardation, and **g**enitourinary and **e**ar anomalies.
  - Lenz's microphthalmos syndrome
  - Goltz focal dermal hypoplasia
  - Basal cell nevus syndrome
  - Warburg's syndrome
  - Aicardi's syndrome
  - Rubinstein-Taybi syndrome
  - Linear sebaceous nevus syndrome
  - Goldenhar's syndrome

CLINICAL FEATURES

- Typical iris colobomas, which by definition occur in the inferonasal quadrant, have the shape of a keyhole, light bulb, or inverted teardrop.
- Typical iris colobomas may be associated with ciliary body, choroid, retina, and optic nerve colobomas.
- Decreased visual acuity, nystagmus, and strabismus may be present if the optic nerve or a large part of the posterior pole is involved.
- Absolute scotomas (blind spots) correspond to retinal colobomas if present.

DIAGNOSIS AND DIFFERENTIAL

- The diagnosis is made on clinical examination.
- The differential includes the following:
  - Aniridia
  - Traumatic sphincter tears
  - Ruptured globe

TREATMENT

- Any associated amblyopia should be treated and vision monitored closely.
- Surgical treatment is rarely indicated. Such indications include the following: a large defect causing significant visual discomfort from halos or glare; a significant cosmetic deformity.

SUGGESTED READINGS

Tripathi BJ, Tripathi RC, Wisdorn J: Embryology of the anterior segment of the human eye. In: Ritch R, Shields MD, Krupin T, eds: *The Glaucomas.* Vol 1. 2nd ed. St Louis: Mosby, 1995.

Wilson ME, O'Neil JW: Pediatric iris abnormalities: In: Wright KW, ed: *Pediatric Ophthalmology and Strabismus.* St Louis: Mosby, 1995:349–365.

OCULOCUTANEOUS ALBINISM

CASE 11

A 17-year-old African American high school senior presents after failing the vision test for his driver's license. He reports no prior medical history. His family history is significant for a brother with lightly colored skin. His best corrected visual acuity is 20/100 in both eyes. His examination is significant for light-colored skin and hair and ocular nystagmus. On slit-lamp examination, he is found to have iris transillumination defects (Fig. 8-14) and foveal hypoplasia in both eyes. Findings of the rest of his examination are within normal limits.

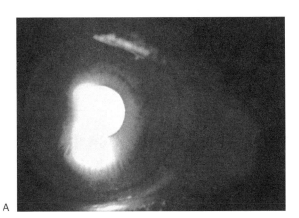

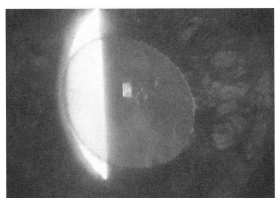

FIGURE 8-14 A and B. Oculocutaneous albinism.

PATHOPHYSIOLOGY

- Albinism is caused by defects in the synthesis of melanin pigment. A congenital reduction or absence of melanin pigment results in specific developmental changes in the optical system.
- The biosynthesis of melanin begins with the hydroxylation of the amino acid L-tyrosine to dihydroxylphenylalanine (DOPA) and the oxidation of DOPA to DOPA quinone by the copper-containing enzyme tyrosinase. The end result is either black-brown eumelanin, or, in the presence of sulfhydryl compounds, red-yellow pheomelanin. Defects of tyrosinase results in albinism.

    Flowchart: L-tyrosine→DOPA–tyrosinase–→ DOPA quinone–→eumelanin (black-brown)\–sulfhydryl compounds→pheomelanin

- The main subdivisions of albinism include the following:
    ○ Oculocutaneous
    ○ Ocular
    ○ Albinoidism (This is the absence of pigment in localized areas and is not as severe as the oculocutaneous or ocular albinism.)
- Oculocutaneous albinism (OCA) is a heterogeneous genetic disorder caused by mutations in several different genes resulting in incomplete melanization of cellular melanosomes.
    ○ OCA involves two regions of the body: the skin/hair and the optic system including the eye and the optic nerves.
    ○ Tyrosinase-positive and tyrosinase-negative oculocutaneous albinism are autosomal recessive. In *tyrosinase-negative* oculocutaneous albinism, the congenital inactivity of the enzyme tyrosinase prevents the cell's use of tyrosine in the formation of the pigment melanin. These patients never produce pigment. In *tyrosinase-positive* oculocutaneous albinism, tyrosinase activity is normal, but there is an inability of the cells to sequester the synthesized melanin into the melanosomes. These patients have some pigment present as adults.
- Ocular albinism is limited to a reduced pigment in the uveal tract and the retinal pigment epithelium of the eye.
    ○ The changes to the optic system associated with hypopigmentation include a reduction in visual acuity resulting from foveal hypoplasia, and disorganization of reticulogeniculate projections at the optic chiasm. Twenty percent of temporal fibers decussate and project to the contralateral dorsal lateral geniculate nucleus rather than the ipsilateral nucleus. These defects create a poor prognosis for binocular function.

CLINICAL FEATURES

- Albinism affects approximately 1 in 17,000 individuals.
- Oculocutaneous as well as ocular albinism exhibits similar ocular and visual dysfunction.
- Patients with oculocutaneous albinism have the following findings:
  - Reduced visual acuity. This is due to macular hypoplasia as well as significant refractive error and astigmatism. Eyes with ocular albinism have variable amounts of uveal pigmentation, and the best acuity among persons with albinism ranges from 20/25 to 20/300. Patients with oculocutaneous albinism exhibit less pigmentation than those with ocular albinism and tend to have lower acuity levels (20/80 to 20/400).
  - Photophobia
  - Strabismus
  - Pendular nystagmus, due to maldevelopment of the macula
  - Transillumination of the iris and globe (this can be seen by placing a pen light or muscle light on the temporal lower or upper eyelid, 8 mm behind the limbus of the opened eye; one may shine the light through the pupil in a dark room and grossly inspect the transillumination defects of the iris and sclera).
  - Blonde fundus with visible choroidal vasculature
  - Macular hypoplasia, due to insufficient uveal pigmentation and poor development of the retinal pigment epithelium; this is always present in patients with albinism
  - Supernormal electro-oculogram (EOG) and electroretinogram (ERG)
- Associated disorders include the following:
  - Hermansky-Pudlak syndrome, an autosomal recessive subtype of tyrosinase-positive oculocutaneous albinism commonly seen in Puerto Rico. These patients have a tendency toward easy bruising and bleeding due to a platelet dysfunction.
  - Chédiak-Higashi syndrome, an autosomal recessive subtype of oculocutaneous albinism. These patients may have a silvery sheen to their skin, with blue to brown irides, an increased susceptibility to infection, and a predisposition to the development of a lymphoma-like condition.

DIAGNOSIS AND DIFFERENTIAL

- The diagnosis is made by physical examination. Molecular analysis can establish the diagnosis for many subtypes of albinism.
- Genetic counseling should be suggested in appropriate cases.

- Laboratory testing for patients may include the following:
  - CBC with differential, PT, PTT, platelet aggregation testing
  - ERG, EOG
  - Tyrosinase testing
- Prenatal diagnosis of albinism is now possible by means of a fetoscope, where a sample of fetal skin can be obtained and analyzed.
- The differential of partial albinism includes the following:
  - Chédiak-Higashi syndrome
  - Hermansky-Pudlak syndrome
  - Prader-Willi syndrome
  - Angelman syndrome
  - Ectodermal dysplasia
  - Choroideremia (is in the differential for the fundus appearance)

TREATMENT

- Currently there is no effective treatment for albinism.
- Visual rehabilitation is advised. Telescopic and microscopic optical devices can provide great improvement in visual function. These optical devices show a magnified retinal image that is viewed over a larger area of the dysplastic macula and retina. This stimulates more photoreceptors than would normally be stimulated, and this quantitative effect allows for an increase in visual acuity.
- Clinically, tyrosinase-positive oculocutaneous albinism exhibits the better prognosis, as pigmentation may increase somewhat throughout life and visual disability is not as severe. The level of visual functioning of the ocular albino varies directly with the level of uveal pigmentation developed.
- Any patient with either ocular or oculocutaneous albinism who exhibits unusual bleeding or susceptibility to bruising should be referred for a hematological consultation.
- Any patient with albinism exhibiting poor bacterial resistance should also be referred for a hematological consultation.
- Persons with albinism have an increased risk of skin cancer, particularly squamous and basal cell carcinoma. However, there is no evidence of increased risk for malignant melanoma.

SUGGESTED READINGS

Albert DM, Jakobiec FA, eds: *Principles and Practice of Ophthalmology.* 2nd ed. Philadelphia: Saunders, 1994.
Yanoff M, Duker J: *Ophthalmology.* New York: Mosby, 1999.

HETEROCHROMIA IRIDIS

CASE 12

A 58-year-old woman is referred for cataract surgery. On examination, however, it can be seen that her right iris is much lighter than her left, which is brown. Even closer examination shows that the right eye has a few small white stellate keratic precipitates scattered diffusely over the endothelium, as well as diffuse iris atrophy. Her best vision is 20/70 OD and 20/30 OS. She has significant nuclear sclerosis of her right eye with only a mild lens change in the left eye (Fig. 8-15). The rest of the findings are normal except for an enlarged cup-to-disc ratio of her right eye

PATHOPHYSIOLOGY

- Heterochromia can be defined as binocular heterochromia (Heterochromia iridum), where each iris differs in color, or as uniocular heterochromia (Heterochromia iridis), where one iris has different colors. In general, most clinicians refer to heterochromia iridum when using the general term heterochromia.
- Heterochromia iridum can be congenital or acquired. It can be a normal variant, though often disorders of the sympathetic system need first to be excluded depending on the patient's history. The affected eye can be hypopigmented (hypochromic) or hyperpigmented (hyperchromic).
- Heterochromia iridis can also be congenital, acquired, or a normal variant. This may be due to the presence of a large nevus, sectoral pigmentation changes, tumor, or previous trauma.

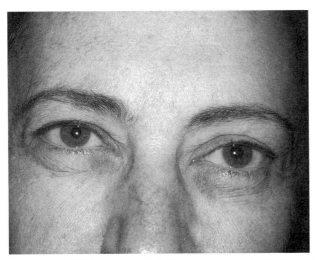

FIGURE 8-15 Heterochromia iridium in a patient with Fuchs' heterochromic iridocyclodialysis.

- The sympathetic nervous system controls iris pigmentation during its development from embryonic development to its completion around two years of age. Congenital heterochromia may be present if a lesion occurs in the sympathetic pathway before the age of two.
- Hypochromic heterochromia occurs when iris melanocytes are deficient in pigment or few in number. The most common cause of hypochromic heterochromia is chronic uveitis and Fuchs' heterochromic iridocyclitis, which causes iris stromal atrophy.
- Hyperchromic heterochromia occurs when iris melanocytes contain more pigment or are more abundant. An increasingly common cause of acquired hyperchromic heterochromia is the use of prostaglandin analogs in the treatment of glaucoma.

CLINICAL FEATURES

- In congenital heterochromia the affected iris remains blue as the other iris changes to brown owing to a defect in the sympathetic system occurring before the age of two. Heterochromia is uncommon in patients with Horner's syndrome acquired later in life.
- The presence of miosis, blepharoptosis, and anhidrosis may help diagnosis subtle heterochromia in a case of congenital Horner's syndrome.
- Patients with congenital oculodermal melanocytosis (nevus of Ota) have extensive slate-gray epibulbar pigmentation and subtle pigmentation of the periocular skin.
- Other ocular signs such as stellate keratic precipitates, mild active iritis, or a unilateral cataract and glaucoma occur in Fuchs' heterochromic cyclitis.
- Other signs, such as previous trauma or ruptured globe, may raise suspicion about an intraocular foreign body.

DIAGNOSIS AND DIFFERENTIAL

- The diagnosis is made by careful physical examination.
- A complete medical history is obtained including a history of a previous intraocular foreign body or ruptured globe, a history of diabetes, a history of cancer, and the use of intraocular medications.
- Categories of heterochromia are congenital heterochromia and acquired heterochromia.
- Congenital hypochromic heterochromia includes the following diagnoses:
  - Horner's syndrome (congenital or early onset); due to abnormalities in sympathetic-innervation dependent melanosome migration. Congenital Horner's is usually due to trauma during delivery.

- Waardenburg's syndrome (hypertelorism, white forelock, white eyelashes, leukoderma, and cochlear deafness)
  - Incontinentia pigmenti
  - Hirschsprung's disease with iris bicolor
  - Parry-Romberg hemifacial atrophy (due to abnormalities in the trophic sympathetic nervous system)
- Congenital hyperchromic heterochromia includes:
  - Oculodermal melanocytosis (nevus of Ota)
  - Ocular melanosis
  - Sector iris pigment epithelial hamartoma
- Acquired hypochromic heterochromia includes:
  - Chronic iritis
  - Fuchs' heterochromic cyclitis
  - Horner's syndrome (chronic)
  - Juvenile xanthogranuloma
  - Metastatic carcinoma
  - Leukemia and lymphoma
- Acquired hyperchromic heterochromia
  - Prostaglandin F2-alpha and prostamide analog drops
  - Diffuse iris nevus or pigmented tumors
  - Melanoma
  - Siderosis or hemosiderosis
  - Rubeosis/iris neovascularization
  - Iridocorneal endothelial (ICE) syndrome
  - Iris ectropion syndrome

TREATMENT

- The underlying cause should be treated if possible.
- Prostaglandin analog drugs (e.g., latanoprost) should be discontinued if necessary.
- Cosmetic contact lenses may be used.

SUGGESTED READINGS

Albert DM, Jakobiec FA, eds: *Principles and Practice of Ophthalmology*, 2nd ed. Philadelphia: Saunders, 1994.
Roy FH: *Ocular Differential Diagnosis*, 3rd ed. Philadelphia: Lea & Febiger, 1984.
Yanoff M, Duker J: *Ophthalmology.* New York. Mosby, 1999.

POLYCORIA/CORECTOPIA

CASE 13

A 34-year-old woman comes to the clinic complaining of blurred vision in her right eye with a change in that eye's appearance (Fig. 8-16) for the last three months. She denies prior trauma. She has no significant past

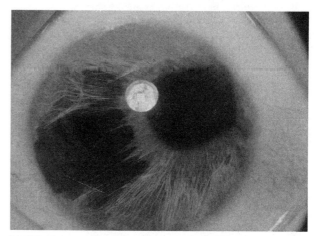

FIGURE 8-16 Iridocorneal endothelial syndrome: essential iris atrophy.

medical or family history. Her left eye is normal. Her IOPs are 26 mmHg OD and 20 mmHg OS. Her right optic nerve has an increased cup-to-disc ratio compared to the left nerve.

PATHOPHYSIOLOGY

- Polycoria is the presence of multiple holes in the iris. Corectopia is pupillary distortion.
- Polycoria may occur from trauma (blunt, surgical, or laser), developmental abnormalities, or prior infections or inflammations.
- In iridocorneal endothelial syndrome, the main abnormality is in the corneal endothelium, which, unlike normal cornea, behaves like epithelium. The endothelium spreads over the trabecular meshwork and the iris, causing glaucoma and iris distortion. The cause is unknown.

CLINICAL FEATURES

- Depending on the etiology, patients may complain of double vision, halos, photophobia, and glare.
- Patients with polycoria from birth or early childhood may have no significant symptoms.
- Slit-lamp examination may reveal new holes in iris stroma or stretch holes. Peripheral anterior synechiae may be present in certain syndromes.

DIAGNOSIS AND DIFFERENTIAL

- The diagnosis is made on previous history of trauma, zoster infection, and a good slit-lamp examination.

- The complete differential includes the following:
  - ○ Iridocorneal endothelial syndrome, i.e. *essential iris atrophy*: prominent polycoria and corectopia is present; *Chandler's syndrome*: mild iris atrophy and corectopia; the corneal endothelium has a hammered metal appearance; and *Cogan-Reese syndrome*: mild iris atrophy with pigmented nodules on the iris surface.
  - ○ Axenfeld-Rieger syndrome: a prominent, anteriorly displaced Schwalbe's line is seen in addition to iris defects such as polycoria, corectopia, and ectropion uvea.
  - ○ Posterior polymorphous dystrophy: an autosomal dominant, bilateral disorder of Descemet's membrane of the cornea. Vesicles form in a linear or grouped pattern with scalloped edges. Other findings include iridocorneal adhesions, corectopia, and secondary glaucoma.
  - ○ Trauma
- Surgical trauma or laser trauma is the most common etiology.
  - ○ Herpes zoster: iris stomal atrophy can occur as a result of associated ischemia.

TREATMENT

- Aggressive treatment of any associated glaucoma, if present, is indicated.
- Endothelial cell counts should be followed if corneal involvement is suspected.
- Cosmetic contact lenses or corneal tattooing may help decrease visual symptoms and cosmetic deformities.
- Surgical repair is rarely indicated in cases of polycoria from iridocorneal endothelial syndrome.
- If prior trauma or surgical trauma is the cause of the polycoria, and the patient has mild complaints of glare, halos, or light sensitivity, a cosmetic contact lens that limits central light rays may be an option. If the patient has significant visual complaints that cannot be corrected with a contact lens, or if the patient is intolerant to contact lenses, surgical correction is an option. An irregular pupil can be surgically corrected with a modified McCannel suture technique with prolene suture.
- If the patient requires cataract surgery in the future, prosthetic iris rings can be inserted into the capsular bag to provide an iris diaphragm.

SUGGESTED READINGS

Albert DM, Jakobiec FA, eds: *Principles and Practice of Ophthalmology*, 2nd ed. Philadelphia: Saunders, 1994.

Hersh P, Zagelbaum B, Lora Cremers S: *Ophthalmic Surgical Procedures*, 2nd ed. New York: Thieme, 2003.

Yanoff M, Duker J: *Ophthalmology.* New York. Mosby, 1999.

PERSISTENT PUPILLARY MEMBRANE

CASE 14

The mother of a 10-year-old girl brings her daughter to the clinic for a routine examination. Her vision is 20/20 in both eyes. Results of her examination are within healthy limits except for a notable pupillary membrane in her left eye (Fig. 8-17).

PATHOPHYSIOLOGY

- Pupillary membranes result from the incomplete involution of the pupillary membrane and anterior vascular capsule of the lens, which is usually completed during the 5th to 6th month of fetal development.
- Persistent pupillary membranes usually undergo considerable atrophy during the first year of life. The remnants tend to atrophy in time and usually present no problem. Because a minimum pupillary diameter of 1.5 mm is sufficient for normal retinal image formation, amblyopia is usually rare. In some cases, however, significant remnants may obscure the pupil and interfere with vision.
- It is not uncommon to see some remnants of the pupillary membrane in newborns, particularly in premature infants. These membranes are nonpigmented strands of obliterated vessels that cross the pupil and may secondarily attach to the lens or cornea.

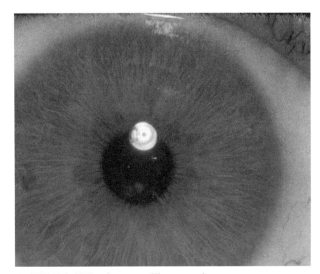

FIGURE 8-17 Persistent pupillary membrane.

CLINICAL FEATURES

- Slit-lamp examination reveals a persistent membrane along the iris border.
- Visual acuity is usually not affected. Rare cases of associated amblyopia have been reported.
- Rarely, blood vessels remain patent within the remnant membrane. Hyphemas may occur from the rupture of these persistent vessels spontaneously or from trauma.

DIAGNOSIS AND DIFFERENTIAL

- The diagnosis is based on clinical examination and history.
- The differential includes the following:
  ○ Foreign body
  ○ Polycoria due to iridocorneal endothelial dystrophy

TREATMENT

- Usually no treatment is needed.
- Rarely, an extensive persistent pupillary membrane in an infant will require treatment to prevent amblyopia. In such cases, mydriatics and occlusion therapy is usually effective. Rarely, laser surgery or intraocular surgery is needed to provide an adequate pupillary aperture.

SUGGESTED READINGS

Albert DM, Jakobiec FA, eds: *Principles and Practice of Ophthalmology*, 2nd ed. Philadelphia: Saunders, 1994.
Yanoff M, Duker J: *Ophthalmology.* New York. Mosby, 1999.

LENS

ABNORMALITIES IN LENS POSITION

CASE 15 (SUBLUXATION)

A 24-year-old professional basketball player presents with blurry vision in his left eye. He has a history of Marfan syndrome. Significantly, examination reveals 20/80 vision in that eye on best-corrected refraction and slit-lamp examination finds a lens dislocated superotemporally (Fig. 8-18).

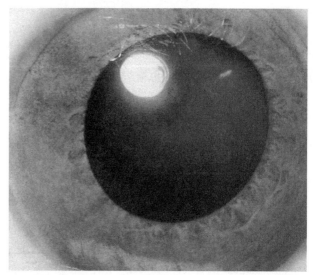

FIGURE 8-18 Subluxation of the lens in a patient with Marfan's syndrome.

PATHOPHYSIOLOGY

- Subluxation is a partial dislocation of the lens with a portion of the lens visible within the pupil.
- Subluxation is due to an abnormality of the zonular attachments with a partial disruption of zonular fibers.
- This may occur in isolation or as part of a systemic condition such as Marfan syndrome, homocystinuria, Weill-Marchesani syndrome, or Ehlers-Danlos syndrome. Lens subluxation can also occur from trauma or in association with the following: uveitis, aniridia, Rieger's syndrome, syphilis, and pseudoexfoliation.

CLINICAL FEATURES

- Visual acuity may be unaffected, but most commonly is decreased below 20/40 on best correction due to the induced prism, astigmatism, or myopic shift caused by the edge of the lens.
- An abnormal red reflex may be appreciated.
- Once a subluxed lens is diagnosed, other clinical signs can determine the underlying cause:
  ○ Patients with Marfan syndrome have an "up and out" lens subluxation, tall stature, arachnodactyly, increased risk of retinal detachment, cardiomyopathy, and aortic aneurysm. It is autosomal dominant.
  ○ Homocystinuria patients have a "down and in" lens subluxation, marfanoid habitus, mental retardation, increased risk of retinal detachment, and systemic thrombosis. It is autosomal recessive.
  ○ Weill-Marchesani syndrome patients have microspherophakia (small round lens), short fingers

and stature, myopia, and seizures. It is autosomal recessive.

DIAGNOSIS AND DIFFERENTIAL

- Diagnosis is based on slit-lamp examination. A dilated slit-lamp examination best shows the dislocation, though iridodonesis and phacodonesis is more apparent on the undilated examination. A significantly subluxed cataractous lens may be viewed with just a penlight.
- Differential: trauma, Marfan syndrome, homocystinuria, Weill-Marchesani, sulfate oxide deficiency.
- Patients with idiopathic lens subluxation should be referred for a metabolic work-up for homocystinuria or sulfate oxide deficiency.

TREATMENT

- Treatment depends on the extent of the subluxation and symptoms. If the patient has minimal symptoms, the dislocated lens can be monitored on follow-up examinations. Glasses or contact lenses that correct for an induced aphakia (lack of lens), myopic shift, astigmatism, or induced prism may initially help. Cycloplegic eye drops to dilate the eye and allow better vision may help in certain cases. Alternatively, miotics to constrict the pupil may help certain patients achieve a pinhole effect and thus better vision.
- Other less commonly used treatments include argon or Nd:YAG iridotomy to further enlarge the aphakic area of the pupillary aperture.
- If the vision is more severely compromised, or if there is a significant risk that the lens may fall into the posterior segment, then surgery is indicated.
- Surgical options depend on the extent of subluxation. If the subluxation is minimal, the lens may be removed by extracapsular cataract extraction or phacoemulsification. An endocapsular ring may be inserted to stabilize the capsular bag in the presence of significant zonular dehiscence. In more advanced cases, a pars plana lensectomy with a pars plana vitrectomy is recommended.

SUGGESTED READINGS

Albert DM, Jakobiec FA, eds: *Principles and Practice of Ophthalmology*, 2nd ed. Philadelphia: Saunders, 1994.

Hersh P, Zagelbaum B, Lora Cremers S: *Ophthalmic Surgical Procedures*, 2nd ed. New York: Thieme, 2003.

Steinert R: *Cataract Surgery: Technique, Complications, & Management*. Philadelphia: Saunders, 1995.

Yanoff M, Duker J: *Ophthalmology*. New York: Mosby, 1999.

CASE 16 (DISLOCATION)

- A 28-year-old boxer comes to the emergency department a few days after being hit in his left eye with a fist. His vision is 20/20 OD and can count fingers at 2 feet OS. His examination is significant for 1+ cell and flare in the anterior chamber. Dilated examination shows an inferiorly cataractous dislocated lens (Fig. 8-19). The vitreous face is intact and the rest of his examination is within healthy limits with no evidence of retinal holes or tears.

PATHOPHYSIOLOGY

- A dislocation is a complete disruption of the zonular fibers. It may be partial or complete, and is usually defined when the lens is displaced out of the pupillary aperture.
- Trauma is the most common cause of lens dislocation.
- The zonules of the lens are stressed to maximal tension and disinserted from their attachments to the lens and/or ciliary body.

CLINICAL FEATURES

- Symptoms include decreased visual acuity, monocular diplopia, increased astigmatism, and impaired accommodation.
- Slit-lamp examination may reveal iridodonesis (movement of the iris with eye motion), and phacodonesis (lens movement with eye motion). Other

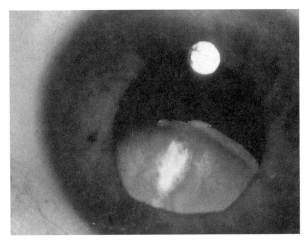

FIGURE 8-19 The viteous face is intact and the rest of the patient's examination is within healthy limits with no evidence of retinal holes or tears.

signs include the loss of the normal reflections of the clear lens on slit-lamp examination, and posterior synechiae formation. If the vitreous body has been violated, the stringy vitreous body may come forward into the anterior chamber. If the vitreous face is intact and the lens has fallen further down into the vitreous cavity, one may only see the dark cavity of the posterior segment or an abnormal red reflex.

• It may be difficult for the novice examiner to appreciate a completely dislocated lens.

DIAGNOSIS AND DIFFERENTIAL

• Diagnosis is based on slit-lamp examination.
• The differential diagnosis includes a subluxation of the lens (see above), previous cataract surgery without placement of an intraocular lens, or couching procedure (where the natural lens is intentionally pushed back into the vitreous cavity to achieve a clear visual pathway).

TREATMENT

• Surgical options depend on the extent of dislocation. If the dislocation is minimal and no vitreous is present in the anterior chamber, the lens may be removed by extracapsular cataract extraction or phacoemulsification. An endocapsular ring may be inserted to stabilize the capsular bag in the presence of significant zonular dehiscence.
• In more advanced cases, a pars plana lensectomy with a pars plana vitrectomy is recommended. A sutured intraocular lens or an anterior chamber intraocular lens can then be placed.
• A nonsurgical option is to fit the patient with a contact lens and leave the dislocated lens in the vitreous cavity. These patients should be monitored for retinal tears or detachments as the result of the initial dislocation. Once stable, the risk of subsequent retinal complications is low.

SUGGESTED READINGS

Albert DM, Jakobiec FA, eds: *Principles and Practice of Ophthalmology*, 2nd ed. Philadelphia: Saunders, 1994.

Hersh P, Zagelbaum B, Lora Cremers S: *Ophthalmic Surgical Procedures*, 2nd ed. New York: Thieme, 2003.

Steinert R: *Cataract Surgery: Technique, Complications, & Management.* Philadelphia: Saunders, 1995.

Yanoff M, Duker J: *Ophthalmology.* New York: Mosby, 1999.

CATARACT

CASE 17

A 72 year-old man presents complaining of hazy vision and difficulty seeing the street signs when driving. His best-corrected vision is 20/50 OD and 20/400 OS. His examination is significant for a moderate nuclear sclerosis in his right eye and a mature cataract in his left eye (Fig. 8-20). The rest of his examination, including a B-scan of his left eye, is within normal limits.

PATHOPHYSIOLOGY

• A cataract is defined as any opacity in the lens regardless of its effect on vision.
• Cataracts usually occur from the aging of the lens. They can occur at birth, develop after trauma (blunt or surgical) or radiation, or develop from inflammation or from a metabolic or nutritional defect.
• Many factors contribute to cataract formation. The following are known mechanisms.
  ○ Protein aggregation: Aging lens crystallins form large aggregates that scatter light and result in the appearance of a white opacity. Nuclear cataracts occur when the aggregates are free in the cytoplasm. Cortical and posterior subcapsular cataracts occur when the aggregates are bound to cell membranes.
  ○ Osmotic stress: Oxygen byproducts such as hydroxyl radicals, super oxide, singlet oxygen, and, most importantly, hydrogen peroxide cause the disruption of membrane structures, deactivation of enzyme systems, protein aggregation, and lens color changes (by forming chromophores).
  ○ Posttranslational protein changes: This includes nonenzymatic glycosylation, racemization, and aggregation.

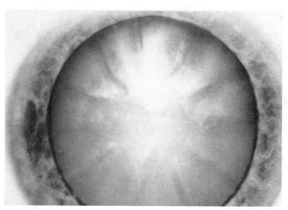

FIGURE 8-20 Cataractous lens. (See Color Plate.)

- In patients with diabetes and galactosemia, sugar is converted by the enzyme aldose reductase to the sugar alcohol sorbitol via the sorbitol pathway. Sorbitol and other sugar alcohols such as galactiol cannot pass through plasma membranes and remain in the cytoplasm. This causes water to enter the cell to neutralize the hyperosmolarity of the cytoplasm. Cells then swell. Intracellular and intercellular changes create light-scattering foci and lens opacities.
- Pathological changes include the following: Initially epithelial and superficial cortical cells undergo vacuolization. This continues with an expansion of intercellular spaces between cortical fibers, which creates cysts, which then coalesce to form vacuoles. This causes the rupture of cell membranes and subsequent biochemical changes as described above.

CLINICAL FEATURES

- A visually significant age-related cataract results in a slow progressive loss of visual acuity (at near or distance) or blurry vision in one or both eyes, usually over months to years.
- Other symptoms depend on the density of the lens and may include the following:
  - Frequent changes in the spectacle prescription required for best vision
  - Difficulty with reading
  - Excessive glare especially with night driving due to oncoming headlights
  - A loss of contrast sensitivity
  - Reduced color perception
  - Monocular double vision due to the cataracts
- Clinically, cataracts appear as a white opacity in the normally clear lens (see Fig. 8-21A, B).
- Cataracts may be classified in many ways:

I. Morphologic Classification
  A. Capsular Cataract
  - Anterior capsular
    a. Congenital: from persistent pupillary membrane
    b. Acquired: pseudoexfoliation syndromes; antipsychotic medications (e.g., chlorpromazine); previous inflammation causing posterior synechiae and an anterior capsular cataract
  - Posterior capsular:
    a. Congenital: in association with persistent hyaloid remnants (Mittendorf's dot)

  B. Subcapsular Cataract
  - Anterior subcapsular
    a. Etiology: acute angle closure glaucoma (glaukomflecken); medications (e.g., amiodarone toxicity, miotics); Wilson's disease

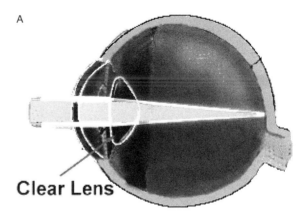

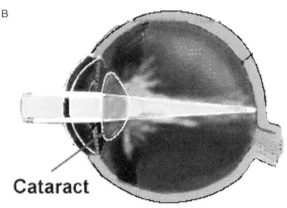

FIGURE 8-21 Illustrations showing a clear lens (A) and one with a cataract (B).

    b. Age related: due to fibrous metaplasia of the anterior lens epithelium
  - Posterior subcapsular
    a. Etiology: diabetes mellitus, myotonic dystrophy, steroids, irradiation
    b. Age related: These are located just in front of the posterior capsule. They are associated with the posterior migration of the anterior epithelium of the lens. Posterior subcapsular cataracts are more symptomatic with complaints of glare and poor near vision compared to anterior cataracts.

  C. Nuclear Cataract
  - Congenital: seen in rubella (Fig. 8-22) or galactosemia
  - Age-related: results from the normal or accelerated aging of the lens nucleus. It is often preceded by the presence of radial water clefts in the cortex. Nuclear cataracts are often associated with myopia owing to the increase in the refractive index. Some patients with nuclear sclerosis may be able to read again without their

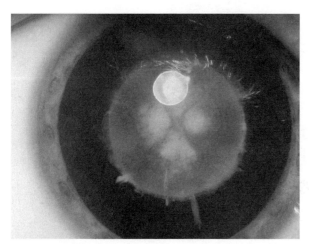

FIGURE 8-22 Congenital cataract.

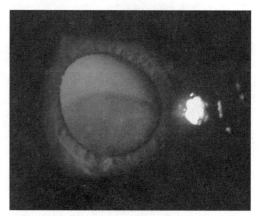

FIGURE 8-23 Morgagnian cataract.

spectacles because of the induced myopia, this explains the "second sight of the aged."

D. Cortical Cataract
These are commonly age-related or congenital. They are spoke-like and can be anterior or posterior. These do not usually interfere with vision.

E. Lamellar Cataract
These are congenital and involve one lamella of the fetal or nuclear zone.

F. Sutural Cataract
These are congenital Y-shaped opacities in the lens nucleus. They are very common and of no clinical significance.

II. Age-Related Classification

A. Immature cataracts have scattered opacities that are separated by clear areas.

B. Mature cataracts have dense anterior cortical changes, which totally obscure the view of the posterior lens and posterior segment of the eye.

C. Intumescent cataracts may be mature or immature. They occur when the lens has become swollen by imbibed water.

D. Hypermature cataracts are mature cataracts that have become swollen with a wrinkled capsule as a result of leakage of water out of the lens.

E. Morgagnian cataracts are hypermature cataracts leading to total liquefaction of the cortex causing the nucleus to sink inferiorly (Fig. 8-23).

III. Classification Based on Age of Onset
   ○ Congenital, infantile, juvenile, presenile, senile

IV. Classification Based on Etiology

A. Age-related: as noted above.

B. Trauma: previous intraocular surgery (e.g., pars plana vitrectomy, prior glaucoma surgery such as trabeculectomy, or laser iridotomy), previous ruptured globe, previous electric shock or lightning injury.

C. Metabolic
   ○ Diabetes mellitus accelerates senile cataract formation. True diabetic cataracts usually have bilateral white punctate or snowflake posterior or anterior subcapsular opacities.
   ○ Galactosemia, galactokinase deficiency, mannosidosis, and hypocalcemic syndromes have multifocal white flakes present within the lens.
   ○ Toxic:
      a. Steroids: systemic steroids are more cataract inducing than topical steroids and usually cause anterior and posterior subcapsular cataracts.
      b. Chlorpromazine causes anterior lens capsular opacities.
      c. Amiodarone causes anterior subcapsular opacities.
      d. Gold (used in rheumatoid arthritis): approximately one half of patients talking gold orally have posterior lens opacities.
      e. Miotics: Chronic use of miotic drops like pilocarpine can cause anterior subcapsular opacities.
   ○ Secondary Cataract:
      a. Chronic anterior uveitis
      b. Status post surgery
   ○ Miscellaneous:
      a. Hereditary fundus dystrophy (e.g., retinitis pigmentosa)
      b. High myopia

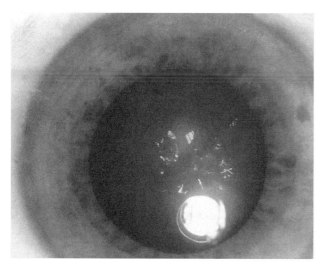

FIGURE 8-24 Christmas tree cataract in a patient with myotonic dystrophy.

c. Acute angle-closure glaucoma attacks can cause anterior capsular or subcapsular opacities in the pupillary zone (Glaukomflecken).
d. Myotonic dystrophy: fine polychromatic granules in the cortex followed later by subcapsular stellate opacities occur in myotonic dystrophy ("Christmas tree" cataract) (Fig. 8-24).
e. Atopic dermatitis is associated with bilateral anterior or posterior stellate opacities
f. Down syndrome
○ Congenital/ intrauterine
a. Congenital rubella:
b. Toxoplasmosis
c. CMV
d. Maternal ingestion of medications (e.g., thalidomide, steroids)
○ Hereditary
a. Usually dominant
b. Congenital to presenile

DIAGNOSIS AND DIFFERENTIAL

- A comprehensive dilated eye exam with slit-lamp examination allows for the accurate diagnosis of a cataract.
- The differential includes causes of leukocoria (a white papillary reflex). In congenital cataracts, one must rule out the following: retinoblastoma; toxocariasis; Coat's disease; PHPV (persistent hyperplastic primary vitreous); retinal detachment due to ROP (retinopathy of prematurity); retinal astrocytoma (associated with tuberous sclerosis); familial exudative vitreoretinopathy; retinochoroidal coloboma. In adults, the differential includes a dense inflammatory membrane or ochre membrane, a fibrotic retinal detachment, and significant uveitis.
- The B-scan ultrasound may be helpful in ruling out underlying retinal abnormalities in a patient with a dense cataract.

TREATMENT

- Treatment depends on the extent of symptoms as they affect the patient. When cataracts progress and begin to limit the patient's ability to perform the activities of daily life, treatment should be considered.
- A fluorescein angiogram may help determine if an underlying macular abnormality is also limiting visual function in the presence of a mild cataract.
- Prescribing new glasses in a few cases may help improve the patient's quality of life until the patient and family are ready for surgical intervention.
- In most cases, however, surgery is the best option.
- Modern cataract surgery involves the use of a microscopic incision either through clear cornea or through sclera with phacoemulsification (in which ultrasound is used to break the cataract into minute pieces and then aspirated through a probe). A small intraocular lens is placed in the eye to replace the focusing power provided by the human lens. This lens, or implant, is permanently affixed inside the eye, cannot be felt, and eliminates the need for thick glasses after surgery. The small incision may be closed with either a few or no sutures.
- Modern cataract surgery is performed almost exclusively on an outpatient basis. The procedure is performed with local anesthesia, and visual recovery is achieved usually within 1–7 days.
- Early research indicates a diet high in antioxidants may help decrease cataract formation.

SUGGESTED READINGS

Hersh P, Zagelbaum B, Lora Cremers S: *Ophthalmic Surgical Procedures*, 2nd ed. New York: Thieme, 2003.
Steinert R: *Cataract Surgery: Technique, Complications, & Management.* Philadelphia: Saunders, 1995.
Yanoff M, Duker J: *Ophthalmology.* New York: Mosby, 1999.

9 GLAUCOMA

Lini S. Bhatia
Teresa C. Chen

EPIDEMIOLOGY

- Glaucoma is the leading cause of blindness among African Americans and Hispanic Americans.[1,2] It is the second leading cause of blindness among Americans aged 18 to 65.[1] An estimated 130,000 Americans are legally blind from glaucoma.[3]
- More than 5.2 million people worldwide are blind from glaucoma, according to the 1995 WHO statistics. Although more commonly seen in the elderly, glaucoma can occur in all age groups.
- Glaucomatous optic neuropathy is associated with a progressive loss of peripheral vision that can lead to total, irreversible blindness. In general, once vision is lost from glaucoma, there is no known treatment to restore the lost vision. However, in nearly all cases, blindness from glaucoma is preventable through early detection. Treatment then focuses on slowing down or stopping this progressive loss of vision.

REFERENCES

1. *American Academy of Ophthalmology*. Preferred practice pattern. Primary open angle glaucoma. San Francisco, 1996.
2. **Rodriguez J, Sanchez R, et al.** Causes of blindness and visual impairment in a population-based sample of U.S. Hispanics. *Ophthalmology* 2002;109(4):737–743.
3. **Quigley HA, Vitale S.** Models of open angle glaucoma prevalence and incidence in the United States. *Invest Ophthalmol Vis Sci* 1997;38:83–91.

DEFINITION

- Glaucoma is not one disease but a group of diseases that, in general, share the following common features: increased intraocular pressure (IOP), optic nerve head damage, and visual field loss. The different types of glaucoma vary in pathophysiology, clinical presentation, and management.

- The common denominator of all types of glaucoma is a characteristic optic neuropathy due to various risk factors, one of which is increased IOP.[4]

REFERENCE

4. **Van Buskirk EM, Ciotti GA.** Glaucomatous optic neuropathy. *Am J Ophthalmol* 113:447,1992.

PATHOPHYSIOLOGY

AQUEOUS HUMOR

- Aqueous humor is secreted by the ciliary body. From the ciliary body, it goes to the posterior chamber (the area between the lens and iris) and then through the pupil to the anterior chamber (AC, the area between the iris and the cornea). The aqueous then drains into the trabecular meshwork and Schlemm's canal. The trabeculocanalicular outflow forms the major draining apparatus of the eye (Fig. 9-1). Some aqueous also drains through a more minor route, the uveoscleral flow. The trabecular meshwork and Schlemm's canal are located in the angle, which is formed at the junction of the peripheral cornea and the base of the iris.
- Intraocular pressure is a balance between the aqueous production, resistance to aqueous outflow, and the episcleral venous pressure. Increased IOP is usually due to resistance in aqueous outflow.

INTRAOCULAR PRESSURE AND ITS EFFECTS

- Intraocular pressure normally varies between 10 and 21 mm Hg.
- Increased IOP is a risk factor for optic nerve damage and for associated retinal nerve fiber layer thinning. These changes typically cause peripheral and later central visual field defects.

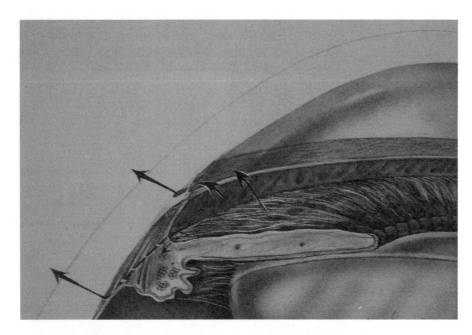

FIGURE 9-1 Aqueous humor leaving the eye by trabeculocanalicular flow and uveoscleral flow. [Used with permission from Stamper RL, Lieberman MF, Drake MV: *Becker–Shaffer's Diagnosis and Therapy of the Glaucomas*, 7th ed. St. Louis: CV Mosby, 1999; Fig. 4-7, p 50.]

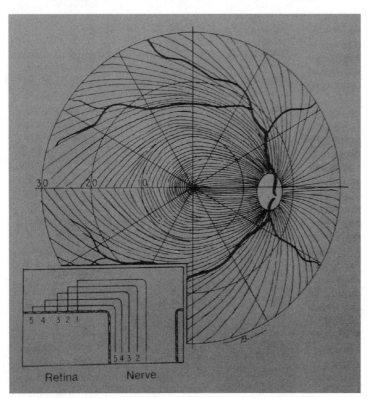

FIGURE 9-2 Distribution of retinal fibers. Note arching above and below the fovea of fibers temporal to the optic nerve head. Inset depicts cross-sectional arrangements of axons, with fibers originating from peripheral retina running closer to the choroid and periphery of the optic nerve, while fibers originating nearer to the nerve head are situated closer to the vitreous and occupy a more central portion of the nerve. [Used with permission from Shields MB: *Textbook of Glaucoma*, 4th ed. Baltimore: Williams & Wilkins, 1998; Fig. 5.5, p 77.]

The retinal nerve fiber layer pattern:

- The retinal nerve fiber layer is arranged in a characteristic pattern which is vital to the understanding of visual field defects in glaucoma (Fig. 9-2). The retinal nerve fibers arise from the ganglion cell layer of the retina and travel to the optic nerve. At the optic nerve head, the nerve fibers bend to leave the globe through a fenestrated canal, the lamina cribrosa, and form the optic nerve. The optic nerve head is also the site of entry of the retinal vessels. The blood supply of the optic nerve head is predominantly from the ciliary circulation.

- The nerve fibers entering the superior and inferior temporal portions of the optic nerve head are the arcuate fibers. They arch above and below the fovea. The fibers from the fovea and the fibers from the nasal

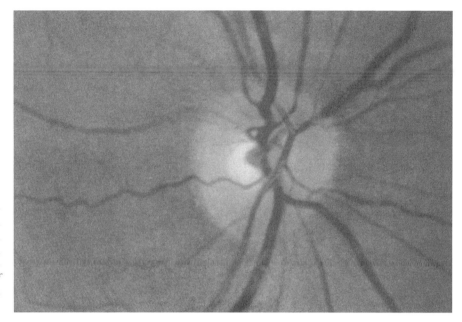

FIGURE 9-3 The morphologic appearance of the normal optic nerve head consists of the central pale depression or cup, which is surrounded by an orange neural rim. [Used with permission from Shields MB: *Color Atlas of Glaucoma*, 4th ed. Baltimore: Williams & Wilkins, 1998; Fig. 110c, pp 20–21.]

retina travel straight without arching to the optic nerve. The arcuate fibers are most susceptible to early glaucomatous damage.[5] Early optic nerve head cupping (i.e., increase in size of the inner white cup relative to the entire optic nerve head) is caused by loss of axonal tissue.[6]

- At birth the optic nerve is largely unmyelinated. Myelination proceeds from the brain to the eye and is complete by 1 month of age, when it stops at the lamina cribrosa. Growth of the optic nerve and disc is largely complete by 1 year of age.

REFERENCES

5. **Dohlman CL, McCormick AQ, Drance SM.** Aging of the optic nerve. *Arch Ophthalmol* 98:2053, 1980.
6. **Quigley HA, Green WR.** The histology of human glaucomatous cupping and optic nerve damage: Clinicopathological correlation in 21 eyes. *Ophthalmology* 86:1803,1979.

CUP-DISC RATIO (CD RATIO)

Optic nerve head:
- When the optic nerve head is visualized through an ophthalmoscope, it is oval and pink in color. The optic nerve head is also called the *disc*. The central portion of the disc is yellow-white and is called the *cup*. The *neural rim* is the tissue between the cup margin and the disc margin. The neural rim consists of axons and is reddish orange in color. The retinal blood vessels exit the cup by crossing the neural rim (Fig. 9-3).

TABLE 9-1   Difference Between a Large Physiological Cup and a Glaucomatous Cup

LARGE PHYSIOLOGICAL CUP	GLAUCOMATOUS CUP
Symmetry in shape and size of the optic nerves between the two eyes.	There may be asymmetry of the CD ratios.
Cup does not change its shape, size and color over time.	Progressive enlargement of the cup and CD ratio occurs due to atrophy of the neural rim tissue.

CD ratio:
- This is the ratio of the horizontal cup radius to the horizontal disc radius. African Americans normally have larger discs and larger CD ratios than Caucasians. High myopes also tend to have larger discs.

Difference between a large physiological cup and a glaucomatous cup:
- It is important to differentiate between a large physiological cup and a glaucomatous cup (Table 9-1).

Changes in the optic nerve in glaucoma are as follows (Fig. 9-4):
- Increase in the cup-disc ratio
- Vertical elongation of the cup
- "Notching" of the neuroretinal rim. This is seen as a focal increase in the cup.
- Deepening of the cup
- Nasalization of the retinal blood vessels
- Optic disc hemorrhage
- As glaucoma advances, the neural rim tissue is lost, eventually leaving a pale disc and a deep cup (Fig. 9-5). This deep cup is sometimes called "bean pot cupping."

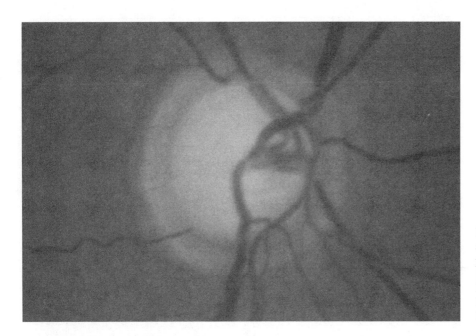

FIGURE 9-4 Glaucomatous optic atrophy: shown here is cupping and pallor with an even peripapillary halo. [Used with permission from Shields MB: *Color Atlas of Glaucoma*, 4th ed. Baltimore: Williams & Wilkins, 1998; Fig. I18a, pp 36–37.]

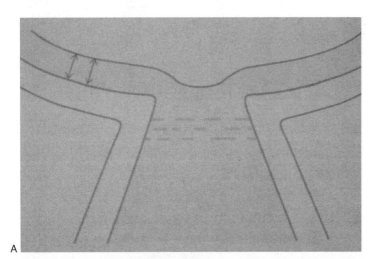

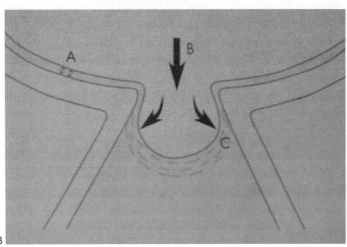

FIGURE 9-5 A. Schematic representation of a normal optic nerve head, with three noteworthy features: the normally thick retinal nerve fiber layer (NFL; arrows), minimal central cup, and orientation of the laminar pores aligned with the curve of the posterior scleral wall. B. Three major alterations of glaucomatous damage are the thinning of the retinal NFL (smaller arrows), posterior excavation and enlargement of the central cup (large black arrow), and outward rotation of the lamina cribrosa with cupping (smaller curved black arrows). [Used with permission from Stamper RL, Lieberman MF, Drake MV: *Becker–Shaffer's Diagnosis and Therapy of the Glaucomas*, 7th ed. St. Louis: CV Mosby, 1999; Fig. 13-4, p 183.]

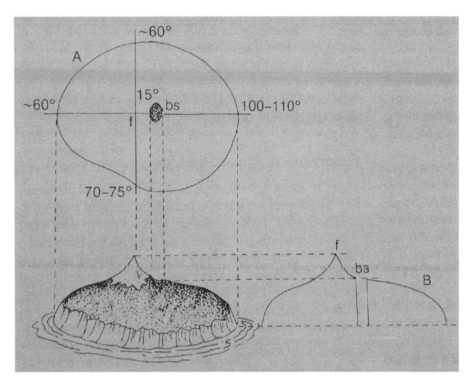

FIGURE 9-6 The normal visual field is depicted as Traquair's "island of vision surrounded by a sea of blindness," with projections showing the peripheral limits (A) and the profile (B). Fixation (f) corresponds to the foveola of the retina, and the blind spot (bs), to the optic nerve head. The approximate dimensions of the absolute peripheral boundary of the location of the blind spot are shown (A). [Used with permission from Shields MB: *Textbook of Glaucoma*, 4th ed. Baltimore: Williams & Wilkins, 1998; Fig. 6.1, p 109.]

VISUAL FIELD

The normal visual field:

- The normal field of vision is described as "an island of vision surrounded by a sea of blindness" (Fig. 9-6). The tallest point in the island corresponds to the fovea (in the macula), which is the area of best visual acuity. The fovea is the point of fixation. The deep pit in the island is the blind spot. This corresponds to the optic nerve head, where there are no photoreceptors and, therefore, no vision. The blind spot is 15° temporal to fixation. Normal peripheral vision extends to about 60° superiorly, 60° nasally, 75° inferiorly and 100–110° temporally (Table 9-2).[7]

Visual fields in glaucoma:

- Optic disc changes precede visual field changes. The appearance of the disc can often be correlated with the visual field changes.
- Nerve fiber layer (NFL) defects also precede and can be correlated with glaucomatous field defects. For example, damage to the temporal nerve fibers that extend from the horizontal raphe and that arch over the fovea to the blind spot can be associated with characteristic arcuate field defects. The nerve fibers from fixation to the blind spot are fairly resistant to increased IOP and are, therefore, damaged later.

Early glaucomatous defects are as follows:

- Generalized depression of the visual field
- Enlargement of the blind spot

TABLE 9-2 The Visual Field

	THE VISUAL FIELD
Superior	60°
Nasal	60°
Inferior	75°
Temporal	100°–110°
Fovea	Point of fixation; best visual acuity
Blind spot	15° temporal to fixation; no vision

- Nerve fiber bundle defects: Nerve fiber bundle defects appear as *scotomas*. The word scotoma is derived from the Greek word "*scoto*," which means darkness. A scotoma (sko-to'mah) is an area of depressed vision in the visual field. There is no perception of light in an *absolute scotoma*, and the perception of light is diminished in a r*elative scotoma*.
  - Paracentral scotoma—a localized defect developing around the point of fixation (Fig. 9-7).
  - Seidel scotoma—a visual field defect that is nasal to and connects with the blind spot (Fig. 9-8).
  - Bjerrum scotoma (beeyer'um)—an arcuate scotoma extending from the blind spot to the horizontal raphe (Fig. 9-9).
  - Double arcuate scotoma—arcuate scotomas are present in both the superior and inferior visual fields (Fig. 9-10).
  - Ronne's nasal step—A step-like defect is created when there is damage to either the superior or inferior nerve fiber layer that meets the horizontal raphe.

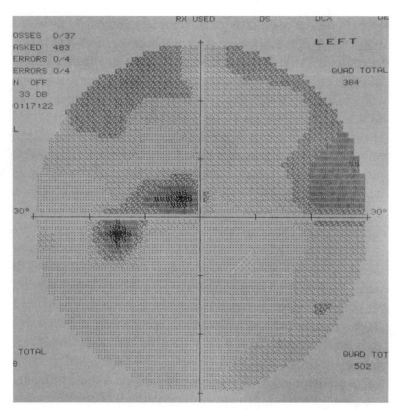

FIGURE 9-7 Computerized perimetry (*bottom*) depicts the paracentral scotoma and nasal step that are demonstrated by Goldmann perimetry. [Used with permission from Stamper RL, Lieberman MF, Drake MV: *Becker–Shaffer's Diagnosis and Therapy of the Glaucomas*, 7th ed. St. Louis: CV Mosby, 1999; Fig. 11-14, p 156.]

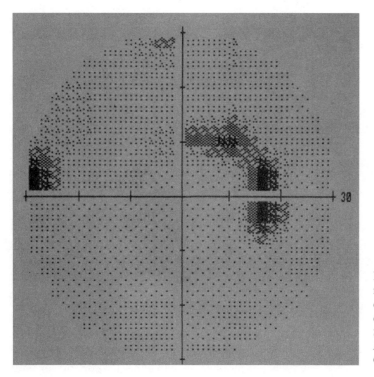

FIGURE 9-8 Chart from the right eye of a patient with normal-tension glaucoma showing a Seidel scotoma extending from the blind spot. There is also a small peripheral superior nasal step defect. [Used with permission from Stamper RL, Lieberman MF, Drake MV: *Becker–Shaffer's Diagnosis and Therapy of the Glaucomas*, 7th ed. St. Louis: CV Mosby, 1999; Fig. 11-9, p 151.]

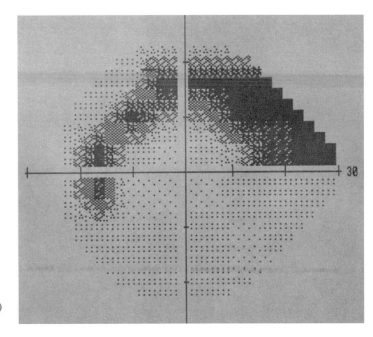

FIGURE 9-9 Superior arcuate scotoma (Bjerrum scotoma) as seen with the Humphrey field analyzer.

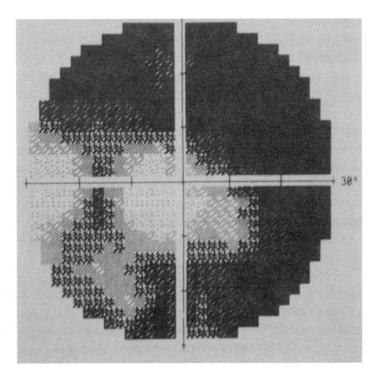

FIGURE 9-10 The superior field (*left eye*) exhibits similar but more advanced loss compared with the inferior field. If the disease is unchecked, both fields will continue to progress. [Used with permission from Stamper RL, Lieberman MF, Drake MV: *Becker–Shaffer's Diagnosis and Therapy of the Glaucomas*, 7th ed. St. Louis: CV Mosby, 1999; Fig. 11-13, p 153.]

For example, when the lower fibers are involved, a superior nasal step is formed (Fig. 9-11).

Late glaucomatous defects are as follows:

• Temporal sector defects occur because of damage to the nasal retinal nerve fibers that traverse a straighter course to the optic nerve.

• Either a small temporal island or a central island of vision can be left in end-stage glaucoma. The patient's central visual acuity may not be affected even when the visual field is limited to a central island of 5°. In some cases, the temporal peripheral vision may remain long after the central vision is lost (Fig. 9-12).

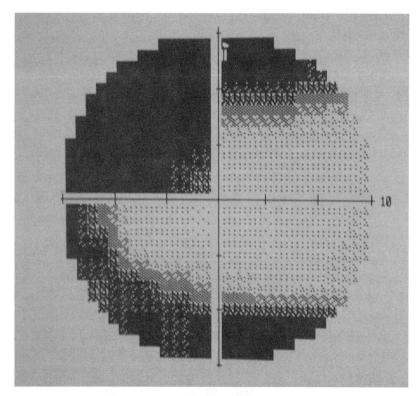

FIGURE 9-11 Central 10° field from the right eye of a patient with advanced glaucoma. The nasal horizontal step (*left side in this figure*) runs all the way to fixation. [Used with permission from Stamper RL, Lieberman MF, Drake MV: *Becker–Shaffer's Diagnosis and Therapy of the Glaucomas*, 7th ed. St. Louis: CV Mosby, 1999; Fig. 11-15, p 148.]

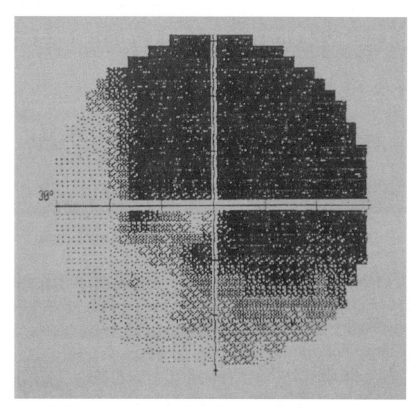

FIGURE 9-12 Central island of a patient's left eye with field defects encroaching on fixation. The temporal field is partially spared. [Used with permission from Stamper RL, Lieberman MF, Drake MV: *Becker–Shaffer's Diagnosis and Therapy of the Glaucomas*, 7th ed. St. Louis: CV Mosby, 1999; Fig. 11-12, p 153.]

- Visual field loss associated with glaucoma is generally irreversible. Minimal improvement in central visual acuity and field of vision may possibly occur if IOP is reduced in the early stages of the disease.

REFERENCES

7. **Harrington DO.** The visual fields. *A Textbook and Atlas of Clinical Perimetry*, 5th ed. St. Louis: CV Mosby, 1981.
8. **Stamper RL, Lieberman MF, Drake MV.** *Becker-Shaffer's Diagnosis and Therapy of the Glaucomas, 7th ed.* St. Louis: CV Mosby, 1999.
9. **Shields MB.** *Textbook of Glaucoma. 4th ed.* Baltimore: Williams and Wilkins, 1998.

THEORIES OF OPTIC NERVE DAMAGE

There are many theories of optic nerve damage:
- Intraocular pressure: IOP is classically associated with glaucomatous optic nerve damage through many mechanisms.
- Vascular theory: Glaucomatous optic atrophy may be secondary to ischemia. Ischemia may be due to either an elevated IOP or an unrelated vascular abnormality.[10]
- Mechanical theory: This theory suggests that there may be direct compression of the optic nerve fibers against the lamina cribrosa. This causes nerve death possibly due to interruption of axoplasmic flow.

- Apoptosis theory: Apoptosis may be an important reason for ganglion cell death. Apoptosis is a genetically programmed death of retinal ganglion cells due to loss of neurotropic signals.[11] It is unclear why glaucoma patients experience apoptosis.
- Neurotoxic theory: Higher levels of glutamate, a neurotoxin, are seen in glaucomatous eyes.[12]
- Other theories: Quigley suggests other mechanisms of glaucomatous nerve damage such as greater susceptibility to damage of glaucomatous ganglion cells or even different connective tissue structure within the optic nerve head.[13]

REFERENCES

10. **Duke Elder S.** Fundamental Concepts of Glaucoma. *Arch Ophthalmol* 42:538,1949.
11. **Glovinsky Y, Quigley HA, et al.** Retinal ganglion cell loss is size dependent in experimental glaucoma. *Invest Ophthalmol Vis Sci* 32:484,1991.
12. **Dreyer EB, Zurakowski D, Schumer RA, et al.** Elevated glautamate levels in the vitreous body of humans and monkeys with glaucoma. *Arch Ophthalmol* 114:299,1996.
13. **Quigley H.** Mechanisms of glaucomatous optic neuropathy. In: Van Buskirk EM, Shields MB, eds: *100 Years of Progress in Glaucoma*. Philadelphia: Lippincott-Raven, 1997.

CLASSIFICATION OF GLAUCOMAS

Glaucoma is divided into primary and secondary glaucomas (Table 9-3).

TABLE 9-3 Classification of Glaucoma, Its Subtypes, and Its Effects

CLASSIFICATION	SUBTYPES	DESCRIPTION
Primary	Primary open-angle glaucoma (POAG)	Increased IOP, optic nerve damage, and visual field loss; cause of trabecular meshwork obstruction unknown.
	Normal tension glaucoma (NTG)	Normal IOP, optic nerve damage, and visual field loss; cause of trabecular meshwork obstruction unknown.
	Primary angle-closure glaucoma (PACG)	Increased IOP, optic nerve damage, and visual field loss; anatomic narrowing of the angle causing obstruction of fluid egress through the trabecular meshwork.
Secondary	Pigment dispersion Pseudoexfoliation Lens-induced Steroid-induced Posttraumatic Postoperative Uveitis Neovascular Intraocular tumor Increased episcleral venous pressure	Increased IOP, optic nerve damage, and visual field loss; trabecular meshwork outflow obstruction due to another ocular or systemic condition.
Congenital	Infantile or primary congenital glaucoma Glaucoma associated with other ocular anomalies Glaucoma associated with other systemic disorders Secondary glaucomas in infants	Increased IOP, optic nerve damage, visual field loss. (e.g., aniridia, anterior segment dysgenesis, etc.) (e.g., Lowe's syndrome, rubella, etc.) (e.g., retinoblastoma, trauma, etc.)

EXAMINATION

Examination of anterior chamber depth using a flashlight:

- An acute angle-closure glaucoma (AACG) attack occurs in a patient with an anatomically shallow AC. A shallow AC can be detected by directing a flashlight from the temporal side of the eye but parallel to the iris. When the AC is of normal depth, the iris does not cast a shadow and the AC is uniformly illuminated on both the temporal and the nasal sides. When the AC is shallow, the iris is bowed forward toward the examiner. Therefore, when the flashlight is shown from the temporal side, it casts a shadow on the nasal side (Fig. 9-13).[14]
- In patients with a shallow AC, pharmacologic pupil dilation, which is routinely done by ophthalmologists to examine the retina, can trigger an acute angle closure attack of glaucoma. A prophylactic laser iridotomy

can prevent an attack of AACG in patients with shallow ACs.

REFERENCE

14. **Vaigas E, Drance SM.** Anterior chamber depth in angle closure glaucoma. Clinical methods of depth determination in people with and without the disease. *Arch Ophthalmol* 90:438,1973.

INTRAOCULAR PRESSURE

- Intraocular pressure (IOP) is measured by tonometry (*tono* = tone, tension). Tonometry works on the principle of measuring the resistance of the eye to an externally applied force (Tension = Force/Area).

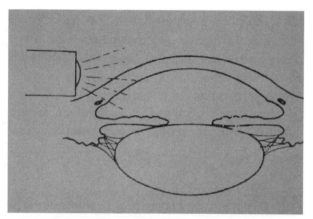
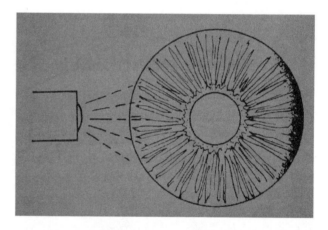
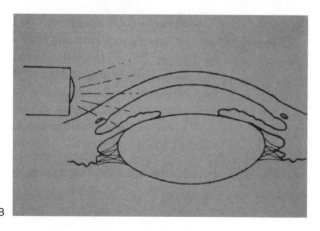
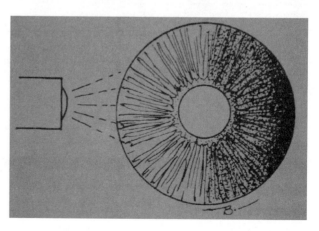

FIGURE 9-13 Oblique flashlight illumination as a screening measure for estimating the anterior chamber depth. A. With a deep chamber, nearly the entire iris is illuminated. B. When the iris is bowed forward, only the proximal portion is illuminated, and a shadow is seen in the distal half. [Used with permission from Shields MB: *Textbook of Glaucoma*, 4th ed. Baltimore: Williams & Wilkins, 1998; Fig. 10.3, p 180.]

The applied force could be two fingers over the eyelids (digital tonometry) or the tips of one of the sophisticated instruments used for measuring IOP. The instruments that measure the IOP are called *tonometers*.

• Tonometers measure the IOP by either flattening the cornea (applanation tonometry) or deforming it (indentation tonometry). The amount of distortion by the tonometer is measured on a calibrated scale which gives the IOP in mm Hg. Most of these instruments need contact with the cornea, whereas some do not.

• Indentation tonometers include the Schiotz tonometer. Applanation tonometers include the Goldmann tonometer, the Perkins tonometer, and the Tonopen. They all require contact with the cornea. An air-puff noncontact tonometer does not require contact with the cornea.

• Various tonometers used clinically are described in Table 9-4.

TABLE 9-4 Tonometers

TONOMETER	DESCRIPTION
Goldmann Applanation (Fig. 9-14)	International standard for measuring IOP. Most accurate and preferred method for regular corneas. Measures the amount of force required to flatten the central cornea. Used with a standard slit lamp.
Schiotz (Figs. 9-15 and 9-16)	Alternative method of measuring the IOP. Used in the clinic, in the emergency department, and at the hospital bedside. Easily used by the primary care physician. Inexpensive, easily available, and portable. Unreliable when the ocular rigidity is altered.
Perkins Applanation (Fig. 9-17)	Hand-held applanation tonometer. Closely resembles the Goldmann applanation tonometer. Portable and can be used in any position. Used for examinations of infants and children, for examinations under anesthesia, and for examinations of patients who cannot sit at the slit lamp. More accurate when the cornea is regular.
Tonopen (Fig. 9-18)	Works on the Mackay-Marg principle. Hand-held electronic applanation tonometer. Useful for scarred or irregular corneas. Has a strain gauge that creates an electrical signal as the footplate flattens the cornea.
Pneumotonometer (Fig. 9-19)	Works on the Mackay-Marg principle. Useful for scarred and irregular corneas.
Air-puff noncontact	Works on the principle of applanation. Cornea is applanated by a puff of room air, which deforms the cornea. No direct contact with the cornea. No need for topical anesthetic. Not as accurate as other methods but may be easier to use.
Digital	IOP can be grossly estimated by palpation of the eyeball with two fingers. When IOP is low, the eye is soft and the palpating fingers feel less resistance. When IOP is high, the eyeball is hard and there is more resistance felt by the palpating fingers. Subject to large errors.

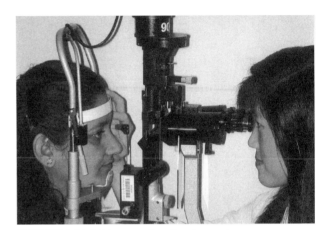

FIGURE 9-14 Goldman applanation tonometry.

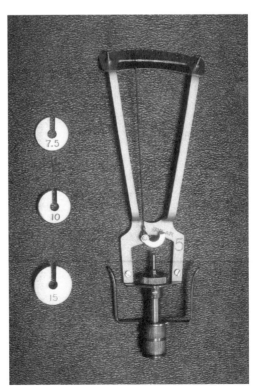

FIGURE 9-15 Schiotz tonometer.

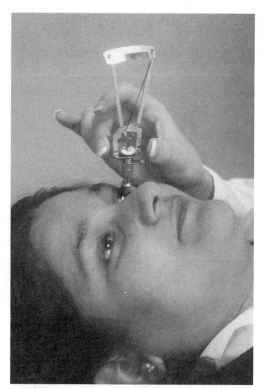

FIGURE 9-16 Schiotz tonometry.

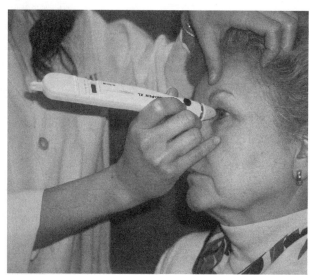

FIGURE 9-18 Tonopen.

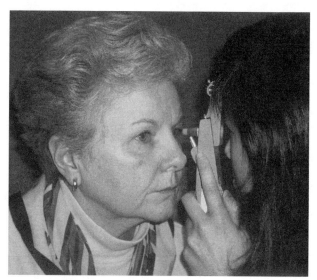

FIGURE 9-17 Perkins tonometry.

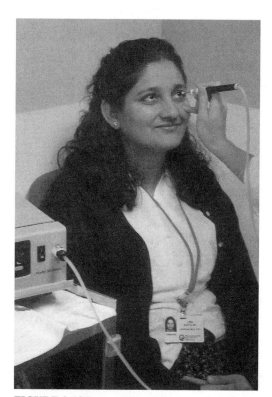

FIGURE 9-19 Pneumotonometry.

VISUAL FIELDS

- Instruments that measure visual fields are called *perimeters*. Perimeters mark the peripheral limits of the visual field.
- Perimeters consist of a background screen and a light target point. The background is usually shaped like a bowl, as in the Goldmann or Humphrey perimeter. The target can vary in size, color, and illumination. The targets can be controlled either manually or automatically.
- There are two ways in which the targets are presented: kinetic (moving) or static (stationary) (Fig. 9-20).
- **Kinetic.** As the patient fixates on a point, targets of varying size and illumination are moved from the peripheral nonseeing area to the central seeing area. A specific visual field, or *isopter*, is mapped for each

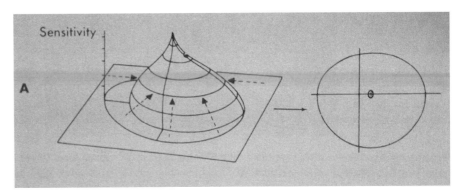

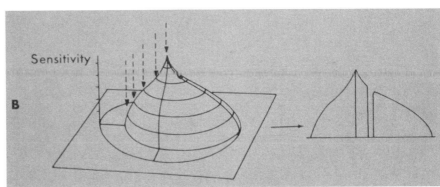

FIGURE 9-20 A. Kinetic perimetry: Test object of fixed intensity is moved along several meridians toward fixation. Points where the object is first perceived are plotted in a circle. B. Static perimetry: Stationary test object is increased in intensity from below threshold until perceived by the patient. Threshold values yield a graphic profile section. [Used with permission from Stamper RL, Lieberman MF, Drake MV: *Becker–Shaffer's Diagnosis and Therapy of the Glaucomas*, 7th ed. St. Louis: CV Mosby, 1999; Fig. 9-1, p 120.]

specific target size or illumination. Many different isopters using different targets are mapped for a single Goldmann visual field test. The Goldmann perimeter has a kinetic target (Fig. 9-21).
- **Static.** As the patient fixates on a point, stationary targets of a specific size but varying light intensity are presented. The light intensity at which the target is spotted 50% of the time is called the *threshold*. Static targets are usually used for automated perimetry. Humphrey automated perimetry (static perimetry) gives computer printouts of the visual field.
- There are various ways to measure the visual fields (Table 9-5).

TABLE 9-5   Various Ways of Visual Field Testing

PERIMETRY	DESCRIPTION
Confrontation visual field (Fig. 9-22)	Simple way of assessing the visual field. Gross defects may be detected. No equipment is required. Assuming the examiner's visual field is normal, the examiner can compare his or her visual field with that of the patient. The examiner can test the patient's right eye by covering his right eye with his right hand. The patient then covers his left eye with his left hand. The examiner can use his or her finger as a target by moving his finger into his own visual field and making sure that the patient first sees the finger at the same time.

TABLE 9-5   (continued)

PERIMETRY	DESCRIPTION
Amsler grid	Measures the central 10° field of vision. Square with sides measuring 10 cm, further divided into smaller squares of 0.5 cm each. Excellent tool for assessing perimacular function. The macula is the area of the retina giving the sharpest, central vision. Missing lines indicate scotomas.
Tangent screen	Measures the central 30° of the visual field. Square black screen mounted on the wall with each side measuring 1 meter. White ball target is mounted at the end of a black pointer.
Goldmann perimeter (Fig. 9-21)	Prototype of the bowl perimeter. Primarily used for kinetic perimetry. Perimeter bowl has a radius of 300 mm. Test object can be changed in size and light intensity. Next best method of evaluating visual fields when the patient is unable to do Humphrey perimetry.
Humphrey perimeter (Fig. 9-23)	Sophisticated automated perimeter. Considered by many to be the gold standard for measuring visual fields in glaucoma. Most sensitive in detecting minute defects in the visual field. Programmable and easily reproducible. Most commonly used automated perimeter.

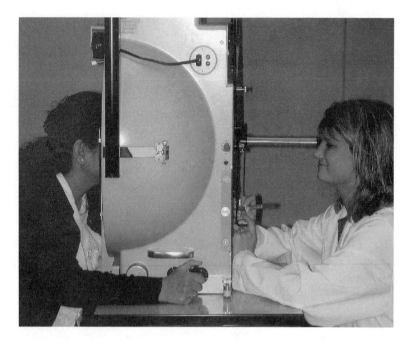

FIGURE 9-21 Goldmann perimetry.

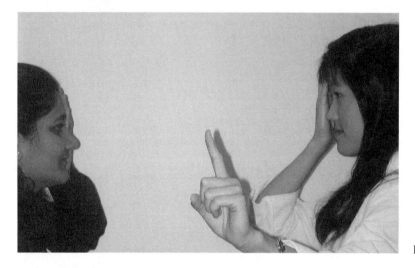

FIGURE 9-22 Confrontation visual field.

GONIOSCOPY

- Gonioscopy is the visualization of structures of the angle of the anterior chamber. Gonioscopy is important in the diagnosis, classification, and management of glaucoma. Special lenses are needed for gonioscopy (Fig. 9-24).
- The structures of the normal angle from posterior to anterior are as follows: ciliary body band, scleral spur, trabecular meshwork, and Schwalbe's line (Fig. 9-25).
- The angle between the iris and the cornea in patients with a deep AC and wide angles is between 20° and 45°. The angle in patients with a shallow AC and narrow angles is generally less than 20°. The ophthalmologist determines whether an angle is open or narrow by gonioscopy (Fig. 9-26).

WHEN TO REFER THE PATIENT

- When glaucoma is suspected, and the following factors are present, the patient should always be referred to an ophthalmologist. This may help in early detection of the disease and ensure proper treatment.

There is a family history of glaucoma

The patient is more than 50 years of age

There is a history of eye trauma

The IOP is more than 22 mm Hg

There is an IOP difference of more than 5 mm Hg between the two eyes

The cup-disc ratio is greater than 0.5

There is significant disc asymmetry

The patient has narrow angles

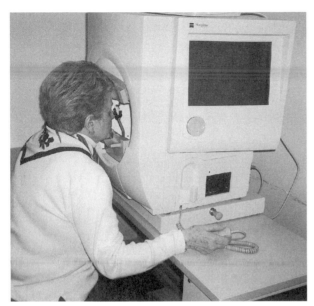

FIGURE 9-23 Humphrey automated perimetry.

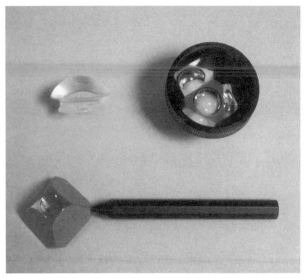

FIGURE 9-24 Gonioscopic contact lenses (clockwise from top left: Koeppe, three-mirror Goldmann, and hand-held Zeiss.)

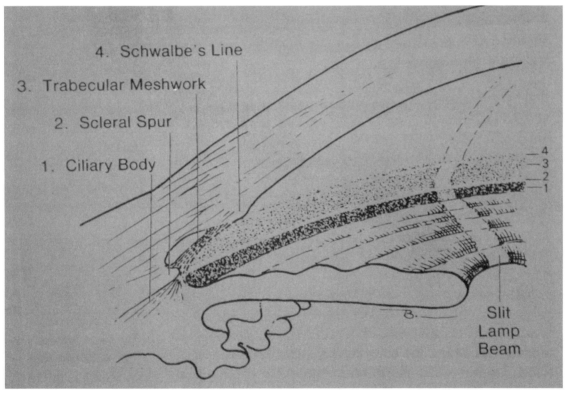

FIGURE 9-25 Normal adult anterior chamber angle showing gonioscopic appearance (*right*) and cross-section of corresponding structures (*left*): 1. Ciliary body band; 2. Scleral spur; 3. Trabecular meshwork; 4. Schwalbe's line. [Used with permission from Shields MB: *Textbook of Glaucoma*, 4th ed. Baltimore: Williams & Wilkins, 1998; Fig. 3.10, p 38.]

The patient presents with signs of acute angle-closure glaucoma (see Primary Angle-Closure Glaucoma section).

An infant has corneal diameters greater than 10 mm or has significant corneal clouding.

SCREENING

Rationale:

- Blindness from glaucoma can be prevented if it is detected early.

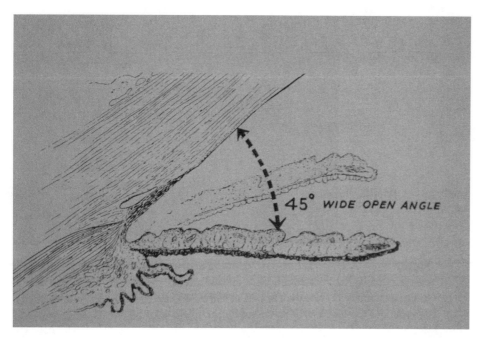

FIGURE 9-26 Narrow angles, 0° to 20°. Wide open angles, 20° to 45°. [Used with permission from Stamper RL, Lieberman MF, Drake MV: *Becker–Shaffer's Diagnosis and Therapy of the Glaucomas*, 7th ed. St. Louis: CV Mosby, 1999; Fig. 7-2, p 93.]

Benefits:

- Half of all patients with glaucoma do not know that they have the disease and therefore receive no treatment.[1] Early diagnosis and management can prevent considerable permanent nerve damage and visual field loss. In general, once vision is lost from glaucoma, it is permanent.

Guidelines:

- Early detection of glaucoma depends on the primary care physician knowing when to refer. A diagnosis of glaucoma must be made by an ophthalmologist.
- Careful history taking, careful examination, and proper referral can lead to early diagnosis.
- Educating the public about glaucoma and the need for early detection is also essential.

GLAUCOMA SUBTYPES AND CLINICAL PRESENTATIONS

PRIMARY OPEN-ANGLE GLAUCOMA

CASE 1

A 65-year-old white man came in for an eye examination. He did not have any specific complaints. He uses only over-the-counter reading glasses and had never visited an ophthalmologist in the past. Visual acuity was 20/40 OU with correction. The anterior segment of both eyes was normal with the exception of very early cataractous changes OU. The IOP was 24 mm Hg OU. Ophthalmoscopy showed a CD ratio of 0.8 OU. Gonioscopy showed open angles. Humphrey visual field testing revealed an inferior nasal step OD and a superior arcuate scotoma OS.

INTRODUCTION AND DEFINITION

- Open-angle glaucoma is the most common form of glaucoma. [*Synonyms*: open-angle glaucoma, chronic open-angle glaucoma (COAG), primary open-angle glaucoma (POAG), idiopathic open-angle glaucoma.] The IOP is usually more than 21 mm Hg, the AC angle is open, and there is characteristic optic nerve head damage and visual field loss. There is no secondary ocular or systemic abnormality that might account for the elevated IOP.

PATHOPHYSIOLOGY

- The increased IOP in open-angle glaucoma is due to a decrease in outflow of aqueous humor. The obstruction is usually located at the level of the trabecular meshwork and the endothelium of Schlemm's canal (Fig. 9-27).

EPIDEMIOLOGY AND GENETICS

- POAG is the predominant form of glaucoma in the United States.
- 2.25 million Americans over 40 years of age are estimated to have POAG.[15] The incidence of POAG in the

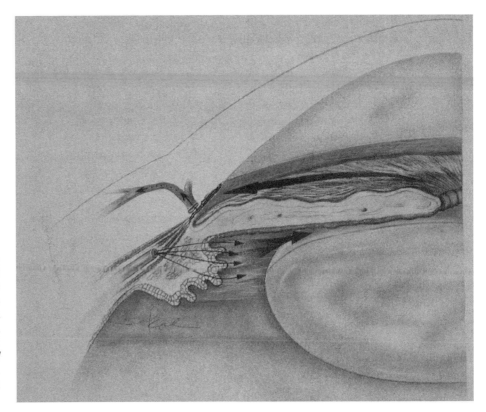

FIGURE 9-27 In open-angle glaucoma, there is impaired flow of aqueous humor through the trabecular meshwork–Schlemm's canal–venous system. [Used with permission from Stamper RL, Lieberman MF, Drake MV: *Becker–Shaffer's Diagnosis and Therapy of the Glaucomas*, 7th ed. St. Louis: CV Mosby, 1999; Fig. 1-3, p 5.]

U.S.A. is 20 per 100,000 persons over age 50, and around 200 per 100,000 over age 80.[3]

- POAG occurs at an earlier age and is more severe in African Americans. The incidence and prevalence of blindness in glaucoma is 8 to 10 times higher among African Americans than among Caucasians in the U.S.A.[16]
- POAG has a multifactorial inheritance pattern.

RISK FACTORS

- See Table 9-6 for POAG risk factors and descriptive commentary.

CLINICAL SYMPTOMS

- POAG is a bilateral disease with a very chronic course. There are usually no symptoms until the patient develops advanced visual field loss. This is why screening is so important in POAG.

SIGNS

- IOP may be increased to above 21 mm Hg. Visual field defects may be documented, and ophthalmoscopy may show typical optic nerve head cupping. Angles are open on gonioscopy.

DIFFERENTIAL DIAGNOSIS

- *Ocular hypertension.* The IOP pressure is more than 21 mm Hg but the optic nerve and visual fields are normal. There is no associated ocular or systemic disease. These patients are at increased risk of developing glaucoma and must be monitored periodically.
- *Normal tension glaucoma.* The IOP is normal, but optic nerve head cupping and visual field loss are present (see Normal Tension Glaucoma).
- Secondary glaucomas.
- Congenital optic nerve defects.
- Optic atrophy from other diseases besides glaucoma.

COURSE AND PROGNOSIS

- Once field loss starts, damage can occur at a lower IOP. Lowering the IOP may either slow the progress of the disease or may arrest it.

WHEN TO TREAT

- When elevated IOP is associated with cupping and field defects
- When there is progressive cupping without field loss
- When there is progressive field loss without cupping
- When there are episodes of acute elevations of IOP

TABLE 9-6   Risk Factors for Primary Open-Angle Glaucoma (POAG)

RISK FACTOR	DESCRIPTION
Increased IOP	Degree of glaucomatous damage may be related to the level of IOP.
Increasing age	Prevalence of POAG increases with age.
Race	POAG occurs at an earlier age in African Americans. POAG is more severe in African Americans. Incidence and prevalence of blindness in glaucoma is 8 to 10 times higher among African Americans than among Caucasians in the U.S.
Family history	Multifactorial inheritance pattern.
Myopia	Increased prevalence of POAG is seen in high myopes. Increased frequency of myopia is seen in patients with POAG.
Diabetes	Prevalence of POAG is higher in the diabetic population.[17]
Steroid sensitivity	Increased response to corticosteroids may be inherited in a similar manner as POAG.[18]

ORDER OF TREATMENT

- The following are aimed at lowering IOP:
  1. *Medical treatment.* The patient is usually treated first with one topical medication. Others are added as needed.
  2. *Laser treatment.* Laser trabeculoplasty is usually done when medical treatment fails.
  3. *Filtration surgery.* When laser treatment fails, filtering surgery or trabeculectomy may be done.
  4. *Tube-shunt surgery.* Tube surgery is done when either previous trabeculectomies have failed or the patient is at high risk for trabeculectomy failure.
  5. *Transscleral cyclophotocoagulation.* This is done as a last resort and only in eyes with poor visual prognosis. It destroys parts of the ciliary body in order to decrease aqueous production.

REFERENCES

15. **Wilson RS.** *Epidemiology of glaucoma.* In: Epstein DL, Allingham RR, Schuman JS, eds. *Chandler and Grant's Glaucoma,* 4th ed., Baltimore: Williams and Wilkins, 1997.
16. **Tielsch JM, Sommer A, Katz J, Quigley HA, et al.** Racial variations in the prevalence of POAG. The Baltimore eye survey. *JAMA* 1991;266:369–374.
17. **Becker B.** Diabetes mellitus and glaucoma. *Am J Ophthalmol* 1971;71:1.
18. **Armaly MF.** Inheritance of dexamethasone; Hypertension and glaucoma. *Arch Ophthalmol* 1967;7:747.

NORMAL TENSION GLAUCOMA

DEFINITION

- In normal tension glaucoma (NTG) (*Synonym:* low tension glaucoma), the IOP is always less than 22 mm Hg, but glaucomatous optic nerve cupping and visual field defects are present. The angles are open and appear normal.

PATHOPHYSIOLOGY

- Many factors may be responsible for the development of normal tension glaucoma; however, the exact cause is unknown. Abnormalities of optic nerve head perfusion may increase susceptibility to optic nerve damage.[19] Some studies suggest increased viscosity and hypercoagulability of blood. IOP is at the upper range of normal. Diurnal variations and postural changes in the IOP may be responsible.

GENETICS

- Normal tension glaucoma may have a genetic basis.

CLINICAL FEATURES

- The clinical features are similar to that of POAG, but the IOP is less than 22 mm Hg. Patients are typically older than 60 years of age. Many studies have shown that women are affected more than men; however, other studies, including the Beaver Dam Eye Study, have shown equal prevalence in both sexes. There is an increased incidence in the Asian population. Since normal tension glaucoma is primarily diagnosed on the basis of cupping, it is often diagnosed late.

DIFFERENTIAL DIAGNOSIS

- Physiologic cupping
- Previous glaucomatous damage (e.g., from steroids, uveitis, trauma, etc.)
- Optic atrophy from other causes (e.g., tumors, sarcoid, syphilis, ischemic optic neuropathy, drugs, retinal or degenerative diseases, etc.)
- Optic nerve abnormalities (e.g., colobomas, optic nerve pits, myopic discs, etc.)
- Optic nerve drusen

WORK-UP

- In NTG, history taking is very important. Any history of corticosteroid use, trauma, inflammation or of any hemodynamic crisis, such as blood loss, anemia, hypotension, or arrhythmia, should be elicited. A diurnal curve, which entails hourly measurements of the IOP throughout the day, may reveal IOP elevations above 21 mm Hg. Pressures higher than 22 mm Hg would suggest primary open-angle glaucoma instead of normal tension glaucoma. A complete cardiovascular system examination including carotid artery auscultation should be performed.

TREATMENT

- The aim is to lower the IOP. Medications, argon laser trabeculoplasty, or surgery does this.
- The most important aspect of managing the patient with low tension glaucoma may be treatment of any cardiovascular abnormalities, gastrointestinal tract lesions, congestive heart failure, arrhythmias, transient ischemic attacks, anemias, etc. This ensures maximum perfusion of the optic nerve head.[20]

REFERENCES

19. **Miller KM, Quigley HA.** Comparison of optic disc features in low tension and typical open angle glaucoma. *Arch Ophthalmol* 110:211,1992.
20. **Chumbley LC, Brubaker RF.** Low tension glaucoma. *Am J Ophthalmol* 81:761,1976.

PRIMARY ANGLE-CLOSURE GLAUCOMA

CASE 2

A 56-year-old woman presented to the emergency department (ED) with sudden loss of vision OD, intense eye pain, headache, abdominal pain, and vomiting. There was no history of any eye problems except for glasses for hyperopia. The visual acuity was counting fingers 1 feet OD and 20/20 OS. The right eye showed circumcorneal injection, diffuse corneal haze, shallow anterior chamber, and a mid-dilated, fixed pupil. The lens was clear. The left eye was normal except for a shallow AC. The IOP was 46 mm Hg OD and 14 mm Hg OS. Fundus examination and gonioscopy OD were not possible because of the corneal haze. Examination of the OS revealed a normal CD ratio of 0.2, and gonioscopy OS revealed a narrow angle.

DEFINITION

- Primary angle-closure glaucoma (PACG) is a condition in which the peripheral iris opposes the trabecular meshwork and obstructs aqueous outflow (Fig. 9-28). Angle-closure glaucoma may be primary or secondary. Primary angle-closure glaucoma is not associated with any other ocular or systemic abnormalities.

PATHOPHYSIOLOGY

- The patient at risk is usually an older person with hyperopia with a shallow AC. There may be a family history of glaucoma.
- An angle-closure attack may be precipitated by pupillary dilation. Factors that cause mydriasis include dim illumination, emotional stress, a prone position, evening hours, and certain medications.

With pupillary block:
- Pupillary block occurs when aqueous cannot flow normally from the posterior chamber, through the pupil, to the AC. There is a functional block at the level of the pupil. This is usually associated with a mid-dilated pupil. Since the aqueous cannot drain into the AC angle, fluid accumulates in the posterior chamber and then causes forward bowing of the peripheral iris, which mechanically closes the angle of the AC.

EPIDEMIOLOGY

- In the United States, angle-closure glaucoma is less common than open-angle glaucoma.
- Primary angle-closure glaucoma (PACG) is the more common type of glaucoma in Asian populations.

RISK FACTORS

- See Table 9-7 for PACG risk factors and descriptive commentary.

STAGES OF PACG

PRODROMAL OR SUBACUTE ATTACK The symptoms are mild. There may be a dull eye ache, slight blurring of vision, and colored halos around lights. The patient may have several such attacks before having an acute attack of angle closure.

ACUTE-ANGLE CLOSURE GLAUCOMA (AACG) The classic scenario is a patient presenting with pain in the eye, corneal edema, and loss of vision. There can be halos around lights, marked ciliary congestion,

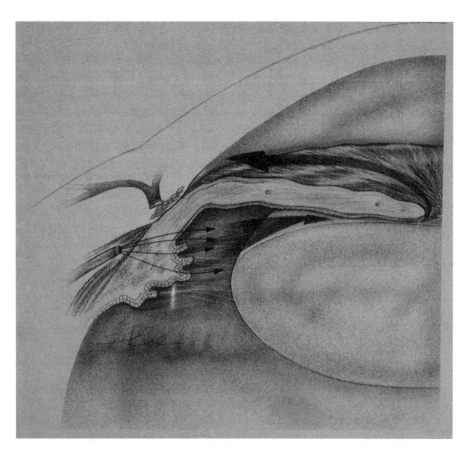

FIGURE 9-28 In angle-closure glaucoma, the peripheral iris covers the trabecular meshwork, obstructing aqueous humor outflow. [Used with permission from Stamper RL, Lieberman MF, Drake MV: *Becker–Shaffer's Diagnosis and Therapy of the Glaucomas*, 7th ed. St. Louis: CV Mosby, 1999; Fig. 1-2, p 5.]

TABLE 9-7   Risk factors for Primary Angle Closure Glaucoma (PACG)

RISK FACTOR	DESCRIPTION
Age	Peak age is 55 to 60 years. The anterior chamber decreases in depth with age due to thickening of the lens.
Sex	Women are 2 to 3 times more susceptible.
Race	Less common among African Americans, higher prevalence in Eskimos and Asians.
Refractive error	More common in hyperopes. They have shallow anterior chambers.
Family history	Potential for angle closure may be inherited.

and a fixed mid-dilated pupil. The patient may have headache, nausea, vomiting, sweating, and bradycardia. This may mimic symptoms of acute abdomen. The IOP is around 40–80 mm Hg.

CHRONIC ANGLE CLOSURE The patient has more episodes of subacute or acute angle-closure glaucoma. There is formation of peripheral anterior synechiae, or scarring of the angle, which leads to chronically elevated IOP.[21]

CLINICAL FEATURES—OCULAR AND SYSTEMIC FINDINGS

- The signs of acute angle-closure glaucoma are increased IOP (40–80 mm Hg), ciliary congestion, cloudy cornea due to corneal edema, shallow AC, a mid-dilated pupil which does not react to light, and profound decrease in vision (Fig. 9-29).

DIFFERENTIAL DIAGNOSIS

- See Table 9-8.

TREATMENT

An acute angle-closure attack of glaucoma is an ophthalmic emergency. If the acute attack is not treated immediately, there may be irreversible angle closure.

IMMEDIATE REFERRAL FOR DEFINITIVE TREATMENT. The acute attack should be managed as follows:
- Reduce the IOP: The IOP is reduced by topical beta-blockers, oral or topical carbonic anhydrase inhibitors, and alpha$_2$ adrenergic agonists. Hyperosmotics may be needed. Miotics are not effective initially, as high IOP causes pupillary sphincter muscle ischemia.

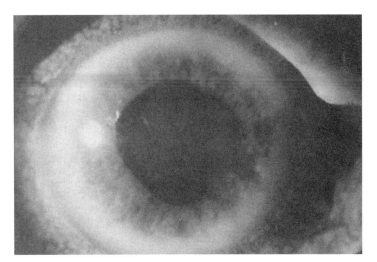

FIGURE 9-29 Acute angle-closure glaucoma: intense conjunctival injection, corneal edema, shallow anterior chamber, and mid-dilated pupil. [Used with permission from Ritch R, Shields MB, Krupin T: *The Glaucomas*, 2nd ed. St. Louis: CV Mosby, 1996; Fig. 38-2, p 824.]

TABLE 9-8   Difference Between Conjunctivitis, Iridocyclitis, and Acute Angle-Closure Glaucoma (AACG)

FACTOR	ACUTE CONJUNCTIVITIS	ACUTE IRIDOCYCLITIS	ACUTE ANGLE-CLOSURE GLAUCOMA
Incidence	Common	Uncommon	Uncommon
Discharge	Copious	None	None
Congestion	Conjunctival congestion	Perilimbal injection	Perilimbal injection
Cornea	Clear	Usually clear	Cloudy
Anterior chamber	Normal	Marked flare and cells Keratic precipitates (KP)	Few flare and cells
Pupil size and shape	Normal	Usually small	Mid-dilated
Pupillary reaction	Normal	May be poor	Not reacting to light
Pain	Little or no pain; discomfort present	Moderately severe	Severe
Photophobia	+/−	Severe	+/−
Visual loss	None	Slight	Severe
IOP	Normal	Normal/low/high	Very high
Systemic symptoms	None	+/−	Nausea, vomiting, sweating, bradycardia
Smear	Causative organism	None	None

- Relieve the angle closure by constricting the pupil. After the IOP is reduced, a miotic can be used to break the peripheral anterior synechiae and break the pupillary block. Pilocarpine 1% is used.
- Reduce the inflammation: A topical steroid may be used to reduce inflammation.
- Pain relief: Systemic analgesics may be needed to relieve the pain.
- Laser peripheral iridotomy: Definitive treatment includes laser iridotomy. If iridotomy does not sufficiently lower the IOP, filtering surgery may be needed.

PROPHYLACTIC LASER PERIPHERAL IRIDOTOMY of the contralateral eye is always done. This will prevent an acute attack of angle-closure glaucoma.

PLATEAU IRIS

- This is a special subtype of narrow angle glaucoma. In plateau iris, the iris is flat in the center but takes a sharp turn posteriorly in the mid-periphery. This creates a narrow angle in the periphery. The AC depth is normal in the center but shallow in the periphery.
- These patients present with angle-closure glaucoma at a younger age (30 to 50 years), there is female predominance, and there may be a family history of angle closure.
- If laser peripheral iridotomy is ineffective, these patients may need chronic miotics and/or argon laser gonioplasty or iridoplasty to prevent an AACG attack.

Gonioplasty or iridoplasty is a laser procedure which photocoagulates the peripheral iris in order to flatten the iris configuration and open the angle.

REFERENCES

21. **Chandler PA, Trotler RR.** Angle closure glaucoma. Subacute types: *Arch Ophthalmol*, 53:305,1955.
22. **Ritch R, Shields MB, Krupin T.** *The Glaucomas*, 2nd ed. St. Louis: CV Mosby, 1996.
23. **Hitchings RA.** Fundamentals in clinical ophthalmology: Glaucoma. *BMJ*, 2000.

CONGENITAL GLAUCOMA

CASE 3

A 5-month-old male infant was brought to the eye clinic by his parents. They said that his eyes had a lot of tearing and that he seemed to be sensitive to bright lights. The mother did note that people often commented on how big and beautiful his eyes were. In the doctor's office, large, edematous and hazy corneas OU were noticed. The IOP was 32 mm Hg OD and 34 mm Hg OS with a Perkins tonometer. Examination under anesthesia later showed angle abnormalities gonioscopically. CD ratios were 0.5 OU.

DEFINITION

• Congenital glaucoma (*Synonyms*: primary congenital glaucoma, infantile glaucoma) is characterized by developmental abnormalities of the aqueous outflow system of the eye. It manifests in childhood and is quite uncommon. Early diagnosis and treatment is very important for a good visual prognosis. There are usually no associated ocular or systemic anomalies.

PATHOPHYSIOLOGY

• Embryologically, there is an arrest in the migration and development of the neural crest cells, which form the angle of the AC. The malformation of the AC leads to aqueous outflow obstruction and high IOP.
• For classification of congenital glaucoma, see Table 9-9.

EPIDEMIOLOGY AND GENETICS

• Primary congenital glaucoma is an uncommon disease. It has an incidence of around 1/10,000–20,000 live births.[24] It commonly presents in the first year of life, is bilateral in 75% of cases, and has a male predominance. Most cases occur sporadically.[25] An autosomal recessive pattern is seen in 10%.[26] A polygenetic pattern of inheritance may be present.[25]

CLINICAL FEATURES

The infant with congenital glaucoma may present with these classic symptoms:
• Epiphora—excessive tearing.
• Photophobia—hypersensitivity to light. The child typically hides his or her face in the pillow in bright light. The photosensitivity is due to the corneal edema secondary to the elevated IOP.
• Blepharospasm—intermittent closure of the eyelids.
Increased IOP may cause the following signs (Figs. 9-30 and 9-31):
• Enlargement of the eye—Increased IOP can cause the eye of a child under 2 years of age to enlarge. This results in *buphthalmos* (literally translated, "cow's eyes").
• Enlarged corneal diameter
• Corneal edema
• Haab's striae—These are caused by tears in Descemet's membrane. Haab's striae are lines oriented horizontally or concentrically in the cornea. In contrast, vertical striae can be caused by birth trauma.
• Progressive myopia—Enlargement of the globe causes an increase in axial length, which causes progressive myopia. The anterior chamber is usually deep.

TABLE 9-9   Classification of Congenital Glaucoma Types

TYPE	CHARACTERISTICS
Primary congenital glaucoma	Maldevelopment of the trabecular meshwork. Iris inserts flatly either at or anterior to the scleral spur. The ciliary body band is not seen.
Primary congenital glaucoma associated with ocular anomalies	Maldevelopment of the trabecular meshwork, iris and/or cornea. Examples include aniridia, Axenfeld-Rieger syndrome, Peter's syndrome, congenital ectropion uveae, microcornea, sclerocornea.
Primary congenital glaucoma associated with systemic anomalies	Examples include Sturge-Weber syndrome, neurofibromatosis, congenital rubella, fetal alcohol syndrome, chromosomal anomalies, Prader-Willi syndrome.
Secondary glaucomas in infants	Acquired glaucoma in childhood. Examples include tumors, aphakic glaucoma (after pediatric lensectomy), inflammation, trauma, persistent hyperplastic primary vitreous, retinopathy of prematurity.

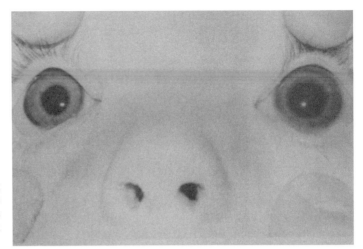

FIGURE 9-30 Infant with congenital glaucoma showing buphthalmos and corneal clouding, both of which are more marked in the left eye. [Used with permission from Shields MB: *Textbook of Glaucoma*, 4th ed. Baltimore: Williams & Wilkins, 1998; Fig. 11.1, p 197.]

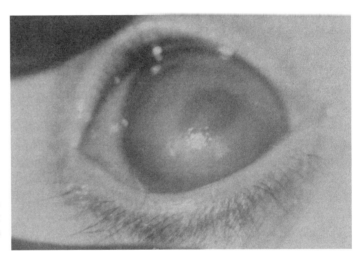

FIGURE 9-31 Dense corneal opacity of newborn with congenital glaucoma. [Used with permission from Shields MB: *Textbook of Glaucoma*, 4th ed. Baltimore: Williams & Wilkins, 1998; Fig. 11.2, p 197.]

- Malformation of the angle may be seen during gonioscopy.
- Cupping—Seen by ophthalmoscopy, cupping proceeds rapidly in infants and is more likely to be reversible if the pressure is lowered early.[27,28]

DIAGNOSIS AND DIFFERENTIAL

- A child with increased IOP, progressive myopia, optic disc changes, and large corneas should arouse a suspicion of congenital glaucoma. Other children in the family of the affected child should be examined. Other causes of epiphora (nasolacrimal duct obstruction), large corneas (megalocornea), and breaks in Descemet's membrane (birth trauma) must be ruled out.
- Long-term treatment is necessary for patients with congenital glaucoma. If untreated, the patient may be left with a blind enlarged scarred eye. These eyes are very susceptible to rupture with minor trauma. Eventually, the eye may become phthisical (Phthisis bulbi is the shrinkage of a sightless, degenerating eye).

TREATMENT

- Surgery done early in the course of the disease has a high success rate. Goniotomy, or surgically incising the trabecular meshwork from an ab interno (or internal) approach, is preferable in younger children who have clear corneas. Trabeculotomy, or surgical opening of the eye's drainage pathways from an ab externo (or external) approach, is preferable in children with hazy corneas. If these fail, trabeculectomy (with or without antimetabolites), drainage implants, or laser cyclodestruction can be tried.

REFERENCES

24. **Miller SJH.** Genetic aspects of glaucoma, *Trans Am Ophthalmol Soc UK* 1962;81:425–34.
25. **Merin S, Morin D.** Heredity of congenital glaucoma. *Br J Ophthalmol* 56:414,1972.
26. **Shaffer RN, Weiss DI.** *Congenital and pediatric glaucoma.* St Louis, CV Mosby, 1970. p 37.

27. **Shaffer RN, Hetherington J Jr.** The glaucomatous disc in infants. A suggested hypothesis for disc cupping. *Trans Am Acad Ophthalmol Otol* 73:929,1969.
28. **Quigley HA.** The pathogenesis of reversible cupping in congenital glaucoma. *Am J Ophthalmol* 84:358,1977.

THE SECONDARY GLAUCOMAS

PIGMENTARY GLAUCOMA

- Pigmentary glaucoma is caused by the dispersion of pigments inside the eye. This causes increased resistance to the outflow of aqueous.
- Pigmentary glaucoma is seen in young (age 20–40 years), myopic Caucasian males.[29,30]
- Pigment is released from the pigmented epithelium of the iris and is deposited on the corneal endothelium, trabecular meshwork, zonules, and other ocular tissues. Exercise can cause an acute release of pigment.
- Clinically, deposition of pigment on the corneal endothelium in the form of a vertical oval spindle pattern is called *Krukenberg's spindle*. Transillumination defects in the mid-peripheral iris in a radial spoke-like pattern is also diagnostic of pigmentary glaucoma. Gonioscopically, a wide dark band of pigment can be seen over the trabecular meshwork.
- Pigment dispersion without glaucoma is called pigment-dispersion syndrome. These patients are at high risk of developing glaucoma, and therefore should be examined regularly.[31]
- The treatment of pigmentary glaucoma is similar to that of POAG.

REFERENCES

29. **Sugar HS, Barbour FA.** Pigmentary glaucoma. A rare clinical entity. *Am J Ophthalmol* 32:90,1949.
30. **Sugar HS.** Pigmentary glaucoma. A 25-year review. *Am J Ophthalmol* 62:499,1966.
31. **Migliazzo CV, Shaffer RN, et al.** Long term analysis of pigment dispersion syndrome and pigmentary glaucoma. *Ophthalmology* 93:1528,1986.

PSEUDOEXFOLIATION GLAUCOMA

- Pseudoexfoliation syndrome is characterized by deposition of protein-like material on the anterior lens capsule, iris, ciliary epithelium, and trabecular meshwork. Increased IOP may be caused by the deposition of this material in the trabecular meshwork. The presence of glaucoma and pseudoexfoliation syndrome is called pseudoexfoliation glaucoma.
- Pseudoexfoliation syndrome is common in older people (age 60–70 years). Women may be affected more than men. It is common in the Scandinavian and Mediterranean populations.
- Clinically it is recognized by the appearance of pseudoexfoliative material in a target-like pattern on the anterior lens surface. The pupil may also have pseudoexfoliative material at its margin and may have a "moth-eaten" appearance due to loss of pigment. Gonioscopy shows open angles and pigment deposition (Sampaolesi's line).
- Treatment is similar to that of POAG. Cataract surgery is associated with a higher rate of complications.

LENS-INDUCED GLAUCOMAS

PHACOMORPHIC GLAUCOMA

CASE 4

A 65-year-old white man came to the ED with a red painful right eye associated with sudden worsening of vision. He said that he had noted gradual decrease in his vision OD over the past year. Examination OD revealed corneal edema, a shallow AC, a semidilated pupil, and a dense, large cataractous lens. The IOP was 46 mm Hg and the angle was closed. The other eye was normal except for a moderate cataract.

- In some eyes with advanced cataract formation, the lens may become swollen and bulge anteriorly. The enlarged lens then causes pupillary block and angle-closure glaucoma.
- Phacomorphic glaucoma is usually unilateral and may be mistaken for PACG. Signs include an intumescent cataract.
- The definitive treatment is cataract extraction. Prior to cataract surgery, medical treatment includes lowering of the pressure and reduction of the intraocular inflammation.

PHACOLYTIC GLAUCOMA

- In a mature or hypermature cataract, lens protein may leak through the intact lens capsule and obstruct the trabecular meshwork. Inflammation results in the phagocytosis of the protein by macrophages.
- When glaucoma occurs, there is an acute onset of pain, redness, increased IOP, and corneal edema. The angle is open and inflammation is seen. There may be a history of chronic decrease in vision from the

cataracts. Bits of fluffy white material may be present in the anterior chamber.

- After initial medical treatment of the IOP, the definitive treatment is removal of the lens.

PHACOANTIGENIC GLAUCOMA

- When patients become sensitized to their own lens protein, phacoantigenic glaucoma occurs. Trauma or extracapsular cataract extraction may be the initiating events. Inflammatory deposits may occlude the trabecular meshwork and increase IOP.
- The inflammation is granulomatous in type, with epithelioid cells, giant cells, lymphocytes, and polymorphonuclear leukocytes.
- The treatment is to reduce the inflammation and the IOP. Residual lens material may need removal.

LENS DISPLACEMENT GLAUCOMA

- A displaced lens may mechanically obstruct the pupil causing pupillary block and secondary angle-closure glaucoma.
- The angle may also be damaged after traumatic lens dislocation. Lens displacement may occur from trauma or from congenital abnormalities such as Marfan's syndrome, homocystinuria, and Weill-Marchesani syndrome.
- The treatment of lens displacement is to initially reduce the IOP with medications. Miotics or mydriatics are given depending on the position of the lens. Cataract extraction is done in many complicated situations.

STEROID INDUCED GLAUCOMA

- Steroids taken by any route, particularly topical or periocular steroids, may cause increased IOP. Patients who have POAG, diabetes, or myopia, or who have a family history of glaucoma are predisposed to steroid responsiveness. The mechanism of steroid-induced glaucoma is not known.
- Steroids with better anti-inflammatory effects tend to have greater incidences of steroid-induced glaucoma. Prednisolone, dexamethasone, and betamethasone are most likely to cause steroid-induced glaucoma. The risk of steroid-induced glaucoma also depends on the dose and duration of the steroid used.
- If steroid-induced glaucoma occurs, the steroid should be stopped. Other anti-inflammatory drugs such as NSAIDs may be used instead, as they do not cause

increased IOP. Even patients on systemic steroids should have eye examinations to screen for glaucoma.

POSTTRAUMATIC GLAUCOMA

BLUNT INJURY

CASE 5

A 13-year-old junior high school student was brought to the ED with a history of trauma to the left eye while playing baseball. He complained of pain and decreased vision in the left eye. The visual acuity was hand movements OS and 20/20 OD. Examination of the left eye showed circumcorneal congestion, a moderately hazy cornea, and blood in the AC. The IOP was 42 mm Hg. Ultrasound of the left eye showed a normal posterior segment. The other eye was normal.

- Blunt or contusion injury may lead to elevated IOP. Many mechanisms may play a role in the development of glaucoma. Early causes may be inflammation, *hyphema* (blood in the AC; see section on hyphema in Chap. 8), a dislocated lens, etc. Progressive scarring of the AC angle may cause late elevation of the IOP.
- Glaucoma can also occur years after blunt injury to the eye. In these cases, there may be a unilateral rise in IOP. Gonioscopy reveals *angle recession*, or the appearance of a wider ciliary body band.

PENETRATING INJURIES

- Penetrating injuries cause elevated IOP through various mechanisms, which include tissue disruption, inflammation, intraocular hemorrhage, peripheral anterior synechiae, and retained intraocular foreign bodies (IOFB). In cases of penetrating injury to the eye, a thorough examination for any retained IOFB is needed.
- Alkali and acid burns involving the eye may also cause increased IOP.

POSTOPERATIVE GLAUCOMA

- Various eye surgeries may also cause elevated IOP. Examples include cataract surgery, penetrating keratoplasty, Argon laser trabeculoplasty, vitrectomy, retinal detachment surgery, retinal photocoagulation, and others.
- Early postoperative elevations in IOP after surgery are due to various causes such as hemorrhage, inflammation, angle closure, pupillary block, AC vitreous, viscoelastic material, etc.

- Late rises in IOP after surgery may be due to peripheral anterior synechiae or damage to angle structures during surgery.
- *Malignant* (*or ciliary block*) *glaucoma* occurs after ocular surgery in the early postoperative period. The mechanism is misdirection of aqueous posteriorly into the vitreous. This pushes the lens forward, causing the AC to flatten and closing the angle. Treatment includes cycloplegics, aqueous suppressants, and sometimes surgery.

UVEITIS

- In most cases of uveitis, aqueous humor formation is reduced and the IOP is low.[32] If the trabecular meshwork is inflamed (*trabeculitis*) and outflow is defective, the IOP can be elevated.

IRIDOCYCLITIS

- Many mechanisms play a role in causing elevated IOP in iridocyclitis.
- Reversible causes include inflammatory deposits, edema of the trabecular meshwork, liberation of prostaglandins, and pupillary block. Other mechanisms include scarring of the angle structures (peripheral anterior synechiae) and neovascularization.
- Treatment generally includes steroids and glaucoma medications.

FUCHS' HETEROCHROMIC IRIDOCYCLITIS

- Mild iritis, iris heterochromia, cataract, and glaucoma characterize this type of secondary open-angle glaucoma. It is usually unilateral and affects young adults (age 30–50 years).
- Gonioscopy may show an open angle with fine vessels over the angle.
- Glaucoma occurs late and can sometimes be controlled medically.

REFERENCE

32. **Krupin T.** Glaucoma associated with uveitis. In: Ritch R, Shields MB, eds.: *The Secondary Glaucomas*. St Louis: Mosby, 1982.

NEOVASCULAR GLAUCOMA

- Ischemia of the retina releases angiogenic factors that cause neovascularization of the iris and the angle.

A fibrovascular membrane may develop on the iris surface and the angle of the AC. This membrane obstructs even an open angle. It may subsequently contract to produce synechiae and secondary angle-closure glaucoma. Neovascularization of the iris is called *rubeosis iridis*.

- *Diabetic retinopathy* is associated with about one-third of cases of neovascular glaucoma, *central retinal vein occlusion* (CRVO) with another third, and other causes such as *carotid occlusive disease* with the remaining third.[33]
- Neovascular glaucoma after CRVO usually develops within 6 months of the CRVO.[34] 30% of patients with CRVO develop neovascular glaucoma.
- Treatment is panretinal photocoagulation (PRP). When a cloudy cornea precludes conventional PRP, cryotherapy (or freezing and subsequent destruction of parts of the retina and the ciliary body) is another treatment option. Glaucoma medications or glaucoma surgery may also be needed.

REFERENCES

33. **Brown GC, Margaral LE, Schachat A, Shah H.** Neovascular glaucoma; etiologic considerations, *Ophthalmology* 91:315, 1984.
34. **Madsen PH.** Rubeosis of the iris and hemorrhagic glaucoma in patients with proliferative diabetic retinopathy. *Br J Ophthalmol* 55:368,1971.

INTRAOCULAR TUMOR

- Primary malignant melanomas of the uvea cause glaucoma by various mechanisms like direct extension, seeding, pigment dispersion, neovascularization, inflammation, and hemorrhage.
- Other diseases that can cause glaucoma include leukemia, lymphoma, medulloepithelioma, retinoblastoma, melanocytoma of the iris, nevus of Ota, Sturge-Weber syndrome, and Von Recklinghausen's disease.

INCREASED EPISCLERAL VENOUS PRESSURE

- Increased episcleral venous pressure raises IOP by increasing resistance to aqueous outflow. Patients can present with chemosis, proptosis, and exophthalmos. The episcleral veins are notably dilated and tortuous.
- Superior vena cava obstruction, thyroid eye disease, cavernous sinus thrombosis, retrobulbar tumors,

TABLE 9-10   Drug Classification.

CLASS	DESCRIPTION
Beta-blockers (Table 9-11)	Most commonly used class of drugs for glaucoma therapy. Effective in lowering IOP in almost any form of glaucoma. Well-defined side effect profile.
Adrenergic agonists (Table 9-12)	Act by stimulation of both alpha$_1$ and alpha$_2$ receptors in the eye. Stimulation of alpha$_2$ receptors causes decrease in aqueous humor formation. Stimulation of alpha$_1$ receptors causes side effects: mydriasis, elevation of IOP, vasoconstriction, eyelid retraction.
Cholinergic stimulators; Parasympathomimetics (Table 9-13)	Simulate the effects of acetylcholine. Topical use of these drugs stimulates the parasympathetic receptors of the iris and ciliary body. Also called miotics. Systemic absorption causes cholinergic effects in the body.
Carbonic anhydrase inhibitors (Table 9-14)	Highly effective in lowering the IOP but have notable systemic side effects. Inhibit the enzyme carbonic anhydrase in the ciliary epithelium and therefore decrease aqueous production.
Prostaglandins (Table 9-15)	Some of the most potent IOP lowering medications. Additive to most anti-glaucoma agents used today.
Hyperosmotic agents (Table 9-16)	Reduce IOP by driving fluid from the eye into the circulation. Used for short-term management of acute glaucoma and pre-operative reduction of IOP. Topical hyperosmotic agents such as glycerin or hypertonic saline are useful in reducing corneal edema for slit-lamp examination and gonioscopy.

Sturge-Weber syndrome, and carotid cavernous fistula are some of the causes of increased episcleral venous pressure.

• The treatment is to treat the cause. Glaucoma medication or surgery may also be needed.

TREATMENT

• Table 9-10 lists and describes six classes of drugs and Tables 9-11–16 provide specific information on each of the six classes.

VISUAL REHABILITATION

• Glaucoma patients with significant permanent loss of vision are good candidates for visual rehabilitation and low vision aids. These devices may help the patient in reading, mobility, and general activities of daily living and vocation.

TABLE 9-11   Beta-blockers and Their Actions

	NONSELECTIVE BETA-BLOCKERS (BETA$_1$ & BETA$_2$)	SELECTIVE BETA-BLOCKERS (BETA$_1$)
Prototypes and other drugs (brand names)	Timolol maleate (Timoptic, Timoptic-XE), levobunolol HCl (Betagan), carteolol (Ocupress), metipranolol (Optipranol).	Betaxolol HCl (Betoptic, Betoptic S).
Mechanism of action	Decreased aqueous production.	Decreased aqueous production.
Physiologic effects	Does not affect pupil size or accommodation.	Does not affect pupil size or accommodation.
Ocular side effects	Burning.	Burning.
Systemic side effects	*Beta$_1$ blockade:* bradycardia, exacerbates sinus bradycardia, heart block, congestive heart failure, syncope, fatigue; check pulse before starting treatment. *Beta$_2$ blockade:* bronchospasm and airway obstruction, exacerbates asthma. Central nervous system: depression, fatigue, confusion.	Cardiovascular and central nervous system side effects are similar to nonselective beta-blockers; betaxolol has fewer pulmonary side effects.
Indications	All forms of glaucoma (open-angle, angle closure, aphakic, secondary, pediatric).	Preferred in patients with bronchial asthma, chronic obstructive pulmonary disease (COPD).
Contraindications	Bronchial asthma, chronic obstructive pulmonary disease (COPD), congestive heart failure, heart block, sinus bradycardia; to be used with caution in patients taking catecholamine-depleting drugs such as reserpine or in patients taking calcium-channel blockers.	Similar to nonselective beta-blockers but may be relatively more safe in patients with pulmonary disease.

TABLE 9-12   Adrenergic Receptor Agonists and Their Actions

	NONSELECTIVE (ALPHA AND BETA) AGONISTS	SELECTIVE ALPHA$_1$ AND ALPHA$_2$ AGONISTS	SELECTIVE ALPHA$_2$ AGONISTS
Prototypes and other drugs (brand names)	Epinephrine HCl (Epifrin, Glaucon), Dipivefrin (Propine).	Apraclonidine (Iopidine).	Brimonidine (Alphagan).
Mechanism of action	Decreased aqueous production Increased outflow of aqueous (dipivefrin is metabolized to epinephrine after absorption into the eye).	Decreased aqueous production.	Decreased aqueous production, increased uveoscleral outflow.
Physiologic effects	Mydriasis.	Mydriasis.	Less mydriasis.
Ocular side effects	Initial vasoconstriction, redness, burning, adrenochrome (pigment) deposits, macular edema.	Follicular conjunctivitis, allergy, conjunctival blanching, lid retraction.	Follicular conjunctivitis, dry eye.
Systemic side effects	Headache, increased blood pressure, tremor, tachycardia, anxiety, palpitation, arrhythmias (less toxicity with dipivefrin).	Dry nose, dry mouth, bradycardia, insomnia.	Hypotension and apnea in children; lethargy, dry mouth.
Indications	POAG; not as commonly used as the selective alpha agonists.	Short-term IOP rise after laser surgeries (e.g., iridotomy, trabeculoplasty, capsulotomy).	IOP rise after laser surgery; POAG.
Contraindications	Angle-closure glaucoma, narrow angles, aphakic and pseudophakic eyes (it may cause cystoid macular edema), cardiac arrythmias, thyrotoxicosis.	Patients with significant cardiac, renal, hepatic, or cerebrovascular disease.	Patients with significant cardiac, renal, hepatic, or cerebrovascular disease; infants and young children; use with caution in patients taking CNS depressants or tricyclic antidepressants.

TABLE 9-13   Cholinergic Agonists - Parasympathomimetics and Their Actions

	CHOLINERGIC DRUGS
Prototypes and other drugs (brand names)	Direct acting (i.e., activate acetylcholine receptors): pilocarpine, carbachol. Indirect acting (i.e., irreversible cholinesterase inhibitors): echothiophate iodide (Phospholine Iodide), demecarium bromide (Humorsol).
Mechanism of action	Increased outflow through the trabecular meshwork in open-angle glaucoma, miosis in angle-closure glaucoma.
Physiologic effects on ocular structures	Miosis, ciliary muscle spasm (i.e., spasm of accommodation).
Ocular side effects	Myopia, cataract, iris cysts, retinal detachment, corneal toxicity.
Systemic side effects	Systemic toxicity is rare with pilocarpine. Side effects are more common with indirect cholinesterase inhibitors and include headache, salivation, diarrhea, bradycardia, sweating, lacrimation, muscle spasm.
Indications	Open-angle glaucoma: to constrict pupil before iridotomy or trabeculoplasty; lower doses may be used for angle-closure glaucoma.
Contraindications	Intraocular inflammation, allergy, peripheral retinal degeneration, retinal holes, high myopes, peptic ulcer, bronchial asthma, hypotension; patients on topical cholinesterase inhibitors need to stop these drops weeks before succinylcholine anesthesia.

TABLE 9-14   Carbonic Anhydrase Inhibitors (CAI) and Their Administration

	ORAL OR INTRAVENOUS	TOPICAL
Prototypes and other drugs (brand names)	Acetazolamide (Diamox), methazolamide (Neptazane).	Dorzolamide (Trusopt), brinzolamide (Azopt).
Mechanism of action	Reduces aqueous humor formation.	Reduces aqueous humor formation.
Ocular side effects	Transient myopia.	Burning, allergy, keratitis.
Systemic side effects	Potassium depletion, abdominal discomfort, paresthesias of the extremities, metabolic acidosis, metallic taste, renal calculi, agranulocytosis, aplastic anemia.	Fewer side effects than systemic CAI.
Indications	To reduce very high IOP in a short time in acute angle-closure glaucoma; long-term treatment of open-angle glaucoma and other glaucomas.	Long-term treatment of open-angle glaucoma and other glaucomas.
Contraindications	Sulfa allergy; renal stones; patients with significant renal, hepatic, pulmonary, metabolic disease.	Sulfa allergy.

TABLE 9-15 Prostaglandins

	PROSTAGLANDIN F_2 ANALOG
Prototypes and other drugs (brand names)	Latanoprost (Xalatan), bimatoprost (Lumigan), travoprost (Travatan), unoprostone (Rescula).
Mechanism of action	Increases uveoscleral outflow.
Physiologic effects	No miosis.
Ocular side effects	Conjunctival hyperemia, darkening of iris color, inflammation, increase in eyelash growth, cystoid macular edema.
Systemic side effects	Myalgias.
Indications	It can be either primary therapy or added to other glaucoma drugs.
Contraindications	Late pregnancy; history of uveitis or cystoid macular edema.

TABLE 9-16 Hyperosmotic Agents and Their Administration

	ORAL	INTRAVENOUS
Prototypes and other drugs (brand names)	Glycerin (Osmoglyn), isosorbide (Ismotic)	Mannitol.
Mechanism of action	Reduces the vitreous volume; decreases aqueous humor production.	Reduces the vitreous volume; decreases aqueous humor production.
Systemic side effects	Nausea, vomiting, headache; glycerin causes increased blood sugar levels.	Cardiovascular overload and pulmonary edema may occur.
Indications	Short-term use for acute rises in IOP (e.g., acute-angle closure glaucoma); reduction in IOP preoperatively or postoperatively; malignant glaucoma.	Short term use for acute rises in IOP (e.g., acute angle-closure glaucoma); reduction in IOP preoperatively or postoperatively.
Contraindications	Glycerin should be avoided in diabetics, other drugs in this group may be used.	

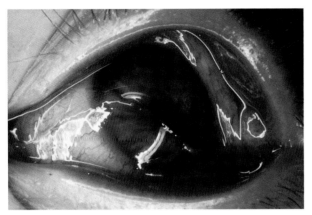

FIGURE 3-3 Ruptured globe. Note flat anterior chamber and oval pupil.

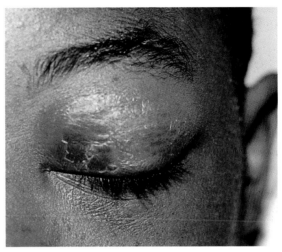

A

FIGURE 3-6A Preseptal cellulitis in a child. There is lid edema and evidence of possible insect bite. Patient is not in distress.

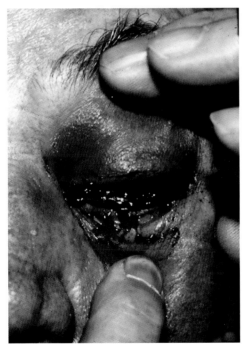

FIGURE 3-5C Orbital abscess in an adult with diabetes.

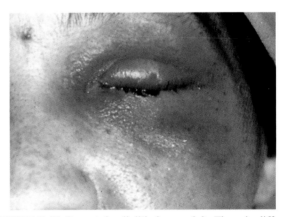

B

FIGURE 3-6B Preseptal cellulitis in an adult. There is diffuse erythema in the periorbital area but there is no proptosis, pain on movement, or decreased vision.

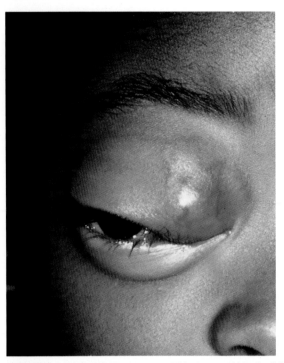

FIGURE 3-7 Rhabdomyosarcoma. This 6-year-old had a lid mass thought to be a chalazion removed 1 week prior to presentation. He now has a large orbital mass with proptosis and downward-outward displacement of the globe.

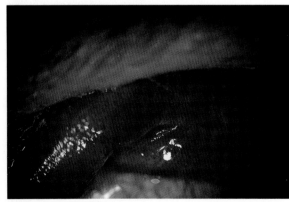

FIGURE 5-15A Sebaceous cell carcinoma of the lid. Note the white lines and pits in the tarsus surrounded by diffusely injected conjunctiva. This patient complains mainly of tearing with discharge.

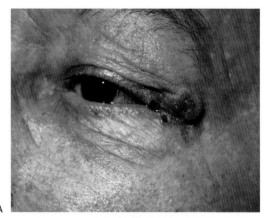

FIGURE 5-16A Basal cell carcinoma of the lid. This lesion involves both the upper and lower lids.

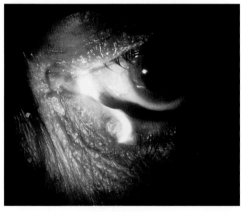

FIGURE 5-16B Basal cell carcinoma of the lid. Note the absence of lash and lack of pigmentation of the lesion.

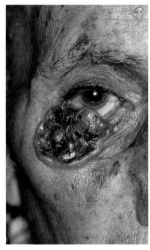

FIGURE 5-16C Basal cell carcinoma of the lid, advanced stage. (Continued)

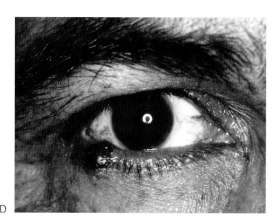

D

FIGURE 5-16D (Continued) Pigmented basal cell carcinoma.

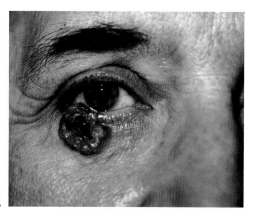

A

FIGURE 5-17A Squamous cell carcinoma of the lid. Lashes are absent.

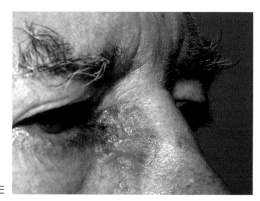

E

FIGURE 5-16E Basal cell carcinoma of the medial canthus.

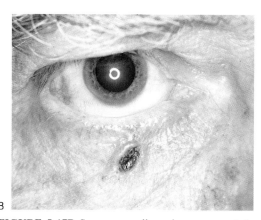

B

FIGURE 5-17B Squamous cell carcinoma presented as a non-healing ulcer.

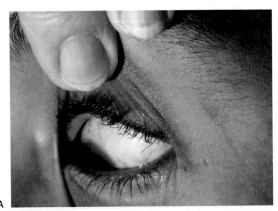

A

FIGURE 6-6A Trachoma. Note pannus on superotemporal cornea.

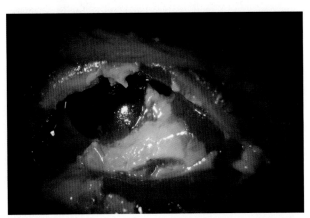

FIGURE 6-7 Munchhausen or self-inflicted injury. This patient gives an inconsistent history. There is no corneal involvement despite extensive conjunctival erosion and maceration.

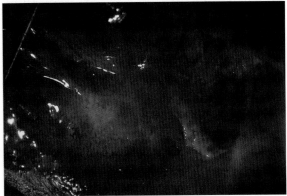

A

FIGURE 6-9A Acute case of Stevens-Johnson syndrome with severe conjunctival injection, chemosis, and pseudomembrane. [Courtesy of Dr. C. Stephen Foster.]

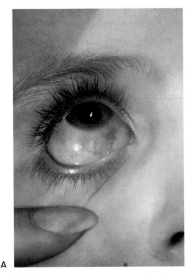

A

FIGURE 6-11A Melanosis bulbi. The pigmentation is in the episclera.

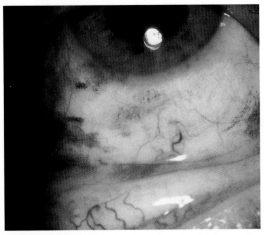

B

FIGURE 6-11B Melanosis of conjunctiva. This may be a primary or an acquired condition.

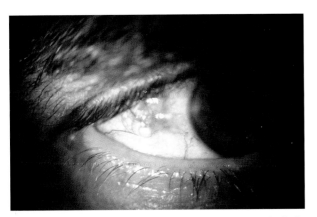

FIGURE 6-12 Conjunctival nevus. Note cysts within the lesion.

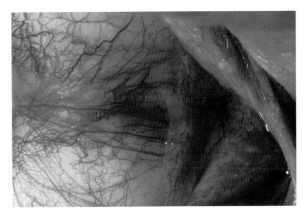

FIGURE 6-16 Squamous cell carcinoma of the conjunctiva.

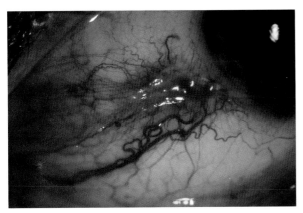

FIGURE 6-15 Conjunctival intraepithelial neoplasm (CIN) at the limbus.

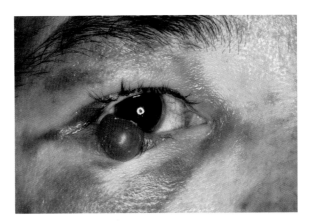

FIGURE 6-17 Kaposi's sarcoma.

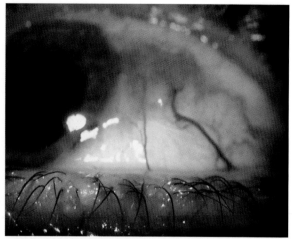

A

FIGURE 6-19A Malignant melanoma of the conjunctiva. Note the relative amelanotic appearance.

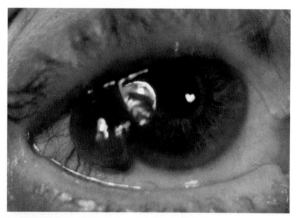

B

FIGURE 6-19B Malignant melanoma of the conjunctiva.

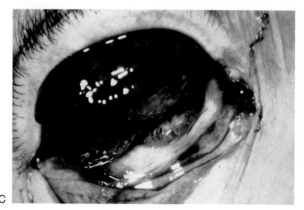

C

FIGURE 6-19C Malignant melanoma of the conjunctiva, advanced stage.

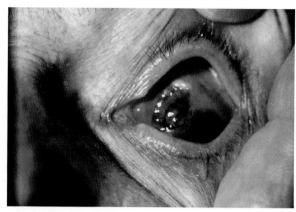

C

FIGURE 6-23C Scleromalacia perforans.

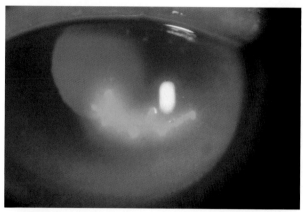

FIGURE 7-3 HSV dendrite.

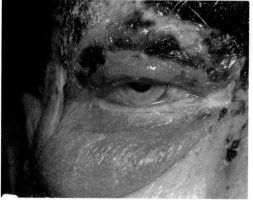

FIGURE 7-5 HZV dermatomal rash.

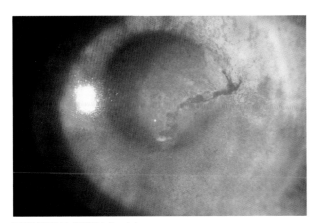

FIGURE 7-6 HZV dendrite.

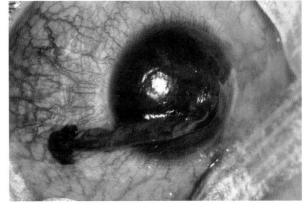

FIGURE 7-10 Open globe.

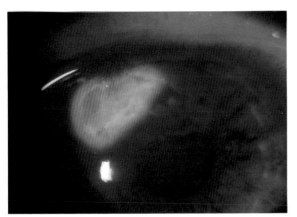

FIGURE 7-9 Corneal abrasion.

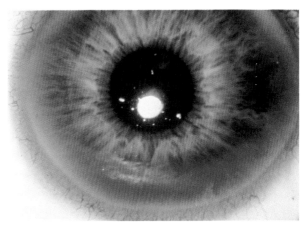

FIGURE 7-20 Kayser-Fleischer ring.

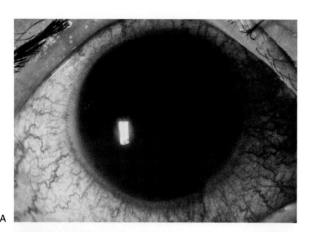

A

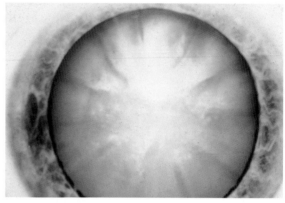

FIGURE 8-20 Cataractous lens.

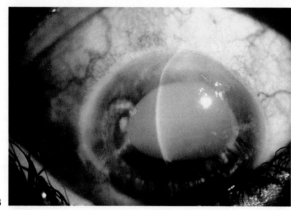

B

FIGURE 8-1 A. Hyphema. B. Corneal staining after a resolving hyphema.

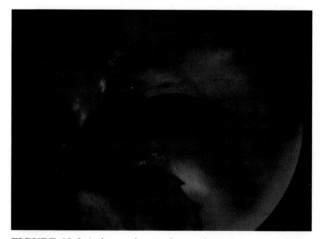

FIGURE 10-3 A dense vitreous hemorrhage in a case of blunt ocular trauma.

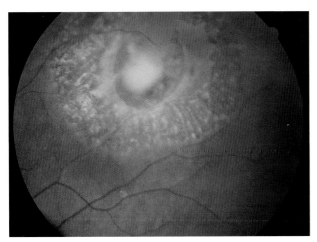

FIGURE 10-4 A horseshoe retinal tear is visible in the upper part of this fundus picture. The tear has an elevated gray flap. There is a small localized retinal detachment around the tear. The localized detachment has previously been surrounded with laser treatment, and the hyperpigmented treatment scars can be seen.

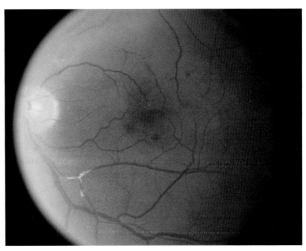

FIGURE 10-6 Hollenhorst plaque. A t-shaped, yellow plaque is visible in the infero-temporal retinal arteriole. Note that the plaque seems even larger than the vessel. This is because the vessel wall is transparent, and we usually see only the blood column.

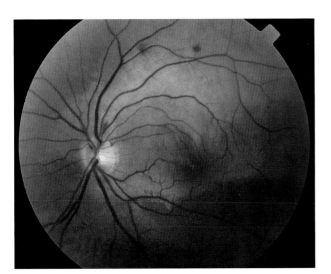

FIGURE 10-5 Commotio retinae. This patient suffered a blunt eye injury from a soccer ball. There is whitening of the retina in the upper 2/3 of the picture. A sharp demarcation between white and normal retina can be seen below the macula. There are two intraretinal hemorrhages near the top of the image.

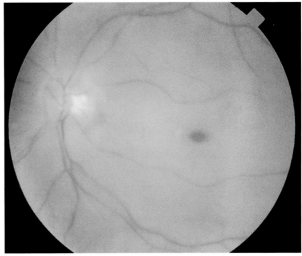

FIGURE 10-7 Central retinal artery occlusion. The retina is diffusely swollen and pale, so choroidal detail cannot be seen. The center of the macula (fovea) retains its normal color, appearing as a cherry red spot in contrast to the pale surrounding retina.

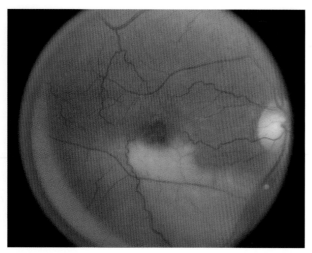

FIGURE 10-8 Branch retinal artery occlusion. The inferior portion of the retina is swollen and pale. A Hollenhorst plaque is visible in the infero-temporal arteriole near the optic disk. The reddish crescent in the far temporal portion of the picture is a photographic artifact.

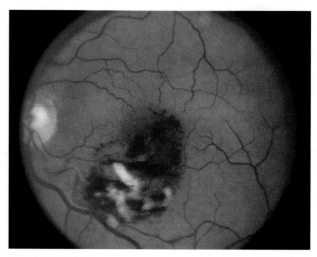

FIGURE 10-10 Branch retinal vein occlusion. There are numerous intraretinal hemorrhages and cotton wool spots confined to one sector of the retina. The occluded vein is obscured by the hemorrhages.

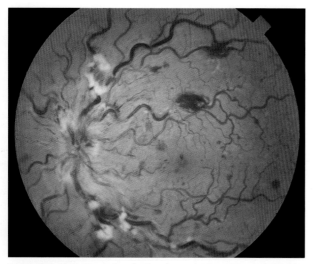

FIGURE 10-9 Central retinal vein occlusion. The retinal veins are dilated and tortuous. There are numerous intraretinal hemorrhages. There are several cotton wool spots (microinfarctions of the retina). The optic disk is hyperemic.

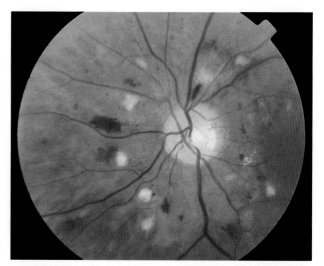

FIGURE 10-11 Hypertensive retinopathy. The retinal arteries are narrow. There are several intraretinal hemorrhages and cotton wool spots. Temporal to the optic disc (on the right side of the photograph) there are a few small hard exudates.

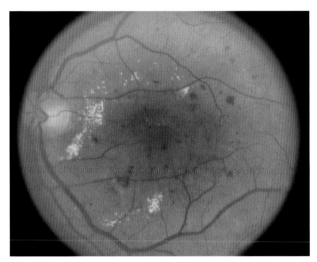

FIGURE 10-12 Nonproliferative diabetic retinopathy. Clinically significant macular edema is present. There are intraretinal hemorrhages and microaneurysms (very small round red dots). There are numerous hard exudates. The macula is swollen (this is difficult to appreciate without a stereoscopic photograph).

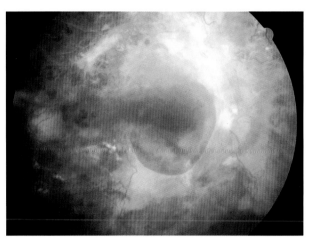

FIGURE 10-14 Proliferative diabetic retinopathy with traction retinal detachment. There is very extensive fibrous proliferation. The central macula is detached. There are numerous hyperpigmented scars from previous laser panretinal photocoagulation. In the supero-temporal fundus (upper left portion of photograph) there are occluded retinal vessels.

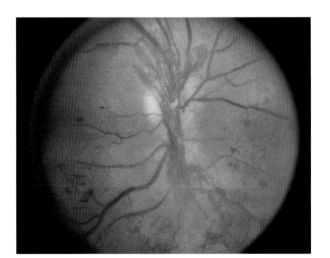

FIGURE 10-13 Proliferative diabetic retinopathy. There is a large sheaf of neovascularization extending off the optic disc. It extends well above and below the disc, as well as anteriorly into the vitreous cavity. There are also intraretinal hemorrhages and microaneurysms, as well as a few small hard exudates (on the left side of the photograph).

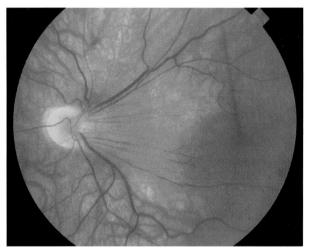

FIGURE 10-15 Retinopathy of prematurity. Left eye. The retinal vessels and macula are "dragged" temporally (by contraction of peripheral fibrosis that is not visible in the photograph). The faint nearly vertical line on the right side of the photograph is a foveal marker, indicating the center of the macula.

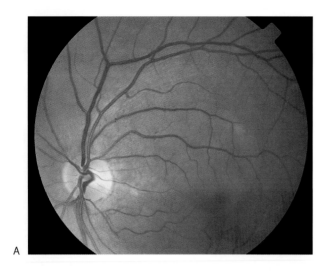

A

FIGURE 10-16 Central serous chorioretinopathy. A. A subtle serous detachment of the retina is visible around the macula.

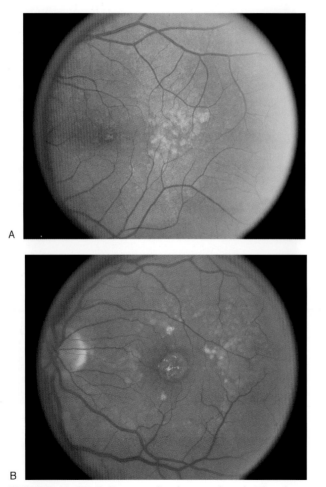

A

B

FIGURE 10-17A,B Dry macular degeneration. A. The photograph is centered temporal to the macula, and the optic disk is not visible. There are numerous drusen (yellow spots). B. A different patient. The central macula shows a circular area of depigmentation of the retinal pigment epithelium (geographic atrophy). There are drusen within this area, and numerous drusen outside it.

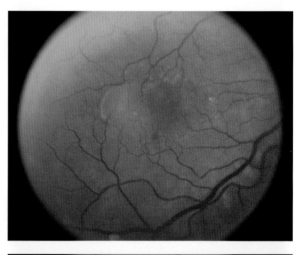

A

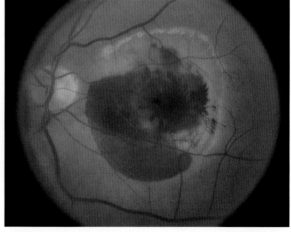

B

FIGURE 10-18A,B Exudative (wet) macular degeneration. A. The photograph is centered just temporal to the macula, and the optic disk is not visible. There is a serous detachment of the retina just temporal to the center of the macula. Drusen are present. B. There is a large subretinal hemorrhage in the macula. There is a serous detachment of the retina superior and temporal to the hemorrhage. There are subretinal hard exudates at the superior border of the serous detachment.

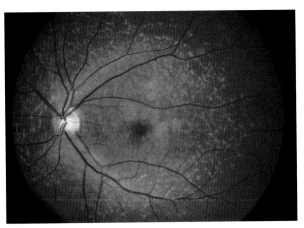

FIGURE 10-19 Stargardt's disease. There is pigment disturbance in the retinal pigment epithelium of the macula, giving a "beaten bronze" appearance. There are numerous yellow fishtail-shaped deep yellow flecks outside the macula.

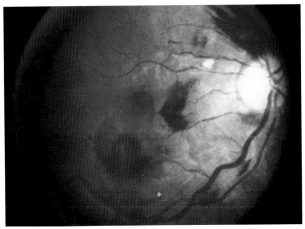

FIGURE 10-21 Retinopathy in a patient with aplastic anemia. There are several intraretinal hemorrhages. There is a preretinal hemorrhage inferior to the macula. There is a cotton wool spot temporal to the 10 o'clock portion of the optic disk.

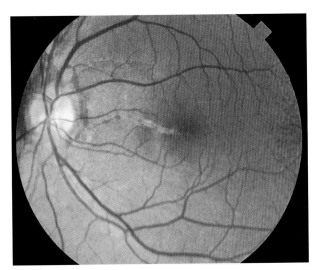

FIGURE 10-20 Angioid streaks. There are several dark angioid streaks around the optic disk. One streak extends from the disk temporally under the macula.

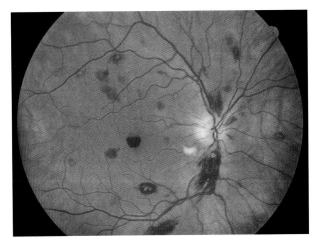

FIGURE 10-22 Retinopathy in a patient with acute myelogenous leukemia. There are numerous intraretinal hemorrhages (some with white centers). There is a single small preretinal hemorrhage in the macula. There is a cotton wool spot infero-temporal to the optic disk.

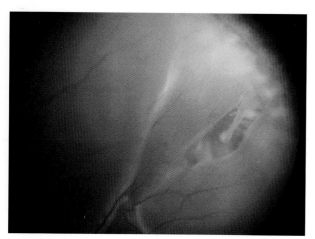

FIGURE 10-23 Retinal detachment. The retina is detached and there are several mobile retinal folds. There is a large horseshoe tear in the retina supero-temporally (in the upper right-hand portion of the photograph).

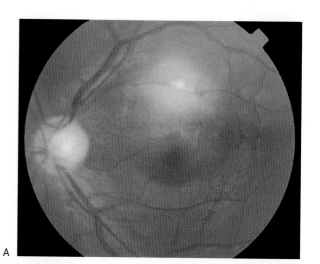

A

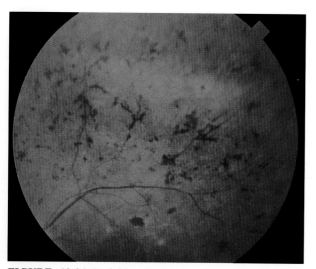

FIGURE 10-24 Retinitis pigmentosa. A photograph of the supero-temporal retina. The optic disk is not seen. The retinal vessels are extremely attenuated. There are numerous areas of hyperpigmentation of the retinal pigment epithelium in a "bone spicule" pattern.

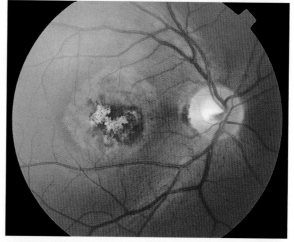

B

FIGURE 10-25A,B Toxoplasmosis chorioretinitis. A. Active toxoplasmosis (*left eye*). The vitreous is clouded from infiltration of white cells. There is an active white retinal infiltrate superior to the macula. B. Healed toxoplasmosis. (*right eye of same patient*). There is a large scar in the macula. The central portion is heavily pigmented. Two irregular white areas are apparent. In these areas, the retinal pigment epithelium and choroid have been totally destroyed, and sclera is visible.

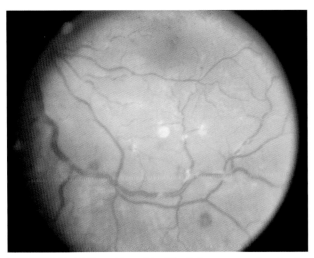

FIGURE 10-26 Sarcoid uveitis. The infero-temporal retina has been photographed. The optic disk is not seen. There are numerous areas of white periphlebitis. There are two intraretinal hemorrhages. The infero-temporal vein is dilated.

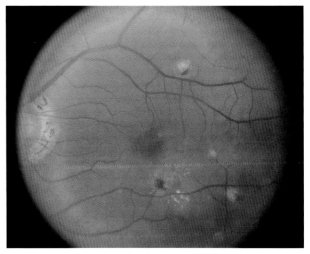

FIGURE 10-28 Ocular histoplasmosis syndrome. There is peripapillary atrophy. There are several small round ("punched out") chorioretinal scars. There are several hard exudates inferior to the macula, suggesting that there is a choroidal neovascular membrane growing from the neighboring scar.

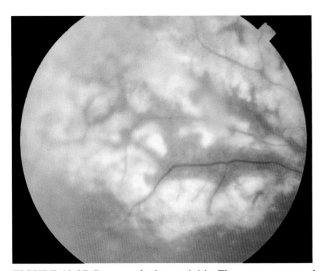

FIGURE 10-27 Cytomegalovirus retinitis. The supero-temporal retina has been photographed. The optic disk is not visible. There are large white retinal infiltrates. Note that the vitreous is relatively clear, despite the extent of retinal involvement. There is a small area of intraretinal hemorrhage in the lower right portion of the photograph.

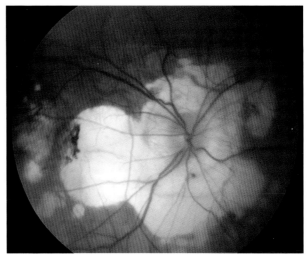

FIGURE 10-29 Pathologic myopia. There are large, white areas representing profound chorioretinal atrophy. The white represents sclera, seen through thinned neurosensory retina. There are several areas of hyperpigmentation representing reactive proliferation of the retinal pigment epithelium.

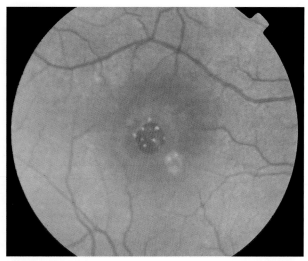

FIGURE 10-30 Macular hole. The optic disk is not visible. There is a large hole in the macula. There are yellow spots from retinal pigment epithelial change within the hole. There is a cuff of localized retinal detachment around the hole. There is a round area of hypopigmentation of the retinal pigment epithelium infero-temporal (down and to the right in this photograph) to the cuff of subretinal fluid.

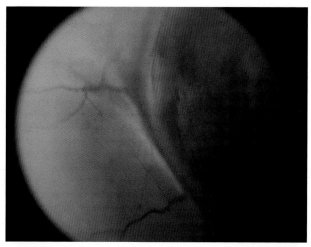

FIGURE 10-33 Choroidal melanoma. There is a large melanoma in the right-hand portion of the photograph. There is an exudative detachment of the retina seen in the left-hand side secondary to leakage from the melanoma.

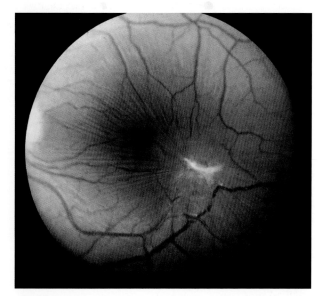

FIGURE 10-32 Epiretinal membrane. An idiopathic epiretinal membrane. There is white fibrous tissue on the retinal surface infero-temporal to the macula. There are numerous retinal folds from traction. The infero-temporal vein is distorted from traction.

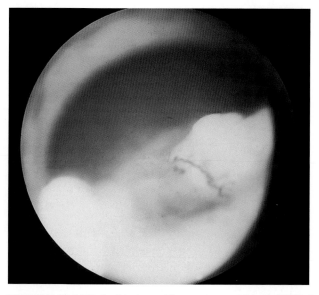

FIGURE 10-34 Retinoblastoma. The eye is more than half filled with a creamy white vascularized mass.

10 VITREOUS, RETINA, AND CHOROID

John I. Loewenstein

VITREOUS

FLOATERS

CASE 1

A 30-year-old myopic graduate student noticed a few translucent, gray irregular spots in front of his eyes. These moved along with his eye movements, but drifted as he began an eye movement or when he stopped. He had no other symptoms. Vision was 20/15 OU (both eyes). Examination showed vitreous degeneration but was otherwise normal.

PATHOPHYSIOLOGY

- Liquefaction of the vitreous, with clumping of collagen fibers that cast shadows on the retina. Myopia, age, trauma, ocular surgery, and uveitis are risk factors. (See Fig. 10-1.)

CLINICAL FEATURES

- The history is characteristic. Spots, irregular lines, "cobwebs," and "flies" are typical descriptions given by patients. The spots are typically gray or black, and are frequently described as translucent.
- Drifting of the opacities in the visual field, particularly as eye movements start or stop, is typical.
- The sudden onset of new floaters, floaters accompanied by photopsia (flashing lights), or floaters accompanied by a visual field defect can be the symptoms of vitreous detachment (collapse) that may be associated with retinal tears or detachment. Patients with these symptoms require urgent referral to an ophthalmologist.
- On examination, some floaters may be seen with ophthalmoscopy, but many are not easily visible.

DIAGNOSIS

- The history and examination are sufficient to make the diagnosis. *Spots that do not drift are not usually floaters.* They may represent scotomas (blind spots). Larger, darker, or red spots may be vitreous hemorrhage.
- A few patients with chronic floaters and no other symptoms may have low-grade uveitis.
- Visual acuity is almost always normal when only benign floaters are present. A careful peripheral retinal exam by an ophthalmologist to rule out retinal tears, detachment, or uveitis is warranted in any patient complaining of floaters.

DIFFERENTIAL DIAGNOSIS

- Vitreous hemorrhage
- Retinal tear
- Retinal detachment
- Posterior uveitis
- Posterior vitreous detachment

TREATMENT

- Typical floaters require no treatment. They may even diminish with time in some patients.
- Vitrectomy surgery has been proposed by some surgeons for patients with bothersome floaters, but the majority of vitreoretinal specialists feel that the risk-to-reward ratio is strongly in favor of no treatment.

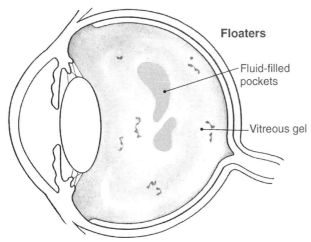

FIGURE 10-1 A diagram of vitreous floaters.

BIBLIOGRAPHY

Sebag J. Vitreous structure. In: Albert D, Jakobiec J,: *Principles and practice of ophthalmology*, 2nd ed. Philadelphia: WB Saunders, 2000, pp 1786–1798.

POSTERIOR VITREOUS DETACHMENT

CASE 2

A 50-year-old myopic banker noticed the sudden onset of a ring-shaped spot in front of her left eye. It moved with eye movement and drifted when starting or stopping eye movement. She had very brief flashes of light at the edge of her field of vision. Examination showed visual acuity of 20/20 OU. There was vitreous liquefaction with a Weiss ring (a ring of collagen fibers on the posterior surface of the detached vitreous, representing the area of previous vitreous attachment to the optic disk). The peripheral retina was normal with scleral depression.

PATHOPHYSIOLOGY

- This is a consequence of liquefaction of the vitreous, with collapse of the vitreous body and separation of the vitreous from the posterior retina (see Fig. 10-2). It is a more severe form of the vitreous degeneration that causes most floaters.
- Photopsia (the hallucination of light flashes) is common in posterior vitreous detachment. It is thought to occur from traction of the vitreous on the retina. This type of photopsia is typically very brief (lasting a second or less), and may be described as resembling a lightning flash or sparkle. It may occur repeatedly, and is often more noticeable in the dark. Photopsia often occurs as part of a migraine (see Chap. 11). In these cases, the photopsia typically is constant for 10 to 15 minutes. It begins near fixation (center of the visual field) and gradually progresses to the periphery. It may or may not be followed by a headache. There are numerous other causes of photopsia, including retinal, optic nerve, and central nervous system disease.
- The denser collagen fibers from the vitreous attachment around the optic nerve typically separate from the nerve, and may cast the shadow of a full or partial ring on the retina.
- Myopia, age, trauma, ocular surgery, and uveitis are risk factors.

CLINICAL FEATURES

- The history is typical. The patient has the sudden onset of new floaters, often accompanied by photopsia. There may be a prominent floater in the shape of a full or partial Weiss ring. Vision is usually normal or only slightly reduced.
- Examination with the slit lamp and a hand-held fundus lens or contact lens shows a detached posterior vitreous, usually with a partial or full Weiss ring.
- A significant proportion (5% or more) of cases are associated with a retinal tear. Patients with these symptoms require urgent referral to an ophthalmologist for a careful dilated fundus examination. (*Fundus* refers to the back, or deepest portion of a hollow organ. In ophthalmology it is usually used to refer to examination of the retina.)

DIAGNOSIS

- History and examination are sufficient to make the diagnosis.
- Careful examination of the peripheral retina by an ophthalmologist is mandatory to rule out a retinal tear or detachment.

DIFFERENTIAL DIAGNOSIS

- Retinal tear
- Retinal detachment

TREATMENT

- Posterior vitreous detachment without retinal tear requires no treatment.

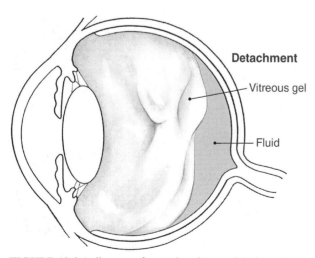

Detachment

Vitreous gel

Fluid

FIGURE 10-2 A diagram of posterior vitreous detachment.

- Symptoms may be annoying but usually improve with time.

BIBLIOGRAPHY

Foos RY, Wheeler NC. Vitreoretinal juncture: Synchysis senilis and posterior vitreous detachment. *Ophthalmology* 96:783, 1983.

Tasman WS. Posterior vitreous detachment and peripheral retinal breaks. *Trans Am Acad Ophthalmol Otolaryngol* 72:217, 1968.

VITREOUS HEMORRHAGE

CASE 3

A 42-year-old truck driver with a 10-year history of diabetes noticed dark streaks in front of his right eye. There was no photopsia. Examination showed vision of 20/200 OD (right eye) and 20/20 OS (left eye). The view of the right fundus was hazy, and the vitreous had a red tinge. The left fundus showed intraretinal hemorrhages and microaneurysms. An ultrasound examination of the right eye showed diffuse echoes in the vitreous, but no evidence of retinal detachment.

PATHOPHYSIOLOGY

- Preretinal neovascularization is the most frequent cause of vitreous hemorrhage.
- Proliferative diabetic retinopathy is the most common etiology of retinal neovascularization. Other proliferative retinopathies such as sickle retinopathy (due to sickle cell anemia) are infrequent.
- Neovascularization after retinal venous occlusion is common.
- These retinopathies share the common feature of retinal capillary closure with resulting ischemia. The ischemic retina produces vascular endothelial growth factor (VEGF), leading to neovascularization.
- Vitreous hemorrhage may also be caused by posterior vitreous detachment, retinal tear, or trauma.

CLINICAL FEATURES

- The history of sudden onset of spots, blotches, or streaks in the field of vision of one eye is typical. Overall blurring of vision in one eye is also a common

history. There may be a red tinge to the whole field or the spots.
- Examination may show reduced vision, depending on the amount of blood in the vitreous.
- The view of the retina may be hazy. The vitreous may look red, but if there is enough blood it will look dark. Older hemorrhages may be tan or gray. (See Fig. 10-3.)

DIAGNOSIS

- Vitreous hemorrhage can be suspected from the history. Examination almost always confirms the diagnosis.
- Urgent referral to an ophthalmologist is indicated to determine the source of the hemorrhage. If photopsia is present, there should be a very high suspicion of a retinal tear or detachment.
- Ultrasonography is indicated in cases of dense hemorrhage, when the retina is not visible, to rule out retinal detachment.

DIFFERENTIAL DIAGNOSIS

- Floaters
- Posterior vitreous detachment
- Posterior uveitis

TREATMENT

- Treatment depends on the cause of the hemorrhage.
- Cases that are due to diabetic or sickle retinopathy, or those associated with neovascularization due to venous occlusion, are treated with panretinal laser photocoagulation (PRP). (See Diabetic Retinopathy.) If there is too much hemorrhage to allow laser, and proliferative retinopathy is suspected, waiting for

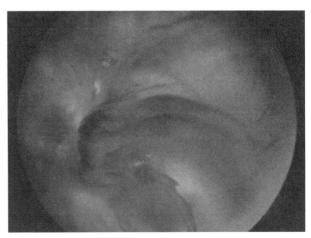

FIGURE 10-3 A dense vitreous hemorrhage in a case of blunt ocular trauma. (See Color Plate.)

spontaneous clearing is generally done. If the hemorrhage shows no sign of clearing over 3 to 6 months, vitrectomy is considered.

- If a retinal tear is found, it is treated with cryopexy (a freezing treatment applied externally) or laser. If a retinal tear is suspected (e.g., if there is photopsia or no other apparent etiology), but the hemorrhage is too dense for thorough examination, the patient should be watched very closely. A few days of bed rest with the head elevated may clear the hemorrhage enough for retinal evaluation.
- See Diabetic Retinopathy and Retinal Tears and Detachment for additional discussion.

RETINA

TRAUMA

RETINAL TEARS

CASE 4

A 12-year-old boy was struck in the left eye with a soccer ball. He experienced blurred vision, light flashes, and dark spots in his vision. On examination he was found to have vision of 20/15 OD and 20/100 OS. Dilated fundus examination showed vitreous hemorrhage OS. A retinal tear was found in the super-temporal fundus (see Fig. 10-4). Cryopexy was performed.
- See Retinal Tears and Detachment for discussion.

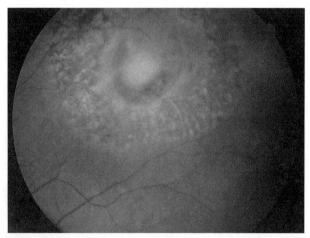

FIGURE 10-4 A horseshoe retinal tear is visible in the upper part of this fundus picture. The tear has an elevated gray flap. There is a small localized retinal detachment around the tear. The localized detachment has previously been surrounded with laser treatment, and the hyperpigmented treatment scars can be seen. (See Color Plate.)

COMMOTIO RETINAE

CASE 5

A 27-year-old man was struck in the right eye with a softball. He had pain, blurred vision, and swelling of his lids. Examination showed vision of 20/200 OD and 20/15 OS. The lids OD showed ecchymoses and edema. There was subconjunctival hemorrhage. The intraocular pressure (IOP) was normal. Pupils were normal. Dilated fundus examination revealed a white appearance to the posterior retina, with a few intraretinal hemorrhages. OS was normal.

PATHOPHYSIOLOGY

- Blunt ocular injuries may lead to shearing of the photoreceptor outer segments. The involved area of retina has diminished function and appears white.
- Hemorrhages are often present. Recovery may or may not occur. (See Fig. 10-5.)

CLINICAL FEATURES

- There is a history of blunt trauma.
- The vision may be affected if the area of commotio involves the macula. The patient may describe a visual field defect if the area is outside the macula.

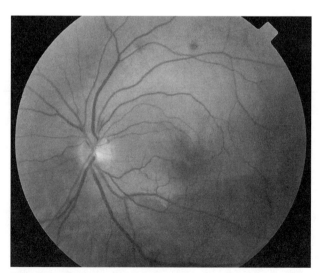

FIGURE 10-5 Commotio retinae. This patient suffered a blunt eye injury from a soccer ball. There is whitening of the retina in the upper 2/3 of the picture. A sharp demarcation between white and normal retina can be seen below the macula. There are two intraretinal hemorrhages near the top of the image. (See Color Plate.)

- The ophthalmoscopic appearance shows characteristic whitening of the retina, frequently with associated intraretinal hemorrhages.

DIAGNOSIS

- The history of trauma is important in making the diagnosis.
- The appearance of the retina is characteristic.
- Rupture of the globe must be ruled out by examination. Retinal tears must be ruled out.

DIFFERENTIAL DIAGNOSIS

- Myelinated nerve fibers
- Cotton wool spots
- Viral retinitis

TREATMENT

- There is no proven treatment.
- Some patients recover full vision, but many do not.

BIBLIOGRAPHY

Sipperley JO, Quigley HA, Gass JDM. Traumatic retinopathy in primates: the explanation of commotio retinae. *Arch Ophthalmol* 96:2267,1978.

VASCULAR DISEASES

AMAUROSIS FUGAX

CASE 6

A 74-year-old man noticed his vision "gray out" in his right eye while he was watching television. He covered his left eye, and found he had no vision at all in the right. He became alarmed, but within a minute, the vision came back. He had no pain. He told his son about it that evening, and an appointment with the ophthalmologist was arranged. The ophthalmic examination was essentially normal. Nevertheless, a visit to the internist and testing was scheduled.

PATHOGENESIS

- Amaurosis fugax is usually caused by embolization of the central retinal artery. The embolus typically breaks up and vision returns within a minute or so.

- The ipsilateral carotid or heart valves are the most common sources of the emboli. If the embolus does not break up, central retinal artery occlusion results (see below).
- Temporal arteritis may also produce unilateral transient obscurations due to optic nerve ischemia.

CLINICAL FEATURES

- The diagnosis is based on the history. Transient monocular blindness lasting a minute or so is characteristic. Vision is typically normal when the patient is seen. This condition is painless.
- In some eyes, residual emboli (Hollenhorst plaques) may be seen in retinal arterioles (see Fig. 10-6).
- Carotid disease may be suspected from carotid bruits or poor pulses.
- The typical history alone, though, should prompt referral to an internist for carotid and cardiac evaluation.

DIAGNOSIS

- As noted above, the history of painless unilateral visual loss, recovering in a minute or so, is sufficient to make the diagnosis.

DIFFERENTIAL DIAGNOSIS

- Transient ischemic attack (visual loss is usually hemianopic, lasts longer, and is accompanied by other symptoms).

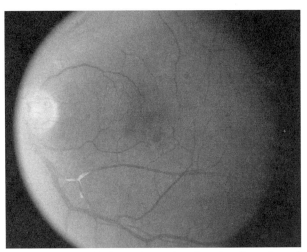

FIGURE 10-6 Hollenhorst plaque. A t-shaped, yellow plaque is visible in the infero-temporal retinal arteriole. Note that the plaque seems even larger than the vessel. This is because the vessel wall is transparent, and we usually see only the blood column. (See Color Plate.)

- Migraine (visual loss is usually hemianopic, lasts longer, and is often followed by headache and nausea).
- Transient obscurations of vision secondary to papilledema (usually last seconds).
- Temporal arteritis.

TREATMENT

- The episode itself does not require treatment as vision returns. Work-up for carotid atherosclerosis and cardiac valvular disease (and temporal arteritis if there are suggestive symptoms or signs) should be performed promptly.

BIBLIOGRAPHY

Burde RM. Amaurosis fugax, an overview. *J Clin Neuroophthal* 9:185,1989.
Fisher CM. Observations of the fundus oculi in transient monocular blindness. *Neurology* 9:333,1959.

ARTERIAL OCCLUSIONS

CENTRAL RETINAL ARTERY OCCLUSION

CASE 7

An 84-year-old woman was playing cards when she noticed the vision had become "dim" in her left eye. She felt well otherwise and had no pain. After a few minutes, she told her companions, and they brought her to an emergency room (ER). Vision was limited to light perception OS, but OD was 20/25. There was a left afferent pupillary defect. The fundus OS showed narrowed vessels with "boxcarring." Most of the retina was abnormally pale, and the macula showed a "cherry red spot."

PATHOGENESIS

- Most central retinal artery occlusions are caused by emboli from the ipsilateral carotid or cardiac valves.
- Temporal arteritis is a nonembolic cause.
- The inner retinal neurons (particularly ganglion cells) undergo cloudy swelling from ischemia. Since the foveal ganglion cells are displaced, the fovea (center of the macula) remains the normal orange-red fundus color, giving the appearance of a cherry red spot.

- "Boxcarring" refers to a segmentation of the blood column in retinal vessels. It resembles a string of boxcars on a train.

DIAGNOSIS

- The retinal findings are characteristic (see Fig. 10-7). If there is uncertainty, fluorescein angiography may be helpful. This test typically shows delayed and incomplete filling of retinal arterioles and increased circulation time.

DIFFERENTIAL DIAGNOSIS

- Ischemic optic neuropathy
- Central retinal vein occlusion
- Retinal detachment

TREATMENT

- There is no proven treatment. Usually attempts are made to lower the IOP abruptly to dislodge the embolus. This may be done by ocular massage, paracentesis of the anterior chamber, and/or use of topical or systemic pharmacologicals.
- Work-up for carotid atherosclerosis, cardiac valvular disease, and temporal arteritis should be performed promptly.

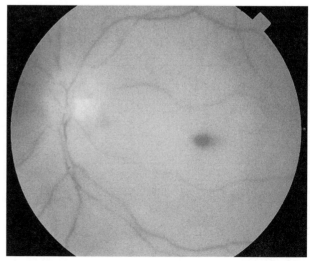

FIGURE 10-7 Central retinal artery occlusion. The retina is diffusely swollen and pale, so choroidal detail cannot be seen. The center of the macula (fovea) retains its normal color, appearing as a cherry red spot in contrast to the pale surrounding retina. (See Color Plate.)

BIBLIOGRAPHY

Brown GC. Arterial obstructive disease and the eye. *Ophthalmol Clin North Am* 3.3:373,1990.

BRANCH RETINAL ARTERY OCCLUSION

CASE 8

A 58-year-old policeman noticed the sudden onset of a "shadow" in his superior field of vision of the left eye. He saw an ophthalmologist urgently. Visual acuity was 20/20 OU. The inferior temporal retina was white. A Hollenhorst plaque (see Amaurosis Fugax above) could be seen in the infero-temporal artery near the optic disc. A carotid work up was initiated.

PATHOGENESIS

- Identical to that for central retinal artery occlusion (see above).

DIAGNOSIS

- The fundus appearance is characteristic (see Fig. 10-8). Fluorescein angiography is occasionally helpful.

DIFFERENTIAL DIAGNOSIS

- Central retinal artery occlusion
- Viral retinitis

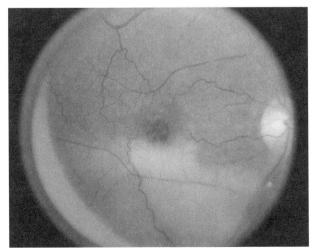

FIGURE 10-8 Branch retinal artery occlusion. The inferior portion of the retina is swollen and pale. A Hollenhorst plaque is visible in the infero-temporal arteriole near the optic disk. The reddish crescent in the far temporal portion of the picture is a photographic artifact. (See Color Plate.)

TREATMENT

- Similar to central retinal artery occlusion (see above). If the macula is uninvolved, invasive treatment (e.g., paracentesis) is usually not undertaken.
- The evaluation is identical.

BIBLIOGRAPHY

Brown GC. Arterial obstructive disease and the eye. *Ophthalmol Clin North Am* 3.3:373,1990.
Ros MA, Magargal LE, Uram M. Branch retinal artery occlusion: a review of 201 eyes. *Ann Ophthalmol* 3:103,1989.

RETINAL VEIN OCCLUSIONS

CENTRAL RETINAL VEIN OCCLUSION

CASE 9

A 70-year-old man noted blurred vision when he lay down on a couch, and a pillow covered his left eye. He sat up and realized the right eye could hardly see. He had no pain or associated symptoms. His ophthalmologist found vision of 20/400 OD and 20/30 OS. Fundus examination OD showed dilated, tortuous retinal veins with many intraretinal hemorrhages in all quadrants. The right disk was swollen. There was an early cataract OS, but the fundus was normal.

PATHOGENESIS

- Central retinal vein occlusion is due to clot formation in the central retinal vein.
- Risk factors include those for vascular disease (e.g., hypertension, hypercholesterolemia, diabetes), clotting disorders (e.g., hyperhomocystinemia), hyperviscosity (polycythemia, leukemia, dysproteinemia), and glaucoma. It is not unusual for cases to occur with no known risk factors.
- Eyes with retinal ischemia, from a variety of causes, are thought to produce VEGF. This factor, probably along with others, leads to growth of abnormal blood vessels in the eye. These may grow on the retina or optic nerve. VEGF may also diffuse anteriorly, where it can lead to vascular growth in the angle. These vessels, and the fibrous tissue that accompanies them, may lead to angle closure. (See Chap. 9.)

DIAGNOSIS

- Fundus appearance is characteristic. (See Fig. 10-9.)

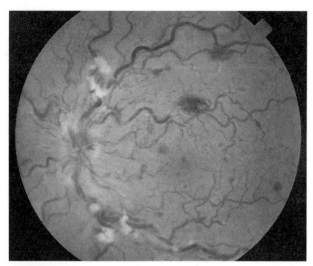

FIGURE 10-9 Central retinal vein occlusion. The retinal veins are dilated and tortuous. There are numerous intraretinal hemorrhages. There are several cotton wool spots (microinfarctions of the retina). The optic disk is hyperemic. (See Color Plate.)

- If there are hemorrhages or other vascular abnormalities in the fellow eye, a prompt and thorough systemic evaluation is important.

DIFFERENTIAL DIAGNOSIS

- Ischemic optic neuropathy
- Central retinal artery occlusion
- Diabetic retinopathy

TREATMENT

- There is no proven treatment. Anticoagulation, use of antifibrinolytics, and laser treatment have all been studied but not shown to be of value.
- Patients should be monitored by an ophthalmologist for development of neovascular glaucoma.
- Systemic evaluation is tailored to the individual patient.

BIBLIOGRAPHY

Central Retinal Vein Occlusion Study Group: Evaluation of grid pattern photocoagulation for macular edema in central vein occlusion. *Ophthalmology* 102:1425,1995.
Central Retinal Vein Occlusion Study Group: A randomized clinical trial of early panretinal photocoagulation for ischemic central vein occlusion. *Ophthalmology* 102:1434,1995.

BRANCH RETINAL VEIN OCCLUSION

CASE 10

A 60-year-old woman complained of a blurred area in her central vision of the left eye. When she saw her ophthalmologist, her vision was 20/25 OD and 20/100 OS. The supero-temporal sector of the retina, including the macula, was edematous with multiple flame-shaped intraretinal hemorrhages. The super-temporal branch vein was occluded at an arterio-venous (A-V) crossing.

PATHOGENESIS

- Branch vein occlusions occur at A-V crossings, typically where an artery crosses over a vein. It is thought that the arteriole wall thickens and hardens (arteriolosclerosis) and compresses the vein. This leads to turbulent flow and clot formation.
- Hypertension is present in two-thirds of patients. The resulting increased pressure in the veins and capillary bed causes hemorrhage and edema. If the macula is involved, vision is reduced.
- Many cases show improvement as remodeling of the vasculature occurs. Some cases develop retinal neovascularization.

DIAGNOSIS

- The diagnosis is based on the fundus appearance (see Fig. 10-10). Occasionally fluorescein angiography is helpful.

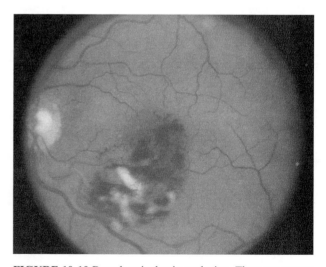

FIGURE 10-10 Branch retinal vein occlusion. There are numerous intraretinal hemorrhages and cotton wool spots confined to one sector of the retina. The occluded vein is obscured by the hemorrhages. (See Color Plate.)

DIFFERENTIAL DIAGNOSIS

- Central retinal vein occlusion
- Diabetic retinopathy
- Hypertensive retinopathy

TREATMENT

- If vision is reduced and macular edema is present, and there is no spontaneous improvement over 3 months, laser treatment is performed. The treatment reduces macular edema and may yield a modest improvement in vision.
- If neovascularization occurs, laser treatment is performed to cause regression of the new vessels and prevent vitreous hemorrhage. If vitreous hemorrhage occurs (a rare complication) and does not clear spontaneously, vitrectomy may be helpful.

BIBLIOGRAPHY

Branch Retinal Vein Occlusion Study Group: Argon laser photocoagulation for macular edema in branch retinal vein occlusion. *Am J Ophthalmol* 98:271,1984.

HYPERTENSIVE RETINOPATHY

CASE 11

A 38-year-old man had mild blurring of vision, and saw an ophthalmologist because he thought he needed a change of glasses. Vision was 20/20 OU. The fundi showed intraretinal flame hemorrhages, cotton wool spots, and arteriolar narrowing. The blood pressure was 170/110 mmHg.

PATHOGENESIS

- Arteriolar narrowing occurs owing to contraction of smooth muscle in the vascular wall in response to high pressure.
- Cotton wool spots are microinfarctions of the retina, due to closure of precapillary arterioles.
- Flame hemorrhages occur in the nerve fiber layer of the retina, following the course of these fibers.
- More severe hypertension can cause optic disk swelling.
- Hypertensive retinopathy is generally reversible with control of blood pressure. In severe cases, there may be irreversible visual loss due to retinal damage.

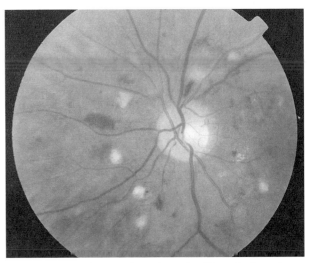

FIGURE 10-11 Hypertensive retinopathy. The retinal arteries are narrow. There are several intraretinal hemorrhages and cotton wool spots. Temporal to the optic disc (on the right side of the photograph) there are a few small hard exudates. (See Color Plate.)

DIAGNOSIS

- Arteriolar narrowing is an important feature.
- The fundus appearance and the blood pressure level usually make the diagnosis. (See Fig. 10-11.)

DIFFERENTIAL DIAGNOSIS

- Diabetic retinopathy
- Retinopathy of anemia or leukemia
- Bilateral retinal vein occlusions

TREATMENT

Control of blood pressure

BIBLIOGRAPHY

Klein R, Klein BEK, Moss SE, Wang Q. Hypertension and retinopathy, arteriolar narrowing, and arteriovenous nicking in a population. *Arch Ophthalmol* 112:92–98,1994.

DIABETIC RETINOPATHY

CASE 12

A 40-year-old woman had had diabetes for 20 years. On her annual ophthalmic visit, hard exudates were noted along with retinal edema adjacent to the left macula.

Her vision was 20/20 OD and 20/25 OS. Laser treatment was recommended.

PATHOGENESIS

- Diabetes damages retinal capillaries. The mechanism is still a subject of investigation and debate.
- Recent evidence suggests that diabetes leads to changes in white blood cells. Early in the disease, leukocytes adhere to the retinal vasculature. This occurs, in part, via intercellular adhesion molecule-1. Leukocyte adhesion causes endothelial cell injury and blood-retinal barrier breakdown.
- Early clinical manifestations of retinopathy include microaneurysms and dot intraretinal hemorrhages. Leakage from microaneurysms and incompetent capillary walls may lead to retinal edema and lipid deposit; the latter forms hard exudates (see Fig. 10-12).
- If there is edema or lipid in the macula, vision will be reduced. These changes are the findings of nonproliferative retinopathy.
- In proliferative retinopathy, blood vessels grow on the surface of the retina or optic disk (see Fig. 10-13). They may be accompanied by fibrous proliferation. Vitreous hemorrhage may occur. The fibrous tissue may contract and lead to retinal traction detachment (see Fig. 10-14).

DIAGNOSIS

- The fundus appearance is virtually characteristic. A history of diabetes for at least several years is almost

always obtained. Fluorescein angiography is useful in selected cases.

DIFFERENTIAL DIAGNOSIS

- Hypertensive retinopathy
- Retinopathy of anemia or leukemia
- Bilateral venous occlusions

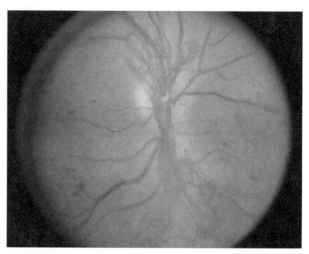

FIGURE 10-13 Proliferative diabetic retinopathy. There is a large sheaf of neovascularization extending off the optic disc. It extends well above and below the disc, as well as anteriorly into the vitreous cavity. There are also intraretinal hemorrhages and microaneurysms, as well as a few small hard exudates (on the left side of the photograph). (See Color Plate.)

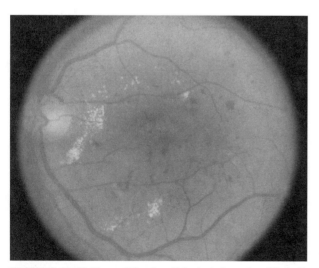

FIGURE 10-12 Nonproliferative diabetic retinopathy. Clinically significant macular edema is present. There are intraretinal hemorrhages and microaneurysms (very small round red dots). There are numerous hard exudates. The macula is swollen (this is difficult to appreciate without a stereoscopic photograph). (See Color Plate.)

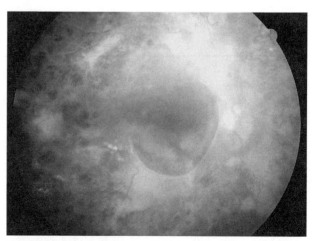

FIGURE 10-14 Proliferative diabetic retinopathy with traction retinal detachment. There is very extensive fibrous proliferation. The central macula is detached. There are numerous hyperpigmented scars from previous laser panretinal photocoagulation. In the supero-temporal fundus (upper left portion of photograph) there are occluded retinal vessels. (See Color Plate.)

TREATMENT

- Macular edema and proliferative retinopathy are treated with laser photocoagulation. Control of blood sugar, blood pressure, and lipids is also important.
- Macular edema is treated if it is "clinically significant," as defined by the Early Treatment Diabetic Retinopathy Study. The criteria are: thickening of the retina at or within 500 microns of the fovea, or hard exudates (associated with thickening) at or within 500 microns of the fovea, or thickening of the retina within one disk diameter (about 1500 microns) of the fovea if the area of thickening is one disk area or greater. A grid pattern of laser is usually administered to the thickened retina, avoiding the area near the fovea. Treatment reduces the risk of visual loss by 50%. Twenty percent of treated patients experience some improvement in vision.
- The Diabetic Retinopathy Study showed that panretinal laser treatment improves the visual outcome in cases of proliferative retinopathy with "high risk characteristics." Treatment reduces the risk of severe visual loss by 50%. The Early Treatment Diabetic Retinopathy Study showed that treatment before high risk characteristics develop leads to results similar to waiting and treating when these characteristics appear. The study described three high-risk characteristics: (1) neovascularization of the optic disk covering an area greater than about one third of the disk surface, (2) any neovascularization of the disk accompanied by preretinal or vitreous hemorrhage, or (3) any neovascularization away from the disk accompanied by preretinal or vitreous hemorrhage. Many retinal specialists now treat proliferative retinopathy if there is any active neovascularization.
- Complications of proliferative retinopathy such as nonclearing vitreous hemorrhage and traction retinal detachment involving the macula are treated with vitrectomy.

BIBLIOGRAPHY

Adamis AP. Is diabetic retinopathy an inflammatory disease? *Br J Opththalmol* 86:363,2002.

Diabetic Retinopathy Study Report Number 2: Photocoagulation of proliferative diabetic retinopathy. *Ophthalmology* 85:82, 1978.

Early Treatment Diabetic Retinopathy Study Report Number 1: Photocoagulation for diabetic macular edema. *Arch Ophthalmol* 103:1796,1985.

The Diabetes Control and Complications Trial Research Group. The effect of intensive treatment of diabetes on the development and progression of long-term complications in insulin-dependent diabetes mellitus. *N Engl J Med* 329:977,1993.

RETINOPATHY OF PREMATURITY

CASE 13

A premature infant was delivered weighing 900 grams. An ophthalmologist who screens premature infants in the neonatal intensive care unit (NICU) examined the child, and noted peripheral neovascularization in the temporal periphery of both eyes. Laser treatment was performed.

PATHOGENESIS

- In premature infants, the peripheral retina may not be vascularized at birth. Ischemia of the nonvascularized retina may lead to production of vasoproliferative factors, and to neovascularization at the junction of vascular and avascular retina.
- The neovascular tissue is accompanied in some cases by fibrosis and contraction (see Fig. 10-15), leading to traction retinal detachment.
- Some cases of early retinopathy of prematurity regress spontaneously.

DIAGNOSIS

- The fundus appearance is virtually characteristic, although the rare hereditary condition familial exudative vitreoretinopathy may be similar. A history of significant prematurity with low birth weight is

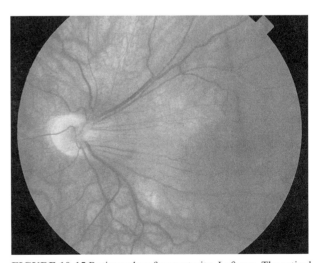

FIGURE 10-15 Retinopathy of prematurity. Left eye. The retinal vessels and macula are "dragged" temporally (by contraction of peripheral fibrosis that is not visible in the photograph). The faint nearly vertical line on the right side of the photograph is a foveal marker, indicating the center of the macula. (See Color Plate.)

almost always obtained, although there are rare cases occurring at full term with normal birth weight.

DIFFERENTIAL DIAGNOSIS

* Familial exudative vitreoretinopathy
* Persistent hyperplastic primary vitreous

TREATMENT

* Screening examination shortly after birth by an ophthalmologist with experience in this condition is very important.
* Prophylaxis of certain early-stage cases with laser or cryopexy reduces the likelihood of visual loss.
* Surgery is done for advanced cases with retinal detachment.

BIBLIOGRAPHY

Cryotherapy for Retinopathy of Prematurity Cooperative Group: Multicenter trial of cryotherapy for retinopathy of prematurity. One year outcome—structure and function. *Arch Ophthalmol* 108:1408,1190.

Hunter DG, Mukai S, Hirose T. Advanced retinopathy of prematurity. In: Albert DM, Jakobiec FA: *Principles and Practice of Ophthalmology*, 2nd ed. Philadelphia: WB Saunders, 2000, p 1936.

CENTRAL SEROUS CHORIORETINOPATHY

CASE 14

A 35-year-old trial lawyer complained of one week of blurred vision in his right eye. He awoke one day, and felt like "a flashbulb went off" in front of that eye. He now sees a disk-shaped area of discoloration centrally, and objects in this area are distorted. On examination, his vision was found to be 20/25 OD and 20/15 OS. A subtle serous detachment of the macula was present OD.

PATHOGENESIS

* The cause of central serous retinopathy is unknown. There is a strong association with so-called Type A personality and stress.
* Corticosteroids can bring on or exacerbate an episode. The mechanism is unknown.

* Focal areas of fluid leakage from the choroid underneath the retina produce the localized exudative retinal detachment.

DIAGNOSIS

* While the history and findings are often typical, fluorescein angiography is usually performed to rule out choroidal neovascularization. The fluorescein typically shows a small leak under the serous retinal detachment (see Fig. 10-16A, B).
* Findings can be subtle and easily missed. Patients may be misdiagnosed with optic neuritis or functional visual loss.

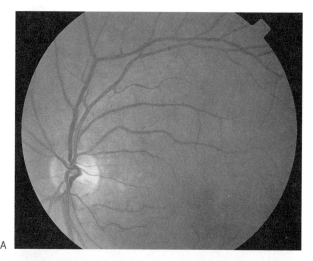

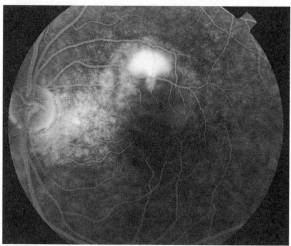

FIGURE 10-16A, B Central serous chorioretinopathy. A. A subtle serous detachment of the retina is visible around the macula. (See Color Plate.) B. Fluorescein angiogram of the same eye. A plume of fluorescent dye is visible, leaking from choroidal vessels into the serous retinal detachment.

DIFFERENTIAL DIAGNOSIS

• Choroidal neovascular membranes (due to a variety of causes)
• Posterior uveitis
• Optic neuritis

TREATMENT

• This condition is often episodic, and each episode almost always resolves spontaneously. The visual outcome is usually very good. Treatment is therefore rarely indicated.
• Laser has been used to close the leak producing the detachment. Although laser shortens the duration of an episode, it does not improve the visual outcome. It also does not prevent recurrences.
• Laser carries a risk of permanent visual loss if treatment is done to a leak close to the fovea. Choroidal neovascularization can also occur from laser treatment scars. Treatment is therefore usually reserved for cases of very long duration, or where occupational needs require rapid resolution.

BIBLIOGRAPHY

Gass JDM. Pathogenesis of disciform detachment of the neuroepithelium. II: Idiopathic central serous choroidopathy. *Am J Ophthalomol* 63:587,1967.
Haimovici R, Gragoudas ES, Duker JS, Sjazda RN, Eliott DC. Central serous chorioretinopathy associated with inhaled or intranasal corticosteroids. *Ophthalmol* 104:1652,1997.

MACULAR DEGENERATION

AGE-RELATED MACULAR DEGENERATION

CASE 15

An 80-year-old woman noticed a dark "blob" in front of her right eye. Her ophthalmologist found her vision was 20/400 OD and 20/30 OS. She had early cataracts. The right fundus revealed a subretinal hemorrhage at the macula. The left showed macular drusen. Fluorescein angiography was performed.

PATHOGENESIS

• The cause of macular degeneration is unknown. It typically results in loss of central vision, sparing the periphery.
• Macular degeneration may have "dry" (nonexudative) and "wet" (exudative) manifestations. In the dry type, yellow lesions called *drusen* may be present under the retina. Atrophy may also occur. (See Fig. 10-17A, B.)
• Drusen are presumably exudative lesions that deposit on Bruch's membrane. Histologically they may be hyalinized or occasionally calcified. In the wet type, neovascularization originates from the choroidal circulation, and typically occurs in the macula (although it may also occur in the periphery on occasion). It may

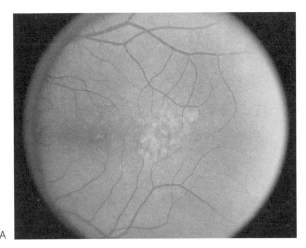

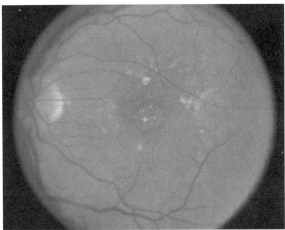

FIGURE 10-17A, B Dry macular degeneration. A. The photograph is centered temporal to the macula, and the optic disk is not visible. There are numerous drusen (yellow spots). (See Color Plate.) B. A different patient. The central macula shows a circular area of depigmentation of the retinal pigment epithelium (geographic atrophy). There are drusen within this area, and numerous drusen outside it. (See Color Plate.)

bleed or lead to exudation. This leads to serous and/or hemorrhagic detachment of the retinal pigment epithelium and/or neurosensory retina. (See Fig. 10-18A, B.) Fluorescein angiography is used to characterize and localize subretinal neovascularization, and to determine suitability for treatment.

DIAGNOSIS

• The fundus appearance is characteristic. Drusen are almost always present. Fluorescein angiography may occasionally help in making the diagnosis, although

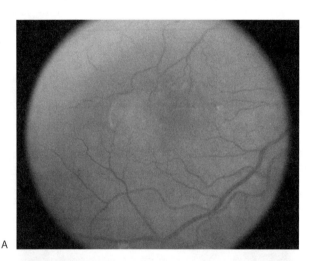

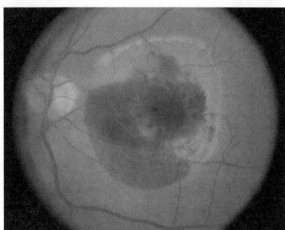

FIGURE 10-18A, B Exudative (wet) macular degeneration. A. The photograph is centered just temporal to the macula, and the optic disk is not visible. There is a serous detachment of the retina just temporal to the center of the macula. Drusen are present. (See Color Plate.) B. There is a large subretinal hemorrhage in the macula. There is a serous detachment of the retina superior and temporal to the hemorrhage. There are subretinal hard exudates at the superior border of the serous detachment. (See Color Plate.)

it is used mainly for planning treatment of the wet type.

DIFFERENTIAL DIAGNOSIS

For wet type:
• Other causes of subretinal neovascularization including myopic degeneration, macular scars due to previous inflammatory disease.
• Retinal macroaneurysm with hemorrhage.

For dry type:
• Foveomacular dystrophy
• Juvenile forms of macular degeneration

TREATMENT

• *Dry type*: The recent Age Related Eye Disease Study trial suggests that a combination of nutritional supplements may slow the progression of dry age-related macular degeneration (AMD), and may prevent progression to wet AMD. This effect was found only in cases with moderate to advanced dry AMD. The supplements used in the study included vitamin C, vitamin E, beta carotene, zinc, and copper. The mechanism by which these supplements work is unknown.
• *Wet type*: Argon laser treatment or photodynamic therapy are used for wet type, depending on the type and location of the neovascularization. For neovascular membranes outside the fovea, argon laser is preferred. Photodynamic therapy is used for subfoveal neovascularization. Many cases of wet AMD are poor candidates for treatment, as the area of neovascularization is often poorly defined.
• Argon laser treatment acts as a cautery. It destroys the full thickness of the retina and usually the choroid in the area of treatment, leading to a scotoma.
• Photodynamic therapy relies on a photochemical interaction between low-power laser light and a photosensitizer to damage the endothelium of choroidal neovascularization. The photosensitizer dye is given intravenously, and about 5 minutes after the dye infusion, laser is applied.
• A variety of other therapies are under investigation for treatment of exudative AMD, including surgical procedures and use of inhibitors of vascular endothelial growth factor.
• Patients should be given an Amsler grid to monitor their vision at home. This grid resembles a piece of graph paper. The patient looks at a dot in the center of the grid with one eye at a time. Distortion of the grid lines (metamorphopsia) can be an early warning sign of exudative disease.

BIBLIOGRAPHY

Gass JDM. Age-related macular degeneration. In: *Stereoscopic Atlas of Macular Diseases*, 4th ed. St. Louis: Mosby, 1997, p 70.

Macular Photocoagulation Study Group. Argon laser photocoagulation for senile macular degeneration: results of a randomized clinical trial. *Arch Ophthalmol* 100:912,1982.

Treatment of Age-related Macular Degeneration with Photodynamic Therapy (TAP) Study Group: Photodynamic therapy of subfoveal choroidal neovascularization in age-related macular degeneration with verteporfin: one-year results of 2 randomized clinical trials—TAP report. *Arch Ophthalmol* 117:1329.1999.

JUVENILE ONSET MACULAR DEGENERATION

CASE 16 (STARGARDT'S DISEASE)

A 10-year-old boy was brought to an optometrist by his father because he could not read the scoreboard at a baseball game. The optometrist could not improve the boy's vision with refraction, and he was referred to an ophthalmologist. There was no previous history or family history of significant eye disease. Vision was 20/100 OU. Anterior segment examination findings were normal. The maculas showed abnormal pigment, resembling "beaten bronze." There were yellow subretinal flecks in the paramacular area of both eyes. The result of electroretinography was normal, and fluorescein angiography showed characteristic changes ("dark choroid"). A diagnosis of Stargardt's disease was made.

PATHOGENESIS

* Mutations of the ABCA4 gene are associated with Stargardt's disease. This is a hereditary autosomal recessive disorder in most pedigrees.
* Patients are affected in the first or second decade of life.
* Vision usually declines to 20/200, and peripheral vision is generally spared.

DIAGNOSIS

* The fundus findings of a "beaten bronze" macula with surrounding yellow flecks is characteristic, although not seen in all cases. (see Fig. 10-19)
* Electroretinography is usually normal, and distinguishes Stargardt's disease from some other causes of

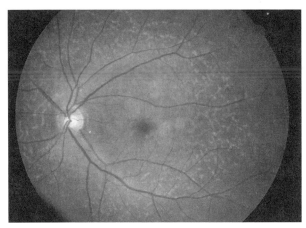

FIGURE 10-19 Stargardt's disease. There is pigment disturbance in the retinal pigment epithelium of the macula, giving a "beaten bronze" appearance. There are numerous yellow fishtail-shaped deep yellow flecks outside the macula. (See Color Plate.)

juvenile macular degeneration such as juvenile X-linked retinoschisis and cone dystrophy.
* Fluorescein angiography usually shows hyperfluorescence in the macula and the yellow subretinal flecks, with hypofluorescence of the rest of the fundus ("dark choroid").

DIFFERENTIAL DIAGNOSIS

* Juvenile X-linked retinoschisis
* Cone dystrophy
* Central areolar dystrophy
* North Carolina dystrophy
* Partial and complete achromatopsia
* Blue cone monochromatism

TREATMENT

* There is no treatment at present. Patients may benefit from vision rehabilitation (use of low-vision aids).
* Genetic counseling.

BIBLIOGRAPHY

Gass JDM. Heredodystrophic disorders affecting the pigment epithelium and retina. In: *Stereoscopic Atlas of Macular Diseases*, 4th ed. St. Louis: Mosby, 1997, chap. 5, p 303.

Reichel E, Sandberg M. Heredofamilial macular degenerations. In Albert DM, Jakobiec FA, eds. *Principles and Practice of Ophthalmology*, 2nd ed. Philadelphia: WB Saunders, 2000, p 2301.

ANGIOID STREAKS

CASE 17

A 30-year-old woman noted the sudden onset of blurred vision and distortion in her right eye. Examination disclosed vision of 20/80 OD, and 20/20 OS. The anterior segments were normal. Fundus examination OD showed subretinal blood and fluid at the macula. There were irregular red-brown streaks under the retina, originating near the disk in both eyes. Fluorescein angiography showed a choroidal neovascular membrane under the macula. The streaks were hyperfluorescent. Examination of the skin of the neck showed a "plucked chicken" appearance. The patient was referred to a dermatologist, who did a skin biopsy. This confirmed the diagnosis of pseudoxanthoma elasticum.

PATHOGENESIS

- Angioid streaks are cracks in Bruch's membrane, the collagenous/elastic membrane that separates the retinal pigment epithelium from the choriocapillaris of the choroid.
- These streaks appear spontaneously or with minor trauma in susceptible eyes.
- Choroidal neovascularization is common if the streaks extend near or under the macula.
- Fluid leakage and/or bleeding from choroidal neovascularization impairs vision.

DIAGNOSIS

- Angioid streaks have a characteristic appearance on fundus examination and fluorescein angiography (see Fig. 10-20).
- Work-up for the underlying cause is important. Patients with pseudoxanthoma elasticum may have premature calcification of large arteries and be prone to gastrointestinal (GI) bleeding.

DIFFERENTIAL DIAGNOSIS

For cause of angioid streaks:
- Pseudoxanthoma elasticum is the most common cause
- Ehlers-Danlos syndrome
- Sickle cell disease
- Paget's disease

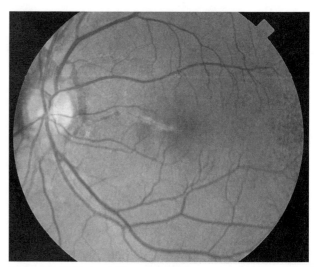

FIGURE 10-20 Angioid streaks. There are several dark angioid streaks around the optic disk. One streak extends from the disk temporally under the macula. (See Color Plate.)

Condition that may mimic angioid streaks:
- Traumatic choroidal rupture

TREATMENT

- No treatment is available for the streaks. Cases that develop neovascularization are treated in a fashion similar to cases of exudative macular degeneration.

BIBLIOGRAPHY

Clarkson JG, Altman RD. Angioid streaks. *Surv Ophthalmol* 26:235,1982.

Sheilds JA, Federman JL, Tomer TL, Annesley WH Jr. Angioid streaks. I: Ophthalmoscopic variations and diagnostic problems. *Br J Ophthalmol* 59:257,1975.

RETINOPATHY OF BLOOD ANOMALIES

ANEMIA

CASE 18

During an admission physical, an intern noted retinal hemorrhages in a patient with severe anemia. Ophthalmology consultation revealed multiple flame hemorrhages OU with a few cotton wool spots. The retinal vessels were somewhat dilated. Vision was 20/20 OU.

PATHOGENESIS

- The combination of anemia and thrombocytopenia can lead to a retinopathy, with venous dilation and tortuosity, retinal hemorrhages and edema, and cotton wool spots.
- The pathogenesis of these retinal changes in anemia are not completely understood. The retina may be relatively hypoxic from the anemia, leading to vascular dilation. This increases the transmural pressure. This increase in pressure, along with hypoxia, is thought to damage vessel walls. Thrombocytopenia may contribute by retarding healing.

DIAGNOSIS

- The findings of bilateral retinal hemorrhages with or without cotton wool spots, and with no significant retinal dilation, should raise the suspicion of anemia. A combination of anemia and thrombocytopenia is usually found, but severe anemia alone may give the same picture. (See Fig. 10-21.)

DIFFERENTIAL DIAGNOSIS

- Hypertensive retinopathy (arteriolar narrowing and high blood pressure are found)
- Diabetic retinopathy (microaneurysms and diabetes are invariably present)
- Bilateral retinal venous occlusions (significant retinal venous dilation is found)

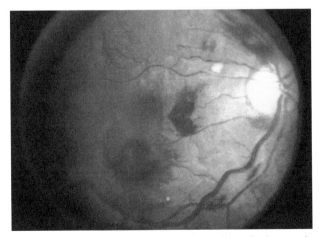

FIGURE 10-21 Retinopathy in a patient with aplastic anemia. There are several intraretinal hemorrhages. There is a preretinal hemorrhage inferior to the macula. There is a cotton wool spot temporal to the 10 o'clock portion of the optic disk. (See Color Plate.)

TREATMENT

- Treatment of the underlying anemia and thrombocytopenia.

BIBLIOGRAPHY

Loewenstein JI. Retinopathy associated with blood anomalies. In: Albert DM, Jakobiec FA, eds. *Principles and Practice of Ophthalmology*, 2nd ed. Philadelphia: WB Saunders, 2000, p 2186.

Rubenstein RA, Yanoff M, Albert DM. Thrombocytopenia, anemia, and retinal hemorrhage. *Am J Ophthalmol* 65:435, 1968.

LEUKEMIC RETINOPATHY

CASE 19

A 28-year-old man developed blurred vision in his left eye. He was just beginning treatment for acute lymphocytic leukemia. Ophthalmology consultation revealed vision of 20/15 OD and 20/100 OS. The right fundus showed flame-shaped intraretinal hemorrhages and cotton wool spots. The left fundus showed similar findings, with a preretinal hemorrhage at the macula.

PATHOGENESIS

- The anemia and thrombocytopenia that accompany leukemia lead to microvascular damage. Flame-shaped hemorrhages and cotton wool spots are common in acute leukemias. Preretinal hemorrhages and leukemic infiltrates are less common. Hyperviscosity may also occur, and can lead to vascular dilation, tortuosity, or venous occlusion.

DIAGNOSIS

- The fundus findings, along with the presence of leukemia, are used to make the diagnosis (see Fig. 10-22).

DIFFERENTIAL DIAGNOSIS

- Retinopathy associated with anemia
- Diabetic retinopathy
- Hypertensive retinopathy
- Bilateral retinal venous occlusions

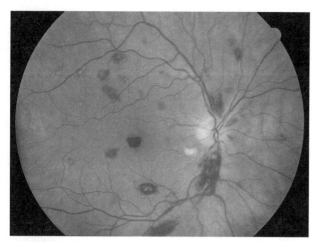

FIGURE 10-22 Retinopathy in a patient with acute myelogenous leukemia. There are numerous intraretinal hemorrhages (some with white centers). There is a single small preretinal hemorrhage in the macula. There is a cotton wool spot infero-temporal to the optic disk. (See Color Plate.)

TREATMENT

• Treatment of the underlying leukemia.

BIBLIOGRAPHY

Loewenstein JI. Retinopathy associated with blood anomalies. In: Albert DM, Jakobiec FA, eds. *Principles and Practice of Ophthalmology*, 2nd ed. Philadelphia: WB Saunders, 2000, p 2186.

Schachat AP, Markowitz JA, Guyer DR, et al. Ophthalmic manifestations of leukemia. *Arch Ophthalmol* 107:697,1989.

RETINAL TEARS AND DETACHMENT

CASE 20

At the airport on his way to a vacation, a 41-year-old myopic car salesman noted dark spots in front of his left eye. He then saw brief but intense flashes of white light in his peripheral vision. He boarded the plane and went on his trip. After a few days, he saw a small dark shadow in his peripheral vision. When it enlarged, he changed his flight and rushed home. He went to the ER of an eye hospital. By the time he arrived, his central vision was blurred. Examination showed vision of 20/20 OD and 20/400 OS. A large retinal detachment involving the macula was found. Scleral buckling was planned.

PATHOGENESIS

• The retina is normally held in place mainly by a pressure gradient (essentially suction) created by ion pumps in the pigment epithelium. The vitreous, when it remains a gel, also provides support for the retina.
• Vitreous liquefaction and collapse may cause retinal tears. This results in both loss of the support of intact gel and loss of continuity in the retina, so that the suction provided by the pigment epithelium is broken. Fluid from the liquefied vitreous goes through the tear and separates the neurosensory retina from the pigment epithelium.
• Myopia is an important risk factor.
• A retinal detachment may occur from any break in the retina. It is more common, however, from "horseshoe" tears, which are tractional tears in the retina that lead to detachment. These tears look horseshoe-shaped on examination, with a flap of torn retina pulled up out of the plane of the retina by vitreous traction. Atrophic holes less commonly lead to detachment. These holes are round and have no flap or visible vitreous traction.

DIAGNOSIS

• The fundus appearance is characteristic. (See Fig. 10-23.)

DIFFERENTIAL DIAGNOSIS

• Vitreous hemorrhage
• Retinal tear without detachment
• Retinal vascular occlusion

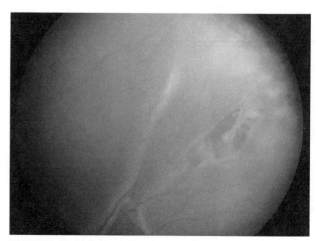

FIGURE 10-23 Retinal detachment. The retina is detached and there are several mobile retinal folds. There is a large horseshoe tear in the retina supero-temporally (in the upper right-hand portion of the photograph). (See Color Plate.)

TREATMENT

- Many retinal tears without detachment do not require treatment. Symptomatic horseshoe tears do require prompt treatment, since they are very likely to lead to retinal detachment. These may be treated with laser or cryopexy. (See Fig. 10-2.)
- Retinal detachments are treated with surgery. Scleral buckling, pneumatic retinopexy, and vitrectomy are used, depending on the situation.
- Scleral buckling is the oldest of these methods, but is highly successful and still widely used. In this procedure, cryopexy is placed around the retinal breaks. The cryopexy will cause pigment epithelial healing that will permanently seal the edges of the retinal break. Scleral sutures are placed to hold an exoplant of silicone rubber to the exterior of the eye, over the breaks. Subretinal fluid is often drained, and when the scleral sutures are then tied, the silicone exoplant indents the eye wall under the breaks, closing them.
- Pneumatic retinopexy is useful in selected cases. The break has to be located in the upper half of the retina, so that it can be readily tamponaded by an intraocular gas bubble. This technique is usually used when there is only one break and the view of the retina is good. Cryopexy is placed over the retinal break. A small bubble of poorly soluble gas (perfluoropropane or sulfur hexafluride) is injected into the vitreous cavity. Oxygen and nitrogen (dissolved in the body fluids) diffuse into the bubble, expanding it (the poorly soluble gas takes days to weeks to dissolve in the ocular fluids). The patient is then instructed to position his- or herself so that the bubble tamponades the retinal break. The retinal pigment epithelium then pumps the subretinal fluid out, reattaching the retina. As with a scleral buckle, the cryopexy leads to permanent sealing of the edges of the break.
- Vitrectomy technically refers to removal of the vitreous gel from the eye. During vitrectomy procedures, however, a wide variety of other intraocular maneuvers may be performed. These include cutting, peeling, and removal of scar tissue, removal of subretinal fluid, placement of intraocular gas or silicone oil tamponades, and laser treatment. Vitrectomy techniques are typically used for unusual or difficult retinal detachment cases, such as giant retinal tears, detachments complicated by proliferative vitreoretinopathy, detachments accompanied by significant vitreous hemorrhage, or detachments caused by very posterior retinal breaks. With advances in vitrectomy techniques and instruments, some surgeons are beginning to use vitrectomy for primary repair of uncomplicated detachments.
- The overall success rate of reattachment is 90%.

- Visual results vary. For cases where the macula did not detach, vision of 20/50 or better is obtained in 70% or more of cases. If the macula is detached preoperatively, the likelihood of 20/50 or better vision falls to 40% or less. Thus, cases where the detachment is close to, but not involving the macula (macular "threatening" detachments) are usually treated urgently.

BIBLIOGRAPHY

Young LHY, D'Amico DJ. Retinal detachment. In: Albert DM, Jakobiec FA, eds. *Principles and Practice of Ophthalmology*, 2nd ed. Philadelphia: WB Saunders, 2000, p 2352.

RETINITIS PIGMENTOSA

CASE 21

A 17-year-old girl had difficulty driving at night when she received a learner's permit. There was no family history of night blindness. Examination by an ophthalmologist showed vision of 20/15 OU. Visual fields were constricted. The fundi showed narrow retinal arteries. The peripheral retina showed pigmentation shaped like "bone spicules." An electroretinogram was ordered, and it showed markedly diminished signals.

PATHOGENESIS

- This is a degeneration of the outer retina. A variety of genetic defects may cause retinitis pigmentosa. Inheritance may be autosomal dominant or recessive, or X-linked. Rare varieties are caused by mitochondrial defects.

DIAGNOSIS

- The fundus appearance is highly suggestive. (See Fig. 10-24.) An electroretinogram (ERG) should be obtained for confirmation. The ERG is usually markedly reduced or nonrecordable ("extinguished") in retinitis pigmentosa.

DIFFERENTIAL DIAGNOSIS

- Congenital stationary night blindness
- Rubella retinopathy

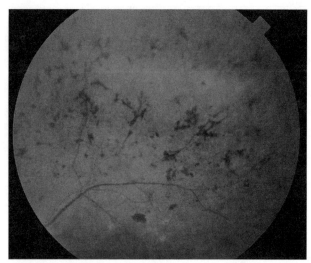

FIGURE 10-24 Retinitis pigmentosa. A photograph of the supero-temporal retina. The optic disk is not seen. The retinal vessels are extremely attenuated. There are numerous areas of hyperpigmentation of the retinal pigment epithelium in a "bone spicule" pattern. (See Color Plate.)

- Congenital syphilis
- Choroideremia
- Gyrate atrophy of the choroid

TREATMENT

- One study suggests vitamin A therapy may slow the degeneration slightly. Low-vision aids may be helpful.

BIBLIOGRAPHY

Berson EL. Retinitis pigmentosa: the Friedenwald lecture. *Invest Ophthalmol Vis Sci* 34:1659,1993.

Dryja TP, McGee TL, Hahn LB, et al. Mutations within the rhodopsin gene in patients with autosomal dominant retinitis pigmentosa. *N Engl J Med* 323:1302,1990.

POSTERIOR UVEITIS

TOXOPLASMOSIS

CASE 22

A 27-year-old woman experienced blurred vision and saw many tiny dots in front of her right eye. She had mild photophobia. Examination disclosed vision of 20/200 OD and 20/15 OS. There was mild injection of the conjunctiva OD. The right pupil was slightly smaller than the left and light reaction was sluggish. There were cells and flare in the anterior chamber OD. Dilated fundus examination showed vitreous haze. There was a fluffy white intraretinal lesion near the macula. At the border of the white lesion, there was a heavily pigmented chorioretinal scar. The left eye was normal.

PATHOGENESIS

- *Toxoplasma gondi* is the responsible organism. It is carried by cats or in contaminated meat.
- Infection may be congenital or acquired. The organisms survive in dormant cysts in retinal scars, and may reactivate at any time, usually without apparent cause. Reactivation may occur in immunosuppressed individuals.
- Toxoplasmosis is the most common cause of posterior uveitis.

DIAGNOSIS

- Fundus appearance is characteristic. Fluffy white lesions with overlying vitreous haze, usually occurring on the border of pigmented scars, are the typical picture. (See Fig. 10-25A, B.) A serum toxoplasmosis titer is helpful, but not absolutely confirmatory.

DIFFERENTIAL DIAGNOSIS

- Sarcoidosis
- Viral retinitis
- Bacterial emboli to the choroid

TREATMENT

- For macular or optic nerve–threatening lesions, treatment consists of sulfadiazine, pyrimethamine, leukovorin, clindamycin, and prednisone. Other lesions may require less aggressive therapy. Treatment is typically carried out for 4 to 6 weeks. Immunosuppressed patients require long-term treatment.

BIBLIOGRAPHY

Foster CS, Vitale AT. *Diagnosis and Treatment of Uveitis.* Philadelphia: WB Saunders, 2002, p 385.

Smith RE, Nozik RA. Toxoplasmic retinochoroiditis. In: *Uveitis, a Clinical Approach to Diagnosis and Management.* Baltimore: Williams & Wilkins, 1989, p 128.

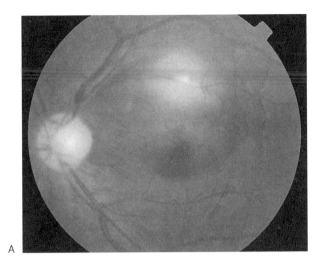

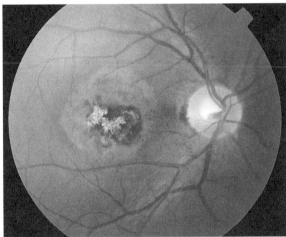

FIGURE 10-25A, B Toxoplasmosis chorioretinitis. A. Active toxoplasmosis (*left eye*). The vitreous is clouded from infiltration of white cells. There is an active white retinal infiltrate superior to the macula. (See Color Plate.) B. Healed toxoplasmosis. (*right eye of same patient*). There is a large scar in the macula. The central portion is heavily pigmented. Two irregular white areas are apparent. In these areas, the retinal pigment epithelium and choroid have been totally destroyed, and sclera is visible. (See Color Plate.)

Tamesis RR, Foster CS. Toxoplasmosis. In: Albert DM, Jakobiec FA, eds: *Principles and Practice of Ophthalmology*, 2nd ed. Philadelphia: WB Saunders, 2000, p 2113.

SARCOIDOSIS

CASE 23

A 30-year-old woman developed photophobia, conjunctival injection, and blurred vision OU. Examination showed vision of 20/50 OU. The conjunctivae were injected. There were "mutton fat" keratic precipitates on the corneas. The anterior chambers showed cells and flare. There were a few vitreous cells OU. The fundi showed white infiltrates along retinal veins. A chest x-ray showed bilateral hilar adenopathy, and the serum angiotensin-converting enzyme titer was elevated.

PATHOGENESIS

• Sarcoidosis is a chronic granulomatous disease of unknown origin.

DIAGNOSIS

• Granulomatous iritis is suggestive of sarcoidosis, and the finding of retinal periphlebitis along with uveitis is highly suggestive (see Fig. 10-26). Keratic precipitates are commonly seen. These are usually of the "mutton fat" variety (large and greasy looking).
• Supporting evidence includes hilar adenopathy, elevated angiotensin-converting enzyme, and elevated serum calcium. A gallium scan may be helpful. Biopsy of the conjunctiva or affected nonocular tissues is not usually done if the disease seems confined to the eyes and is clinically characteristic.

DIFFERENTIAL DIAGNOSIS

• Syphilitic uveitis
• Tuberculous uveitis
• Viral retinitis

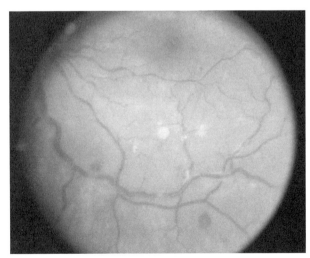

FIGURE 10-26 Sarcoid uveitis. The infero-temporal retina has been photographed. The optic disk is not seen. There are numerous areas of white periphlebitis. There are two intraretinal hemorrhages. The infero-temporal vein is dilated. (See Color Plate.)

TREATMENT

- Topical and systemic steroids depending on the location and severity of disease.

BIBLIOGRAPHY

Aaberg TA. Editorial. The role of the ophthalmologist in the management of sarcoidosis. *Am J Ophthalmol* 103:99,1987.
Foster CS, Vitale AT. *Diagnosis and Treatment of Uveitis.* Philadelphia: WB Saunders, 2002, p 710.
Jabs DA, Johns CJ. Ocular involvement in chronic sarcoidosis. *Am J Ophthalmol* 102:297,1986.

CYTOMEGALOVIRUS

CASE 24

A 43-year-old man with AIDS stopped taking his medications and did not see his physician for several months. He developed blurred peripheral vision. Ophthalmic examination showed vision of 20/20 OU. There were a few vitreous cells OU. There was peripheral retinal scarring, and at the posterior border of the scars, there were white retinal infiltrates. There were retinal hemorrhages near the infiltrates. The CD4 count was 11.

PATHOGENESIS

- Cytomegalovirus is ubiquitous, but generally nonpathogenic. It may infect the retina, kidneys, and other organs of immunocompromised hosts.

DIAGNOSIS

- Retinal appearance is characteristic (see Fig. 10-27). Cytomegalovirus titers may be helpful.

DIFFERENTIAL DIAGNOSIS

- Acute retinal necrosis
- Progressive outer retinal necrosis
- Diffuse toxoplasmosis retinitis

TREATMENT

- Gancyclovir IV is usually the initial treatment. Recent studies suggest that oral pro-drug forms of gancyclovir may also be adequate.

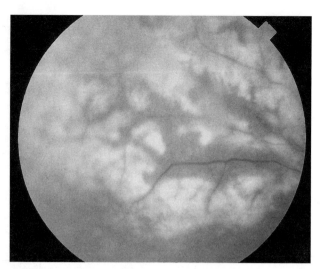

FIGURE 10-27 Cytomegalovirus retinitis. The supero-temporal retina has been photographed. The optic disk is not visible. There are large white retinal infiltrates. Note that the vitreous is relatively clear, despite the extent of retinal involvement. There is a small area of intraretinal hemorrhage in the lower right portion of the photograph. (See Color Plate.)

- Intraocular injections or ganciclovir implants are used in selected cases.
- Foscarnet or cidofovir may be helpful in cases of ganciclovir resistance.
- Controlling immunosuppression may allow cessation of therapy.

BIBLIOGRAPHY

Bachman DM, Rodrigues MM, Chu FC, et al. Culture-proven cytomegalovirus retinitis in a homosexual man with the acquired immunodeficiency syndrome. *Ophthalmology* 89:797,1982.
Morinelli EN, Dugel PU, Lee M, et al. Opportunistic intraocular infections in AIDS. *Trans Am Ophthalmol Soc* 90:97,1992.

HISTOPLASMOSIS SYNDROME

CASE 25

A 30-year-old woman noted blurred vision and distortion in her left eye while driving. Ophthalmic examination disclosed vision of 20/20 OD and 20/80 OS. There was subretinal blood and fluid in the macula. There was peripapillary atrophy in both eyes, along with small atrophic scars in the midperiphery OU. A retinal specialist was consulted, and a fluorescein angiogram was done. This showed a subfoveal choroidal neovascular membrane. Photodynamic therapy was performed.

PATHOGENESIS

- Although the etiology is unproven, the distribution of this condition in the United States follows the geographic area where histoplasmosis is endemic. Studies of skin testing for histoplasmosis also show that those with the triad (see below) are more likely to have positive tests.
- Choroidal neovascularization commonly develops in the macular scars. Leakage of fluid and bleeding from these vessels leads to central visual loss.

DIAGNOSIS

- The triad of peripapillary atrophy, small "punched out" midperipheral chorioretinal scars, and a macular scar is characteristic of the presumed ocular histoplasmosis syndrome (see Fig. 10-28).
- Skin testing is usually not done.
- Fluorescein angiography is performed in cases with suspected neovascular membranes.

DIFFERENTIAL DIAGNOSIS

- Multifocal choroiditis
- Idiopathic choroidal neovascularization

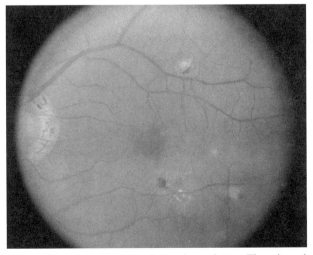

FIGURE 10-28 Ocular histoplasmosis syndrome. There is peripapillary atrophy. There are several small round ("punched out") chorioretinal scars. There are several hard exudates inferior to the macula, suggesting that there is a choroidal neovascular membrane growing from the neighboring scar. (See Color Plate.)

TREATMENT

- Only cases with choroidal neovascularization are treated.
- Argon laser photocoagulation is done if the neovascularization is outside the fovea.
- Photodynamic therapy is the only modality shown to be beneficial in a randomized trial for subfoveal neovascularization.
- Results of a randomized trial of surgical removal of subfoveal membranes are pending.

BIBLIOGRAPHY

Ciulla TA, Piper HC, Xiao M, et al Presumed ocular histoplasmosis syndrome: update on epidemiology, pathogenesis, and photodynamic, antiangiogenic, and surgical therapies. *Curr Opin Ophthalmol* 12:442,2001
Macular Photocoagulation Study Group: Argon laser photocoagulation for ocular histoplasmosis. *Arch Ophthalmol* 101:1347, 1983.

PATHOLOGIC MYOPIA

CASE 26

A 40-year-old woman complained of sudden deterioration of vision in her left eye. Neither eye had ever been correctable to 20/20. She had worn very thick glasses since childhood. Examination disclosed vision of 20/40 OD and 20/100 OS. Her right fundus showed areas of atrophy around the optic disk and at the macula. Her left eye showed similar findings, but in addition, there was a subretinal hemorrhage at the macula.

PATHOGENESIS

- Pathologic myopia is thought to be hereditary. The etiology is unclear.
- Eyes with pathologic myopia are elongated, and the sclera, choroid, and retina are thinned.
- There are frequently areas of chorioretinal atrophy which commonly involve the macula.
- Cracks often develop in Bruch's membrane. These may lead to acute subretinal hemorrhage with visual loss, or choroidal neovascularization with hemorrhage and visual loss.
- Lattice degeneration of the retina is more common in myopia. In this condition, there are patches of thinning in the retinal periphery.

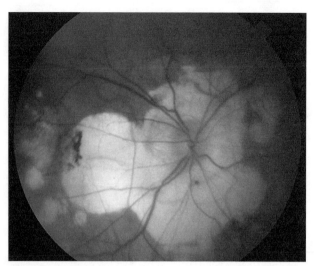

FIGURE 10-29 Pathologic myopia. There are large, white areas representing profound chorioretinal atrophy. The white represents sclera, seen through thinned neurosensory retina. There are several areas of hyperpigmentation representing reactive proliferation of the retinal pigment epithelium. (See Color Plate.)

DIAGNOSIS

- The fundus appearance is characteristic (see Fig. 10-29).
- The patient's refraction is usually −10 diopters or greater.

DIFFERENTIAL DIAGNOSIS

- Other causes of chorioretinal atrophy include age-related macular degeneration and other hereditary retinal degenerations.
- Other causes of subretinal neovascularization include age-related macular degeneration, ocular histoplasmosis syndrome, angioid streaks, etc.

TREATMENT

- See Chap. 2 for treatment of the refractive error.
- There is no treatment available for the atrophy except low-vision aids.
- Choroidal neovascularization is treated as in ocular histoplasmosis syndrome.

BIBLIOGRAPHY

Miller DG, Singerman LJ. Natural history of choroidal neovascularization in high myopia. *Curr Opin Ophthalmol* 12:222,2001.

IDIOPATHIC MACULAR HOLE

CASE 27

A 70-year-old woman presents with a 2 week history of distortion and visual loss in her right eye. Her vision is 20/80 OD and 20/25 OS. She had early nuclear cataracts in both eyes. There is a red, round hole at the right macula.

PATHOGENESIS

- Degeneration of the vitreous with traction on the macula is thought to lead to macular holes. They presumably occur at the fovea since this is the thinnest part of the retina.
- They usually represent a pulling open (dehiscence) at the fovea, with no loss of tissue.
- There is still debate about the exact mechanism.
- There are different stages of hole formation that can be identified clinically. Stage 1 holes are also called "impending" holes. They appear as a small yellow dot or ring in the macula. Stage 2 holes are frank dehiscences of the fovea, with the hole less than 400 microns in diameter. Stage 3 holes are larger than 400 microns. Stage 4 holes are associated with a posterior vitreous detachment.

DIAGNOSIS

- The appearance of the hole is usually characteristic (see Fig. 10-30).
- Early-stage holes may be difficult to diagnose. Fluorescein angiography and ocular coherence tomography (OCT) may be helpful.

DIFFERENTIAL DIAGNOSIS

- Pseudohole of the macula.
- Macular cyst.

TREATMENT

- Macular holes may be treated with vitrectomy and instillation of intraocular gas tamponade.
- Surgery closes 80 to 90% of holes.
- Visual results of surgery are usually modest, with most patients recovering 2 or more lines of visual acuity.

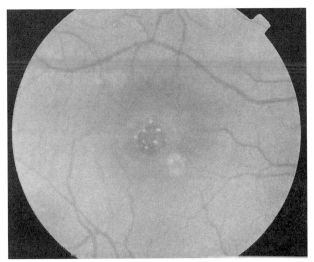

FIGURE 10-30 Macular hole. The optic disk is not visible. There is a large hole in the macula. There are yellow spots from retinal pigment epithelial change within the hole. There is a cuff of localized retinal detachment around the hole. There is a round area of hypopigmentation of the retinal pigment epithelium infero-temporal (down and to the right in this photograph) to the cuff of subretinal fluid. (See Color Plate.)

BIBLIOGRAPHY

Gass JDM. Reappraisal of biomicroscopic classification of stages of development of a macular hole. *Am J Ophthalmol* 119:752,1995.

Kelly NE, Wendel RT. Vitreous surgery for idiopathic macular holes; results of a pilot study. *Arch Ophthalmol* 109:654,1991.

CYSTOID MACULAR EDEMA

CASE 28

A 73-year-old man had uneventful cataract surgery OS, and recovered vision of 20/20 at 2 weeks postoperatively. Over the next few weeks, his vision declined. When he saw his surgeon at 6 weeks, vision OS was 20/60. The surgeon found nothing abnormal except for a slight yellow spot at the macula. A fluorescein angiogram demonstrated cystoid macular edema. There was also fluorescein leakage into the optic disk.

PATHOGENESIS

- The pathogenesis of cystoid macular edema is not clear.
- It occurs in about 0.5 to 1% of uncomplicated cataract operations.

- It may also occur after other eye surgery, with uveitis, or with retinal vascular disease.
- There is leakage of fluid from retinal vessels. This fluid accumulates in the outer plexiform layer of the retina, forming cysts at and around the fovea in a characteristic petaloid pattern. Vessels in the optic disk often show leakage as well.

DIAGNOSIS

- In some cases, the characteristic cystoid pattern at the macula may be visible clinically.
- Fluorescein angiography demonstrates the leakage and petal-shaped cystic pattern (see Fig. 10-31).

DIFFERENTIAL DIAGNOSIS

- Diabetic macular edema
- Macular hole
- Age-related macular degeneration
- Epiretinal membrane

TREATMENT

- Many cases of postcataract cystoid macular edema resolve spontaneously.
- Treatment with topical steroids and nonsteroidal anti-inflammatory agents may be helpful.
- Peribulbar steroid injections may be helpful if topical therapy fails.

BIBLIOGRAPHY

Gass JDM, Norton EWD. Cystoid macular edema and papilledema following cataract extraction; a fluorescein fundoscopic and angiographic study. *Arch Ophthalmol* 76:646,1966.

EPIRETINAL MEMBRANES

CASE 29

- A 40-year-old executive complained of several months of decreased vision and distortion in his right eye. Examination disclosed a posterior vitreous detachment in that eye. There were subtle folds in the retina at the macula, and there was white tissue overlying the macula.

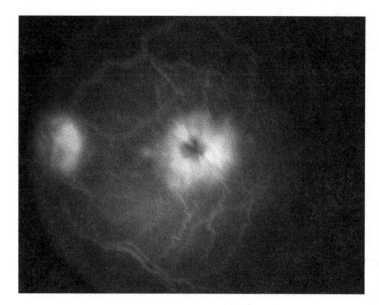

FIGURE 10-31 Cystoid macular edema. A late frame from a fluorescein angiogram in a patient with cystoid macular edema following cataract surgery. There is hyperfluorescence (white) from leakage of fluorescein into the cystic spaces around the central macula, forming a petaloid pattern. Note that the optic disk also shows hyperfluorescence from dye leakage.

PATHOGENESIS

- Epiretinal membranes may be caused by posterior vitreous detachment, retinal holes or retinal detachment, uveitis, injuries, or retinal vascular disease.
- The membranes are formed by glial cells and/or metaplastic retinal pigment epithelial cells, and collagen fibers.
- Breaks in the internal limiting membrane of the retina may allow glial cells to migrate onto the retinal surface.
- Full-thickness breaks in the retina allow retinal pigment epithelial cells to migrate onto the retinal surface, where they may undergo metaplasia into fibroblast-like cells.
- Contraction of the membranes distorts the retina.
- In some cases, there may be a hole over the fovea. This usually results in good vision. This "pseudohole" may be mistaken for a true hole in the macula (see Idiopathic Macular Hole).

DIAGNOSIS

- The diagnosis can usually be made on ophthalmoscopy. Fine retinal folds and epiretinal white tissue are seen (see Fig. 10-32).
- Occasionally fluorescein angiography or OCT is useful.

DIFFERENTIAL DIAGNOSIS

- Cystoid macular edema
- Cotton wool spots
- Age-related macular degeneration

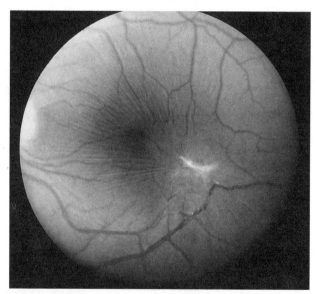

FIGURE 10-32 Epiretinal membrane. An idiopathic epiretinal membrane. There is white fibrous tissue on the retinal surface infero-temporal to the macula. There are numerous retinal folds from traction. The infero-temporal vein is distorted from traction. (See Color Plate.)

- Central serous retinopathy
- Macular hole

TREATMENT

- In cases with significant visual reduction, vitrectomy with peeling of the epiretinal membrane may be useful.
- About 70% of cases have modest visual recovery (2 lines or more) with vitrectomy.

BIBLIOGRAPHY

Michels RG. Vitreous surgery for macular pucker. *Am J Ophthalmol* 92:628,1981.
Wise GN. Clinical features of idiopathic preretinal macular fibrosis. *Am J Ophthalmol* 79:363,1975.

TUMORS

CHOROIDAL MELANOMA

CASE 30

A 50-year-old nurse's aide had an intravenous solution splash into her eyes when a bottle was dropped. She had mild burning, and the employee health service referred her to ophthalmology. Examination disclosed 20/20 acuity OU. Anterior segments were normal. Dilated fundus examination revealed normal OD, but showed a large pigmented peripheral mass under the retina OS.

PATHOGENESIS

• Choroidal melanomas arise from choroidal melanocytes. The pathogenesis is unclear.

DIAGNOSIS

• Patients should be referred to a very experienced clinician, usually an ocular oncologist, as the diagnosis is made mainly based on the fundus appearance on indirect ophthalmoscopy. (See Fig. 10-33) Biopsy is usually not done. Ultrasonography and fluorescein angiography may be helpful.

DIFFERENTIAL DIAGNOSIS

• Choroidal metastasis
• Choroidal hemangioma
• Choroidal hemorrhage
• Choroidal nevus

TREATMENT

• Proton beam irradiation or episcleral radioactive plaque therapy is performed in most cases. Enucleation (removal of the eye) is usually reserved for very large lesions.
• The prognosis depends primarily on the size, location, and cell type of the tumor.

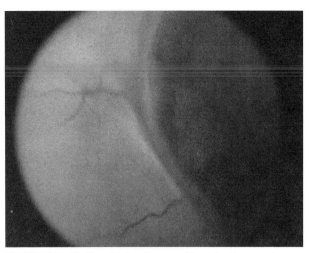

FIGURE 10-33 Choroidal melanoma. There is a large melanoma in the right-hand portion of the photograph. There is an exudative detachment of the retina seen in the left-hand side secondary to leakage from the melanoma. (See Color Plate.)

BIBLIOGRAPHY

Mukai S, Gragoudas ES. Diagnosis of choroidal melanoma. In: Albert DM, Jakobiec FA, eds: *Principles and Practice of Ophthalmology*, 2nd ed. Philadelphia: WB Saunders, 2000, p 3665.
Shields JA, Shields CL. *Intraocular Tumors. A Text and Atlas.* Philadelphia: WB Saunders, 1992, p 117.

RETINOBLASTOMA

CASE 31

A grandmother noticed that her 2-month-old grandchild had an abnormal pupil, "like a cat." The mother had noticed that the same eye occasionally turned in. The pediatrician confirmed leukocoria (a white pupil) and could not see the fundus. A pediatric ophthalmologist was consulted. The child did not fix or follow with the involved eye, but did follow a light with the other eye. Esotropia was present. Dilated fundus examination revealed a creamy white mass. Ultrasonography showed a large intraocular mass, with probable calcification within it. There was no family history of retinoblastoma. The eye was enucleated, and histopathologic examination confirmed a retinoblastoma.

PATHOGENESIS

• Retinoblastomas arise when both copies of a tumor suppressor gene, known as the retinoblastoma gene, are absent or abnormal. The tumors are therefore often hereditary (usually bilateral) but may also be sporadic (usually unilateral).

- Hereditary cases may be associated with pinealoma ("trilateral retinoblastoma").

DIAGNOSIS

- History and examination. A very experienced clinician should be involved in diagnosing and treating these tumors. As with choroidal melanoma, the clinical appearance is very important in making the diagnosis (see Fig. 10-34). Ultrasonography or computed tomography scan may show calcification in the tumor, which is very helpful in confirming the diagnosis. Biopsy is usually not done.

DIFFERENTIAL DIAGNOSIS

- Congenital cataract
- Retinopathy of prematurity
- Coat's disease
- Persistent hyperplastic primary vitreous
- Toxocariasis

TREATMENT

- Large tumors, especially in unilateral cases, are usually treated by enucleation. Smaller lesions may be treated by radiation, cryopexy, or occasionally laser.

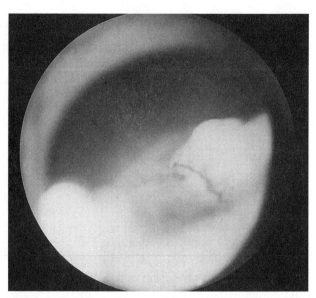

FIGURE 10-34 Retinoblastoma. The eye is more than half filled with a creamy white vascularized mass. (See Color Plate.)

- Chemotherapy may be used to shrink tumors prior to treatment with these modalities.

BIBLIOGRAPHY

Shields JA, Shields CL. *Intraocular Tumors. A Text and Atlas.* Philadelphia: WB Saunders, 1992, p 305.

11 NEURO-OPHTHALMOLOGY

Michael S. Lee

PUPILS

- Pupillary evaluation involves notation of pupil size, direct and consensual response, the swinging flashlight test, and in some cases accommodation.
- Normal size: 2–7 mm and equal in size.
- Evaluate pupil response to a bright light with the patient looking in the distance in a dimly lit room. Both pupils normally react briskly when light is shined in either eye (direct response: same eye, consensual response: opposite eye).
- See Relative *Afferent Pupil* Defect below for swinging flashlight test.
- Pupillary response to accommodation does not need to be tested unless the response to light is sluggish. Asking the patient to fix on a *near* target elicits pupil constriction in normal patients. A brisk response with accommodation and a sluggish response to direct light is known as *light near dissociation* (Fig. 11-1). Causes of light near dissociation are listed in Table 11-1.

ANISOCORIA

- Anisocoria refers to asymmetric pupil sizes.
- A general approach to anisocoria is outlined in Fig. 11-2.

TABLE 11-1 Causes of Light Near Dissociation

Argyll Robertson pupil
Adie's tonic pupil
Dorsal midbrain syndrome
Aberrant regeneration following third nerve palsy
Total optic nerve dysfunction
Diabetes

- The smaller pupil is abnormal if anisocoria is more obvious in the dark and the larger pupil is abnormal if anisocoria is greater in the light. It may be difficult to distinguish if the asymmetry varies between light and dark. Photographing or measuring the pupils with a ruler can quantify the difference.

PHYSIOLOGIC ANISOCORIA

CASE 1

A 32-year-old woman, when putting on makeup, noticed that her left pupil was larger than her right. Her visual acuities were 20/20 in each eye. She had no ptosis and her extraocular motility was normal. The left pupil was consistently 1 mm larger than the right in both light and dark. Both pupils reacted briskly to light and there was no afferent pupil defect.

CLINICAL FEATURES

- Physiologic anisocoria occurs in approximately 20% of normal individuals and is asymptomatic.
- Rarely will the difference in pupil size be greater than 1 mm. The inequality appears the same in both light and dark situations.
- The anisocoria may vary from day to day and may on occasion alternate sides.

DIAGNOSIS AND DIFFERENTIAL

- Diagnosis is made clinically.
- Differential includes Horner syndrome, unilateral tonic pupil, and trauma.

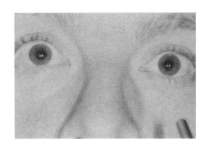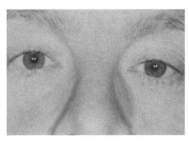

FIGURE 11-1 Light near dissociation. *Left panel*: Poor pupillary response to light with distant viewing. The light source can be seen in the lower right corner. *Right panel*: Pupils constricted to near stimulus.

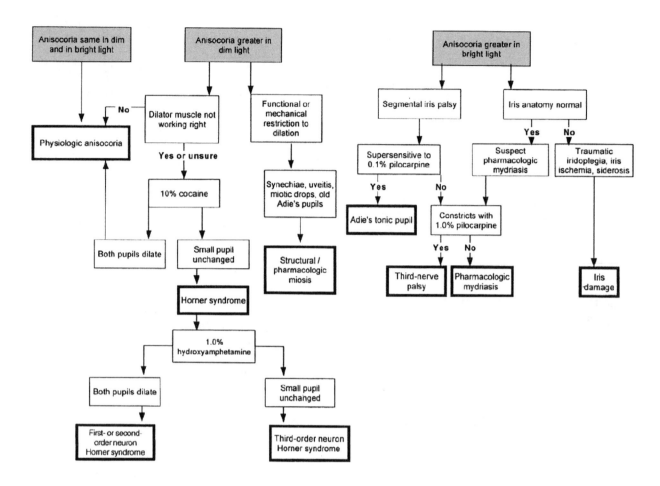

FIGURE 11-2 Flowchart for evaluation of anisocoria. (Reprinted, with permission, from *Neuro-Ophthalmology*. Basic and Clinical Science Course. Section 5. San Francisco: American Academy of Ophthalmology, 2001.)

• If any doubt exists about ptosis of the upper lid in the eye with the smaller pupil, it is reasonable to perform cocaine testing to rule out Horner syndrome.

TREATMENT

• Reassurance.

HORNER SYNDROME

CASE 2

A 59-year-old previously healthy man had noticed 5 weeks prior that his right upper eyelid was drooping, accompanied by a dull ache along the right side of his neck. He denied recent trauma. Visual acuities were 20/20 in each eye. He had 1.5 mm ptosis of the right upper lid. In room light, his right pupil was slightly smaller than the left. This disparity became more obvious in dim light (Fig. 11-3). Axial magnetic resonance imaging

(MRI) demonstrated a comma-shaped, T2-weighted hyperintensity along the right internal carotid artery consistent with dissection (Fig. 11-4).

PATHOPHYSIOLOGY

• Horner syndrome results from an interruption of any one of three neurons in the oculosympathetic chain (Fig. 11-5).
• The 1st order neuron begins in the hypothalamus and descends through the ipsilateral brain stem and spinal cord to synapse with the 2nd order neuron at the ciliospinal center of Budge located from C8 to T2.
• The 2nd order neuron travels over the ipsilateral apex of the lung and subclavian artery and ascends in the neck to synapse with the 3rd order neuron in the superior cervical ganglion located at the bifurcation of the internal and external carotid arteries (at the posterior angle of the mandible).

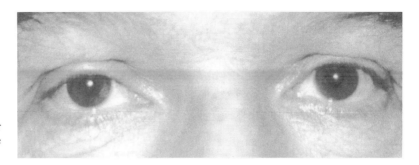

FIGURE 11-3 Horner syndrome. The right upper lid is ptotic and the right pupil is smaller than the left.

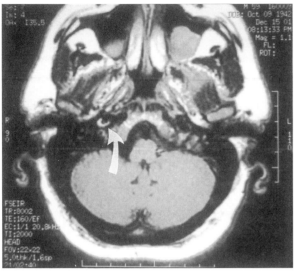

FIGURE 11-4 Axial MRI of the patient in Fig. 11-3. There is a comma-shaped T2 hyperintensity consistent with a right internal carotid artery dissection (*arrow*).

- Postganglionic sweat fibers to the ipsilateral face follow the external carotid artery. The remaining fibers ascend in a plexus surrounding the internal carotid. In the cavernous sinus, fibers destined for the iris join the abducens nerve (VI) briefly and then travel with the first division of the trigeminal nerve (V_1) before entering the eye with the long ciliary nerves. Fibers to the upper and lower lids join the oculomotor nerve (III) in the cavernous sinus.

CLINICAL FEATURES

- Classic triad: unilateral ptosis, miosis, and facial anhidrosis.
- Upper lid is slightly lower (ptosis) and the lower lid is slightly higher (reverse ptosis) giving the illusion of a retracted eye (pseudoenophthalmos).
- Anisocoria is greatest within the first 5 seconds of turning off the lights since the affected pupil does not dilate as quickly as the normal one (dilation lag).

- A smooth plastic object may slide more easily on the affected, dry side of the face than the normal contralateral one. Anhidrosis may be absent with lesions distal to the carotid bifurcation.
- Other clinical findings of disrupted sympathetic input include ipsilateral conjunctival hyperemia, reduced intraocular pressure (IOP), and nasal stuffiness. These may be present initially.
- The affected iris may appear lighter in color (iris heterochromia) in congenital or longstanding Horner syndrome.

DIAGNOSIS AND DIFFERENTIAL

- The diagnosis of Horner syndrome is confirmed with 10% cocaine drops. Cocaine blocks reuptake of norepinephrine at the neuromuscular junction leading to dilation in the normal eye. One drop of cocaine is placed in both eyes followed by another 5 minutes later. After 40 minutes, the affected pupil fails to dilate symmetrically with the normal one. The test is considered positive if there is 1 mm or more difference in the pupil size.
- Forty-eight hours after cocaine testing, hydroxyamphetamine 1% drops can be used to localize the lesion to preganglionic (1st or 2nd order) or postganglionic (3rd order) neurons. Hydroxyamphetamine causes release of norepinephrine, which stimulates the pupillary dilator muscle. Drop administration is the same as for cocaine. In 1st or 2nd order Horner syndrome both pupils dilate. The pupil does not dilate as well as the normal one (1 mm or greater anisocoria) in 3rd order neuron lesions. Causes of Horner syndrome are listed in Table 11-2.
- 1st order Horner syndrome is often accompanied by other neurologic findings such as sensory or motor signs, homonymous hemianopia, and eye movement abnormalities.
- Associated head or neck pain mandates an axial MRI of the neck to evaluate for carotid dissection. Carotid dissections may also be associated with an abnormal taste in the mouth (dysgeusis).

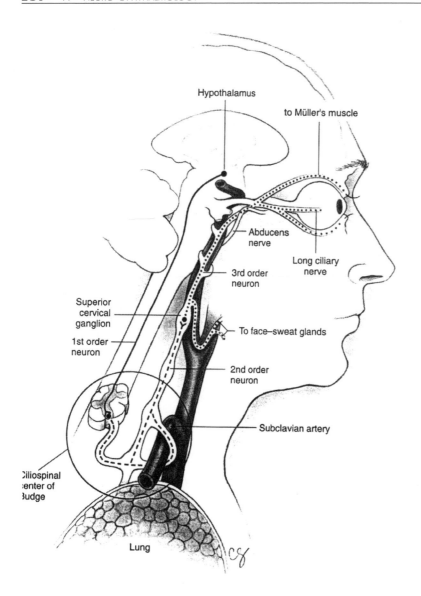

Hypothalamus

to Müller's muscle

Abducens nerve

Long ciliary nerve

3rd order neuron

Superior cervical ganglion

To face–sweat glands

1st order neuron

2nd order neuron

Subclavian artery

Ciliospinal center of Budge

Lung

FIGURE 11-5 Anatomy of the three-neuron sympathetic chain to the pupil. (Reprinted, with permission, from *Neuro-Ophthalmology. Basic and Clinical Science Course. Section 5.* San Francisco: American Academy of Ophthalmology, 2001.)

TABLE 11-2   Causes of Horner Syndrome

1st order	Brain stem stroke
	Demyelination
	Tumor
2nd order	Apical lung tumor (Pancoast)
	Thyroid mass
	Central line placement
	Neck trauma or surgery
	Lymphadenopathy
	Spinal anesthesia
3rd order	Cluster headache
	Carotid artery dissection
	Cavernous sinus tumor
	Idiopathic

- A chest roentgenogram or computed tomography (CT) scan is recommended with a history of smoking to rule out a Pancoast tumor.
- The main differential in young children includes birth trauma and neuroblastoma. Without a history of birth trauma, neuroimaging from the neck to the abdomen should be performed to evaluate the sympathetic chain. Urine screening of vanillymandelic acid and homovanillic acid is recommended.

TREATMENT

- Treatment is based on the cause of the Horner syndrome.

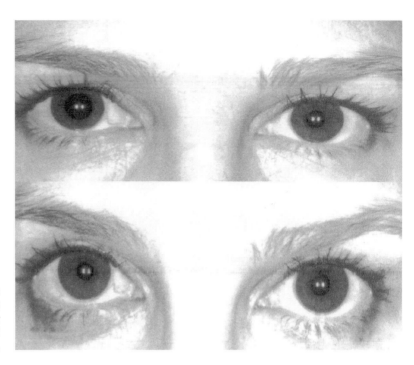

FIGURE 11-6 Adie's tonic pupil. *Top panel*: The right pupil is larger than the left. *Bottom panel*: Example of denervation supersensitivity. After instillation of dilute pilocarpine, the right pupil has constricted, but the left remains the same size.

ADIE'S TONIC PUPIL

CASE 3

A 37-year-old woman began to note while reading that the vision in the right eye was "strained" and "similar to when your eye is dilated." Two weeks later her sister noted that the patient had a dilated right pupil. She had a mild right supraorbital headache. Her visual acuities were 20/20 each eye. She could not read small letters with the right eye when compared to the left. She had no ptosis and her motility was full. The right pupil was larger than the left and did not react well to direct or consensual light. She had a brisk reaction to near stimulus with -slow redilation. After the instillation of 1/8% pilocarpine, the right pupil constricted and the left remained the same (Fig. 11-6).

PATHOPHYSIOLOGY

- The short ciliary nerves originate in the ciliary ganglion and innervate the pupillary sphincter muscle (pupil constriction) and the ciliary muscles (accommodation).
- Damage to the ciliary ganglion leads to pupillary dilation and abnormal accommodation.
- As the short ciliary nerve fibers regrow, they do not uniformly reinnervate the iris, causing segmental contraction separated by areas of sphincter paralysis. Fibers destined for the ciliary muscles may aberrantly innervate the iris instead, leading to significant pupillary constriction to a near stimulus (light near dissociation).

CLINICAL FEATURES

- More common in women and usually unilateral (1% per year risk to other eye).
- May have difficulty with near work but more commonly asymptomatic.
- Initially the involved pupil is larger, but after several years it may become smaller than the normal one.
- Light near dissociation of Adie tonic pupil is present with slow redilation of the pupil after near stimulus.
- Magnified view of pupil margin may reveal irregular constriction and immobility of the iris sectors.
- A tonic pupil together with absent deep tendon reflexes is known as Adie syndrome.

DIAGNOSIS AND DIFFERENTIAL

- The diagnosis is confirmed with dilute (0.125%) pilocarpine. One drop is placed in both eyes, followed by another 5 minutes later. After 40 minutes, the tonic pupil constricts (denervation hypersensitivity) but the normal pupil does not. The tonic pupil may not respond to dilute pilocarpine in the first several weeks.
- Syphilis and, rarely, diabetes can cause bilateral light near dissociation and absent deep tendon reflexes.

TREATMENT

- Reassurance.
- Some patients may want to use dilute pilocarpine to make the pupils appear equal.

PHARMACOLOGIC

CASE 4

A 37-year-old intensive care unit (ICU) nurse developed blurry vision in the right eye and a dilated right pupil while on the job. She denied pain. Her acuities were 20/20 in each eye. Color vision and extraocular motility were normal. Her right pupil was 9 mm in diameter and unreactive to direct light or near stimulus. Her left pupil was 4 mm and her response brisk.

CLINICAL FEATURES

- Nurses or anesthesia personnel may work with atropine. Patients may inadvertently touch their eye after scopolamine patch. Other patients intentionally place dilating drops in their eye.
- Vision may be blurred, especially at near.
- A pupil greater than 7 mm in diameter is rarely non-pharmacologic.
- Pharmacologically dilated pupils do not react to light or near stimulus.
- Extraocular motility should be normal.

DIAGNOSIS AND DIFFERENTIAL

- Diagnosis is confirmed with 1% pilocarpine. One drop is placed in both eyes followed by another 5 minutes later. After 40 minutes, the normal pupil constricts. The pharmacologically dilated pupil remains larger (Fig. 11-7).
- A dilated pupil from neurologic causes will always constrict with 1% pilocarpine.

TREATMENT

- Reassurance.
- The pupil should regain reactivity within a week.

RELATIVE AFFERENT PUPIL DEFECT (MARCUS GUNN PUPIL)

PATHOPHYSIOLOGY

- The anatomy of the pupillomotor pathway is illustrated in Fig. 11-8.

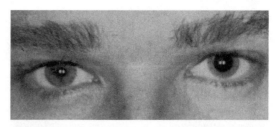
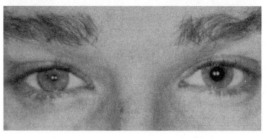

FIGURE 11-7 *Top*: The pharmacologically dilated left pupil is unreactive to direct or consensual light or near stimulus. *Bottom*: After two drops of 1% pilocarpine, the left pupil is still large. Note that the right pupil is extremely miotic.

- The swinging flashlight test: light is shone for 2 seconds in each eye alternately and the pupillary reactions are compared. When light is directed at the normal pupil, both constrict and then enlarge slightly. As the light is swung to the abnormal pupil, there is an asymmetric response.
  - An immediate dilation may occur.
  - Subtle afferent defects may constrict initially, followed by enlargement more rapidly than the fellow pupil.
  - The asymmetric response represents a *relative* imbalance in the amount of afferent input to the Edinger-Westphal nucleus.

CLINICAL FEATURES

- Reduced vision, abnormal color vision (dyschromatopsia), and a visual field defect are often present with ipsilateral optic neuropathy.
- An optic tract lesion may reveal a contralateral homonymous hemianopia and afferent defect (see section on visual field defects in Central Nervous System Disorders).
- Pupils are equal size.

DIAGNOSIS AND DIFFERENTIAL

- Unilateral or asymmetric optic nerve dysfunction.
- Unilateral or asymmetric retinal disease.
- Rarely dense amblyopia and contralateral optic tract lesion.

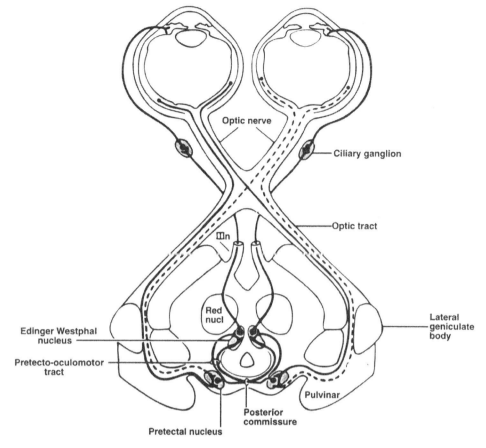

FIGURE 11-8 Pathway of the pupillary light reaction. The signal travels in the optic nerve through the chiasm and along the optic tract. Prior to the lateral geniculate nucleus, it leaves the tract to synapse at the pretectal nucleus. Information is then sent to both the ipsilateral and contralateral Edinger-Westphal nuclei. Finally, the fibers synapse in the ciliary ganglion prior to innervating the ciliary sphincter muscle. (Reprinted, with permission, from *Neuro-Ophthalmology. Basic and Clinical Science Course. Section 5.* San Francisco: American Academy of Ophthalmology, 2001.)

- Cataract and vitreous hemorrhage should not cause an afferent pupil defect (APD).
- MRI of the brain and orbits with gadolinium may reveal the source.

TREATMENT

- Treatment is directed at the underlying cause.

ARGYLL ROBERTSON PUPIL

PATHOPHYSIOLOGY

- The anatomic location of the lesion is not known.

CLINICAL FEATURES

- Slightly irregular pupils that do not react to light well.
- Brisk near response.
- C. Argyll Robertson originally described the pupils as small; however, numerous cases of mid-dilated pupils have been reported.
- Deep tendon reflexes may be absent.

DIAGNOSIS AND DIFFERENTIAL

- Rapid plasma reagent (RPR) and venereal disease research laboratory (VDRL) are screening tests for syphilis. May be negative in neurosyphilis.
- Fluorescent treponemal antibody absorption (FTA-ABS) and microhemagglutinin assay for *Treponema pallidum* (MHA-TP) are more specific for syphilis and are positive in neurosyphilis.
- If the above tests are positive, lumbar puncture should be performed. The cerebrospinal fluid (CSF) may reveal an elevated white blood cell count and protein and positive CSF VDRL.
- Differential includes dorsal midbrain syndrome, bilateral tonic pupils, and diabetes.

TREATMENT

- Intravenous (IV) aqueous penicillin should be given for at least 10 days.
- Unclear whether to give subsequent intramuscular procaine penicillin.

OPTIC NERVE

- The clinical characteristics of optic nerve dysfunction (optic neuropathy) of any cause include visual loss, color vision loss (dyschromatopsia), visual field defect, relative afferent pupil defect (Marcus Gunn pupil), and an optic nerve that may appear normal or abnormal.

OPTIC NEURITIS

CASE 5

A 27-year-old previously healthy woman presented, having become aware of progressive blurring in the vision of her left eye 5 days prior. She noted tenderness and pain with eye movement. The right eye was completely normal. In the left eye, the visual acuity was 20/100 with markedly abnormal color vision. She was found to have a left afferent pupil defect and a central scotoma on visual field testing (Fig. 11-9). Results of her dilated fundus examination were normal. An MRI revealed an abnormal T2 signal and gadolinium enhancement of the left optic nerve (Fig. 11-10). Multiple T2 white matter lesions were present (Fig. 11-11).

PATHOPHYSIOLOGY

- Idiopathic, inflammatory response leads to breakdown of myelin sheaths. Conduction of visual information is then slowed.

CLINICAL FEATURES

- Average age is early thirties with a female-to-male ratio of 3:1. Incidence is 1–6/100,000 per year.

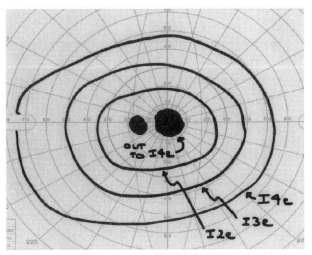

FIGURE 11-9 Goldmann visual field demonstrating a central scotoma of the left eye.

- Vision loss is subacute and progressive over the course of 3–4 days associated with pain exacerbated by touching the eye or moving it (92%).
- Optic nerve appearance is normal in two thirds of cases and swollen in one third.
- The visual nadir occurs by 7 days and the vision begins to improve by 4 weeks (96%).
- Approximately 30% will have a recurrence in either eye.
- There is a strong association with multiple sclerosis (MS).
- Children may have an antecedent febrile illness and develop bilateral optic neuritis.

DIAGNOSIS AND DIFFERENTIAL

- Diagnosis is made clinically. In the typical patient (young adult, subacute optic nerve dysfunction, painful eye movements), blood work and lumbar puncture are not indicated.

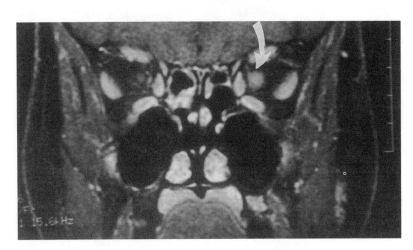

FIGURE 11-10 Post gadolinium, coronal MRI of the orbit shows enlargement and enhancement of the left optic nerve (*arrow*).

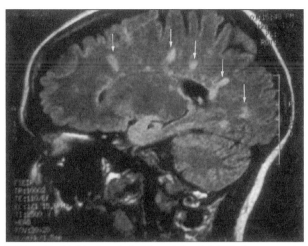

FIGURE 11-11 Saggital T2-weighted MRI demonstrating periventricular white matter lesions (*arrows*).

- MRI is not necessary for diagnosis but is helpful for prognostication. With normal MRI findings, approximately 20% of patients will develop MS in 14 years compared with 88% of patients with T2 white matter lesions.
- A patient with a swollen optic nerve should be observed for lipid accumulation in the macula (neuroretinitis). The main causes are cat scratch, Lyme disease, and syphilis. Neuroretinitis is not associated with MS.
- Atypical features are older age, vision loss for more than 1 week, no improvement by 1 month, and lack of pain. Suggested work-up includes RPR, FTA-ABS, Lyme titer, angiotensin-converting enzyme (ACE), anti-nuclear antibody (ANA), erythrocyte sedimentation rate (ESR), chest roentgenogram, and MRI of the brain and orbits with gadolinium. A lumbar puncture and mitochondrial analysis for Leber's optic neuropathy can be considered.
- The differential diagnosis includes ischemic optic neuropathy (see below), infection (Lyme disease, syphilis, tuberculosis, cat scratch), inflammation (sarcoid, lupus), and compression of the optic nerve.

TREATMENT

- The final visual outcome in optic neuritis is unaffected by treatment, and spontaneous recovery is typical (90% reach 20/40 acuity).
- IV methylprednisolone 1 gram per day for 3 days followed by oral prednisone taper for 14 days has been shown to restore vision more quickly than placebo but to have no effect on final visual outcome. IV corticosteroids have also been shown to reduce the risk of developing MS in the first 2 years. Consider them in patients requiring quick recovery (e.g., monocular patient, airplane pilot) or with T2 white matter lesions.

- Oral steroids alone are contraindicated and may cause an increase in the recurrence of optic neuritis.
- Weekly intramuscular interferon Beta-1a has been demonstrated to reduce the risk of developing MS following an attack of optic neuritis in patients with at least two T2 white matter lesions.

ANTERIOR ISCHEMIC OPTIC NEUROPATHY (AION)

NONARTERITIC

CASE 6

A 64-year-old man with diabetes and hypertension noted sudden, painless vision loss in the left eye that had begun 2 days prior. He denied seeing any positive visual phenomena. His visual acuities were 20/20 right eye and 20/100 left. The right was normal. He missed half of the color plates with the left eye and had a left afferent pupil defect. A left inferotemporal altitudinal visual field defect was found on visual field testing (Fig. 11-12). The left optic disk was swollen with splinter hemorrhages (Fig. 11-13). The right optic disk had almost no cup. He had no other systemic complaints, and his ESR was 4 mm/hr.

PATHOPHYSIOLOGY

- Presumed insufficiency in the circulation to the anterior (intraocular) portion of the optic nerve.
- The exact pathogenesis is unknown, but it has been postulated that microvascular disease and a crowded optic nerve may result in poor perfusion pressure.

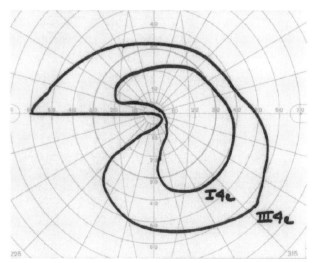

FIGURE 11-12 Left inferior altitudinal defect on Goldmann visual field.

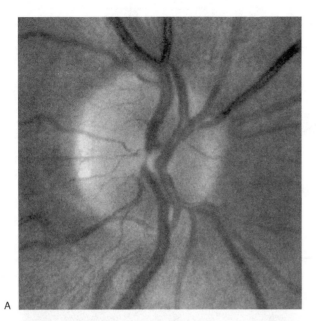

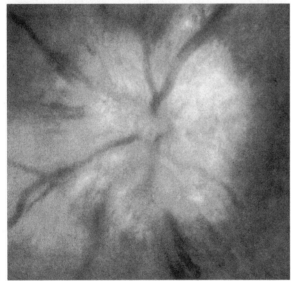

FIGURE 11-13 A. Right optic nerve is normal and has a small cup-to-disk ratio. B. Nonarteritic ischemic optic neuropathy with a swollen left optic nerve associated with hemorrhages.

- Nocturnal hypotension and obstructive sleep apnea may play a role.

CLINICAL FEATURES

- Average age is mid-sixties with slight male predominance. Incidence is 2.3/100,000 per year in patients more than 50 years old.
- Diabetes and hypertension are associated, but carotid disease is not.

- It is a painless (90%) optic neuropathy involving the intraocular portion of the optic nerve. The optic disk by definition is always swollen.
- Visual nadir usually occurs within 3 days. Improvement can occur, with 43% regaining 3 lines or more.
- Approximately 30% will develop contralateral eye involvement, but recurrence in the same is eye is extremely rare.

DIAGNOSIS AND DIFFERENTIAL

- The diagnosis is made clinically. The optic nerve must be swollen, and the fellow optic disk often has a small cup-to-disk ratio.
- There is significant overlap with patients with optic neuritis, and occasionally the differentiation is difficult in the early stages.
- Giant cell arteritis can cause anterior ischemic optic neuropathy and needs to be ruled out (see below in Arteric section).

TREATMENT

- There is no treatment or prophylactic measure to prevent contralateral eye involvement.
- Optic nerve sheath fenestration, aspirin, steroids, and hyperbaric oxygen therapy have been studied and are not effective.

ARTERITIC

CASE 7

A 75-year-old woman presented with a one-day history of painless vision loss in the right eye. Three weeks prior she had experienced a 5-minute episode of horizontal, binocular double vision. She admitted to an unintentional 15 lb weight loss in the past 6 weeks and unexplained fever and malaise. Not normally a headache sufferer, she had had a new right-sided headache for the past 2 weeks. She denied jaw claudication. Her vision was no light perception in the right eye and 20/20 in the left. She had an amaurotic (nonreactive) pupil on the right. Her left eye was normal with a cup-to-disk ratio of 0.5. The right disk was swollen and chalky white (Fig. 11-14). Her ESR was 102 mm/hour. Right temporal artery biopsy revealed an occluded lumen with giant cells in the artery wall (Fig. 11-15).

PATHOPHYSIOLOGY

- Inflammation of the ophthalmic and posterior ciliary arteries leads to narrowed lumen and thrombosis.

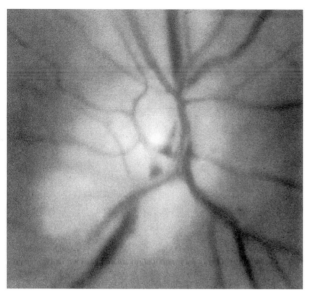

FIGURE 11-14 Arteritic anterior ischemic optic neuropathy. The right optic nerve is swollen and chalky white.

CLINICAL FEATURES

- Female predominance (3:1), and most patients are Caucasian.
- May have premonitory transient monocular blindness or double vision.
- May be accompanied by systemic symptoms (jaw claudication, myalgias, weight loss, headache, neck pain, scalp tenderness, malaise, fever).
- Associated with polymyalgia rheumatica.
- Extremely unusual in a patient under 55. Most patients are 70+.

DIAGNOSIS AND DIFFERENTIAL

- The presence of systemic symptoms and an elevated ESR (>47 mm Hg) or C-reactive protein (>2.45 mg/dl) in a patient older than 55 are suggestive of giant cell arteritis.
- The gold standard is temporal artery biopsy looking for epithelioid cells, thrombosis, and disruption of the internal elastic lamina. The presence of giant cells is not mandatory.

TREATMENT

- Prednisone (60–100 mg/day) is used to prevent damage to the other eye.
- Steroids are then tapered by following the ESR and symptoms.
- Methotrexate may be used as a steroid-sparing agent.

COMPRESSIVE OPTIC NEUROPATHY

CASE 8

An 89-year-old woman with a history of coronary artery disease and hypertension complained of a gradual blur in the left eye for 11 months. She had documented 20/30 vision one year ago. Her visual acuity was 20/25 in the right eye and 20/400 in the left. She could identify the colors of large objects accurately with the left eye but felt they looked less vibrant when compared with the right. There was increased resistance when pushing on the eye. She had a left afferent pupil defect and a

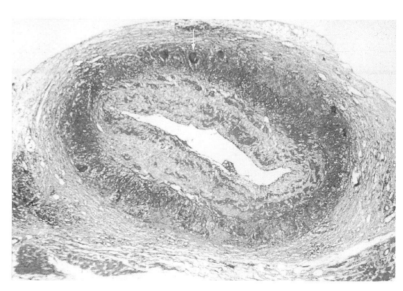

FIGURE 11-15 Light microscopic cross section of right temporal artery. The lumen is narrowed and a giant cell is seen in the wall (*arrow*).

temporal island of visual field. Her left optic nerve was pale with a large cup-to-disk ratio.

CLINICAL FEATURES

- No age or gender predilection.
- Slowly progressive vision loss is common, although acutely expansive lesions may lead to sudden vision loss (e.g., aneurysm, lymphangioma).
- Proptosis, headache, loss of smell, or other cranial neuropathies may be present. Gaze-evoked amaurosis fugax is a classic symptom of optic nerve sheath meningioma.
- The optic nerve may be pale and is typically not swollen.

DIAGNOSIS AND DIFFERENTIAL

- Neuroimaging is mandatory if a compressive lesion is suspected.
- Lesions of the brain and orbits are best imaged with magnetic resonance (MRI). Gadolinium is imperative since some lesions (e.g., meningioma) are isointense to brain and difficult to see until they enhance with gadolinium. Fat-saturated, thin-section MRI of the orbit with axial and coronal views should be obtained.
- A CT scan may demonstrate calcification in the lesion or any changes to orbital bones.
- Compressive lesions of the optic nerve are listed in Table 11-3.

TREATMENT

- Treatment is directed at relieving compression on the optic nerve. Visual recovery is variable depending on lesion type and duration of compression. For example, when pituitary adenomas are resected, visual recovery

TABLE 11-3 Optic Nerve Compressive Lesions

Orbital	Optic nerve glioma
	Optic nerve sheath meningioma
	Schwannoma
	Cavernous hemangioma
	Metastasis
	Invasion from sinus tumor
	Orbital lymphoma
Intracranial	Meningioma—olfactory groove, sphenoid wing, parasellar
	Pituitary adenoma
	Aneurysm—carotid, circle of Willis
	Craniopharyngioma
	Fibrous dysplasia

is often dramatic. In contrast, resection of meningiomas rarely results in visual improvement.

TRAUMATIC OPTIC NEUROPATHY

CASE 9

A 19-year-old woman was a driver without a seat belt in a head-on collision. She struck the steering wheel and sustained multiple bilateral orbital fractures. She was intubated and sedated for 3 days. After regaining awareness, she complained of poor vision in the right eye. Acuities were no light perception right eye and 20/20 left. She had a right pupil unreactive to direct light, but a brisk consensual response. There was an afferent pupil defect. Findings of dilated fundus examination were normal in both eyes.

PATHOPHYSIOLOGY

- Shearing or stretching of the optic nerve within the confines of the optic canal occurs as the head decelerates and the globe continues forward.
- It has been postulated that swelling occurs leading to compression against the walls of the optic canal.

CLINICAL FEATURES

- Features of an optic neuropathy are present after blunt trauma to the forehead or ipsilateral cheek.
- Trauma may even be minor, and consciousness is not necessarily lost.

DIAGNOSIS AND DIFFERENTIAL

- Thin-section, coronal CT scan of the optic canal to rule out canal fracture or intra-sheath hematoma.
- Differential includes malingering in patients with secondary gain, preexisting visual loss, and traumatic retinal detachment.
- Malingerers do not have an afferent pupil defect.

TREATMENT

- Some recovery with optic canal decompression in retrospective studies has been reported, but intervention is considered controversial unless a canal fracture or hematoma with impingement of the nerve is present.

- Megadose or spinal-cord dose steroids may be useful in reducing swelling of the optic nerve. Again, their efficacy has not been proven.

PSEUDOTUMOR CEREBRI (IDIOPATHIC INTRACRANIAL HYPERTENSION)

CASE 10

A 26-year-old obese woman noted loss of vision in both eyes lasting seconds after bending over to pick up a box. She had developed a holocranial headache 2 weeks prior which was variably relieved with Tylenol. She also noted an "ocean sound" in her ears that waxed and waned with her pulse. Her visual acuities were 20/20 in each eye and she had normal color vision. Her visual fields were constricted in both eyes (Fig. 11-16). Both optic disks were extremely swollen with splinter hemorrhages (Fig. 11-17). Findings from MRI of the brain with gadolinium were unremarkable. An opening pressure of 540 cm H_2O was obtained on spinal tap and the constituents were normal. She was begun on acetazolamide 500 mg sequels twice a day for several months with resolution of her symptoms.

PATHOPHYSIOLOGY

- The cause of pseudotumor cerebri is not well understood.
- There may be an endocrinologic role, given the strong relationship to obesity, female gender, and steroid withdrawal.
- Two observations have been made though not universally: increased venous sinus pressure and decreased absorption of cerebrospinal fluid (CSF) by arachnoid villi.

CLINICAL FEATURES

- Average age is in the late twenties to early thirties with a strong female predominance.
- Adult pseudotumor cerebri patients are almost invariably obese. In contrast, weight and gender are not risk factors in pediatric patients.
- There are many alleged associations, but highest likelihood is with steroid withdrawal, hypervitaminosis A, recent weight gain, and tetracycline.

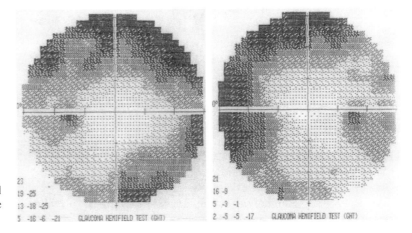

FIGURE 11-16 Automotated (Humphrey) visual field showing peripheral constriction in each eye in a patient with pseudotumor cerebri.

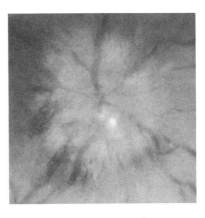
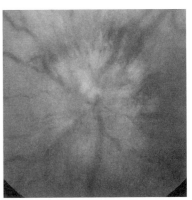

FIGURE 11-17 Bilateral disk edema of the patient in Fig. 11-16.

- Symptoms include headache, transient (seconds) visual obscurations worsened with valsalva, intracranial pulsatile bruit, and double vision.
- Visual field loss is usually peripheral and insidious. Color vision is typically intact.

DIAGNOSIS AND DIFFERENTIAL

- The definition of papilledema is bilateral optic nerve swelling in the setting of *increased intracranial pressure*.
- The diagnostic criteria of pseudotumor cerebri includes the following: (1) signs of increased intracranial pressure (papilledema, headache, nausea, vomiting); (2) normal neuroimaging; (3) spinal tap with a normal CSF constituents and elevated opening pressure (>250 mm H_2O); (4) a normal neurologic examination (excluding unilateral or bilateral 6th nerve palsy).
- Differential diagnosis includes malignant hypertension, intracranial tumor, meningitis, and venous sinus thrombosis.

TREATMENT

- The only adverse sequela of pseudotumor is irreversible vision loss. Patients must be followed with serial automated visual fields and eye examinations.
- As little as 6% weight loss may be beneficial.
- Acetazolamide 500 mg sequel tablets twice a day to begin. This can be increased to a maximum of 3 g/day.
- Lasix in cases of sulfa allergy or intolerance of acetazolamide side effects (paresthesias, kidney stones, nausea).
- Initial severe vision loss may warrant IV methylprednisolone and oral acetazolamide.
- In cases of progressive vision loss despite diuretic therapy, surgical intervention is considered. If headache is significant, lumboperitoneal shunt is recommended. Optic nerve sheath fenestration on the eye with the worse vision is another option.

NUTRITIONAL OPTIC NEUROPATHY

CASE 11

A 45-year-old man presented with a 2-year history of progressive, bilateral blurring of vision. He had a history of Crohn's disease and had undergone several bowel resections. His visual acuities were 20/70 in each eye and his color vision was impaired. His pupils and motility were normal. Visual field testing revealed a scotoma that included his central vision and a blind spot [centrocecal scotoma (Fig. 11-18)] in each eye. The optic disks were slightly pale. Results of MRI of the brain and orbits with gadolinium were normal. Serum B_{12} was markedly reduced. After 3 months of intramuscular B_{12}, the patient's vision improved to 20/30 in both eyes.

PATHOPHYSIOLOGY

- Vitamin B_{12} is found in meat, eggs, and dairy products. It must be ingested, bound to intrinsic factor, and absorbed in the terminal ileum.
- Deficiency of vitamin B_{12} occurs from inadequate dietary intake, lack of or competition for intrinsic factor, or poor ileal absorption.
- Degeneration of the optic nerve myelination that subserves central vision.
- Smoking may worsen the effects of vitamin B_{12} deficiency. It has been postulated that cyanide toxicity may play a role.

CLINICAL FEATURES

- Bilateral, slowly progressive, painless vision loss.
- Dyschromatopsia, centrocecal scotoma.
- Patients at risk for nutritional optic neuropathy include those post–ileocecal resection, alcoholics, those with pernicious anemia, and, rarely, strict vegetarians.
- A peripheral neuropathy (paresthesias, weakness, reduced deep tendon reflexes) may be present.

DIAGNOSIS AND DIFFERENTIAL

- Diagnosis is supported by clinical history.

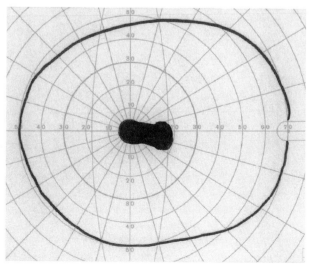

FIGURE 11-18 Centrocecal scotoma on Goldmann visual field.

- Low B$_{12}$ level, high methylmalonic acid, or high homocysteine.
- Megaloblastic anemia may be present.
- Differential includes toxic exposure, Leber's hereditary optic neuropathy, and normal pressure glaucoma.

TREATMENT

- B$_{12}$ supplementation may reverse vision loss.

CENTRAL NERVOUS SYSTEM DISORDERS

VISUAL FIELD DEFECTS

PATHOPHYSIOLOGY

- The visual pathways are illustrated in Fig. 11-19.
- Note that the temporal and nasal retinae are responsible for the nasal and temporal (opposite) visual fields, respectively.
- The nasal fibers (temporal field) cross in the chiasm, which is why lesions of the chiasm classically cause a bitemporal hemianopia. More fibers cross (53%) than do not cross (47%) in the chiasm.
- Posterior to the chiasm, nasal fibers from the contralateral eye and temporal fibers from the ipsilateral eye travel together. Together they represent the contralateral visual field in each eye (e.g., the left optic tract represents the right visual field). They then synapse in the lateral geniculate nucleus (LGN).
- From the LGN the inferior fibers travel forward in Meyer's loop through the temporal lobe before reaching the visual cortex in the occipital lobe. Superior fibers take a more direct route through the parietal lobe.

CLINICAL FEATURES

- In general, visual field defects that respect the vertical meridian (termed hemianopia) are secondary to lesions at or behind the chiasm.
- Defects that respect the horizontal meridian are typically in the eye itself or the prechiasmal optic nerve.
- Visual field characteristics are helpful in localization of lesions. First decide if the visual field defect is monocular or binocular. Monocular field defects are typically due to lesions in front of the chiasm.
- Binocular hemianopias that are on the same side of the vertical meridian are termed *homonymous*. If they

are on opposite sides, they are called either *binasal* or *bitemporal* depending on which fields are involved.
- Homonymous defects should be evaluated for how relatively similar (congruous) they appear to each other (see Fig. 11-20). In the setting of a complete homonymous visual field defect, congruity cannot be assessed. In general, more congruous visual field defects occur from lesions more posterior in the visual pathway. Occipital lesions, for example, tend to be exquisitely congruous.
- Patients with hemianopic defects retain normal visual acuity in each eye.

DIAGNOSIS AND DIFFERENTIAL

- The hallmark of chiasmal compression is a bitemporal hemianopic visual field defect. (See Chiasmal Syndrome below.)
- Tract lesions may present with a contralateral afferent pupil defect. Causes include craniopharyngioma, suprasellar meningioma, and pituitary adenomas.
- Occipital lobe lesions are extremely congruous and may be neurologically isolated. Causes include strokes, vascular malformations, tumors, and trauma.
- Temporal lobe lesions tend to have contralateral visual field defects that are denser superiorly because of Meyer's loop ("pie-in-the-sky"). Lesions may be associated with hallucinations or neurologic deficits (seizures, fluent aphasia, personality change).
- Parietal lobe lesions tend to affect inferior field and may cause an asymmetric optokinetic nystagmus response. Since the parietal lobe is involved in smooth pursuit, the optokinetic response toward the side of the lesion is dampened. They may also be associated with left-sided neglect and memory loss (nondominant) or aphasia and an inability to read or write (dominant).

TREATMENT

- Treatment is directed at the cause of the visual field defect.

CHIASMAL SYNDROME

CASE 12

A 30-year-old woman developed galactorrhea and amenorrhea for 6 months prior to presentation. She denied any visual problems or headache. Her visual acuities were 20/20 in each eye. She had bitemporal visual field defects that respected the vertical meridian. An MRI

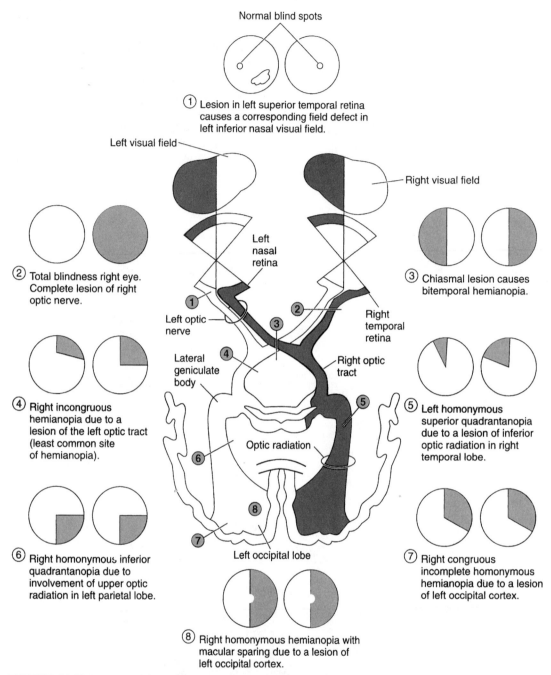

Normal blind spots

① Lesion in left superior temporal retina causes a corresponding field defect in left inferior nasal visual field.

Left visual field

Right visual field

Left nasal retina

② Total blindness right eye. Complete lesion of right optic nerve.

③ Chiasmal lesion causes bitemporal hemianopia.

Left optic nerve

Right temporal retina

④ Right incongruous hemianopia due to a lesion of the left optic tract (least common site of hemianopia).

Lateral geniculate body

Right optic tract

⑤ Left homonymous superior quadrantanopia due to a lesion of inferior optic radiation in right temporal lobe.

Optic radiation

⑥ Right homonymous inferior quadrantanopia due to involvement of upper optic radiation in left parietal lobe.

⑦ Right congruous incomplete homonymous hemianopia due to a lesion of left occipital cortex.

Left occipital lobe

⑧ Right homonymous hemianopia with macular sparing due to a lesion of left occipital cortex.

FIGURE 11-19 Anatomy of the visual pathways and visual field defects due to various lesions. (From Vaughan D, Asbury T, Riordan-Eva P, eds: *General Ophthalmology, 15th ed.* McGraw-Hill, 1999.)

revealed an enlarged sellar mass with suprasellar extension compressing the chiasm. Serum prolactin level was markedly elevated.

PATHOPHYSIOLOGY

• The anatomy of the visual fields is illustrated in Fig. 11-19.

• The chiasm contains the crossing fibers of the nasal retinae from each eye.

• The chiasm is located 10 mm above the sella. Pituitary tumors must therefore be greater than 1 cm in diameter in order to affect the chiasm and are often 3 cm or more.

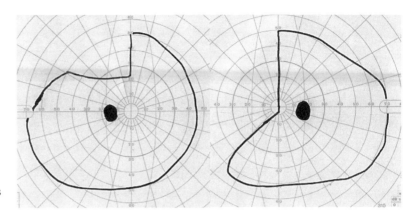

FIGURE 11-20 Incongruous left homonymous hemianopia.

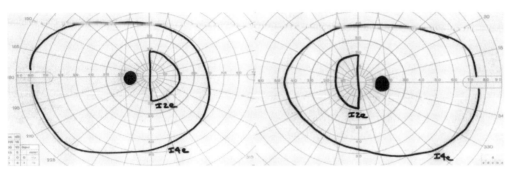

FIGURE 11-21 Bitemporal hemianopia of the smaller, central stimulus (I2e). Goldmann visual field is full to brighter stimulus (I4e).

CLINICAL FEATURES

- Bitemporal hemianopia (Fig. 11-21). A monocular temporal hemianopia localizes to the chiasm as well.
- Visual acuity is typically normal.
- Endocrinological abnormalities such as galactorrhea, amenorrhea, reduced libido, acromegaly, and diabetes insipidus may be present.

DIAGNOSIS AND DIFFERENTIAL

- MRI is the preferred neuroimaging modality for evaluating the chiasm. Magnetic resonance angiography (MRA) should be considered if aneurysms are suspected.
- The most common disorder of the chiasm is from compression (pituitary tumor, meningioma, craniopharyngioma, aneurysm).
- Tilted optic disks in myopia can cause a pseudobitemporal defect. The temporal defect crosses the vertical midline in each eye.
- Ethambutol can cause a chiasmopathy.
- Chiasmal neuritis in MS can also occur.
- Other causes include trauma, lymphocytic hypophysitis, pituitary apoplexy, metastasis, and benign tumors.

TREATMENT

- Some pituitary tumors respond to dopaminergic agonists such as bromocriptine and cabergoline. Others require resection typically via transphenoidal approach through the nose or upper lip. Large tumors may require a craniotomy. Visual prognosis is usually very good.
- Halting ethambutol may or may not resolve the visual field defects.

CORTICAL VISUAL LOSS

CASE 13

A 69-year-old man could not respond or be roused at home. His daughter attempted to resuscitate him until the ambulance arrived 10 minutes later. He was intubated in the field and admitted to the ICU. He was extubated 3 days later when he regained awareness. He noted poor vision in both eyes. Visual acuities were hand movements in each eye. Goldmann visual field testing could not be performed. An MRI of the brain revealed bilateral ischemic changes in the occipital lobes.

PATHOPHYSIOLOGY

- The anatomy of the visual pathways is illustrated in Fig. 11-19.
- Visual acuity is not affected in unilateral damage to the occipital cortex. Bilateral occipital lobe damage is necessary.

CLINICAL FEATURES

- Bilateral complete or almost complete vision loss.
- Patients may deny they are blind (Anton's syndrome).
- Pupils are normal.
- An eye examination finds that structures are normal.

DIAGNOSIS AND DIFFERENTIAL

- If findings from an MRI of the head are normal, consider a positron emission tomography (PET) scan.
- Most commonly, the cause is bilateral occipital lobe stroke (Fig. 11-22).
- Less common causes include trauma, metastases, and tumor.
- Malingering may be difficult to differentiate because pupils are normal in both eyes (see Functional Visual Loss below).

TREATMENT

- Treatment is usually not helpful, but patients should undergo a stroke work-up.

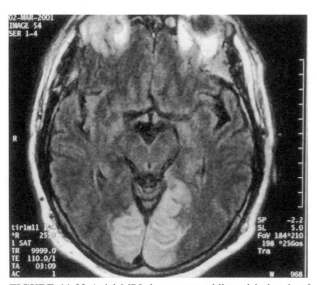

FIGURE 11-22 Axial MRI demonstrates bilateral ischemia of the occipital lobes.

- A low-vision or a blind visual services consultation should be considered.

MIGRAINE

PATHOPHYSIOLOGY

- The trigeminal nerve innervates pain-sensitive arteries, dura, and venous sinuses. Vasodilatation of blood vessels stimulates the trigeminal nerve to relay nociceptive information to higher central nervous system centers where headache is perceived.
- Certain individuals may have a genetic predisposition, with altered thresholds (hyperexcitability) induced by trigger factors.
- Aura may represent a slowly spreading depression of electrical activity across the brain.

CLINICAL FEATURES

- Sixty to 70% are women.
- Auras usually develop before, but may be simultaneous with, headache. Visual symptoms classically begin as scintillating zigzag lines that march around the periphery of a visual field defect but may be manifest as simply blurry vision (Fig. 11-23). Visual disturbances gradually resolve between 15 and 50 minutes.
- Headaches are typically unilateral, throbbing, and on alternate sides with subsequent episodes. Other symptoms include nausea, vomiting, photophobia, phonophobia, and fatigue.
- Rarely, a transient or permanent neurologic deficit may accompany the attack (complicated migraine).
- Family history of migraine is common. There may be a personal history of motion sickness.
- May be precipitated by red wine, chocolate, bright lights, emotional stress, and fatigue.

DIAGNOSIS AND DIFFERENTIAL

- Diagnosis is based on clinical features.
- Work-up, performed for atypical features such as persistent neurologic deficits or pain always on the same side of the head, includes brain MRI with gadolinium.
- Can sometimes be confused with other headache syndromes (cluster, tension, sinus, trigeminal neuralgia).
- Acute angle-closure glaucoma may cause unilateral pain and blurry vision associated with nausea and photophobia. Usually the eye is red and tender to palpation. The pupil is typically mid-dilated and unreactive. (See Chap. 9.)

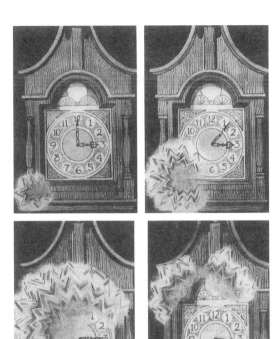

FIGURE 11-23 Artist's rendition of classic scintillating, fortification spectra that march around the periphery of the visual field. [Reprinted from *Survey of Ophthalmology* Vol 33, No 4, 1989, pp 221–236, Hupp et al: Visual disturbances of migraine, © 1989, with permission from Elsevier Science.]

- Amaurosis fugax may present with transient loss of vision lasting approximately 5 minutes.
- Increased intracranial pressure can present with headaches and nausea. Photisms or sparkles of light in the temporal visual field can sometimes be seen. Patients may have bilateral disk edema or even a 6th nerve palsy.

TREATMENT

- Avoid precipitants.
- Nonsteroidal anti-inflammatory agents, ergotamines, or sumatriptan may abort or abbreviate attacks.
- Prophylaxis for frequent headaches includes beta-blockers, calcium channel blockers, and amitriptyline.

FUNCTIONAL VISUAL LOSS (NONPHYSIOLOGIC)

CASE 14

"Ever since the accident the vision has been blurry in my left eye" was the chief complaint of a 45-year-old passenger who was not using a seat-belt when the car was struck from behind. She denied head trauma but was in a soft collar for 2 weeks for "whiplash." Her acuities were 20/20 right eye and counting fingers left eye. She did not have an afferent pupil defect. Results of her entire examination were normal. With both eyes open and the right eye surreptitiously fogged, she was able to read the 20/20 line easily. A small horizontal prism placed in front of the left eye caused both eyes to shift.

CAUSES

- Some patients may deliberately malinger for some external gain.
- Others may exaggerate symptoms to convince the physician something is wrong.
- Stress (poor schoolwork, abuse, family problems) may cause functional vision loss in children.
- True psychiatric illness is rarely the cause.

CLINICAL FEATURES

- Deliberate malingerers may bump into objects as they enter the room. They may discuss lawyers or suggest an accident as the beginning of their problems.
- No ocular abnormalities are found with normal pupils.

DIAGNOSIS AND DIFFERENTIAL

- The most common setting of functional vision loss is when superimposed upon true vision loss.
- The examiner must use "tricks" to deceive the patient into revealing better vision than claimed.
- With profound unilateral vision loss, an afferent pupil defect (APD) should be present.
- An optokinetic tape or drum will induce nystagmus if the true vision is 20/400 or better (Fig. 11-24).
- Visual field testing may reveal unreliable responses or nonexpanding fields to larger stimuli.
- It is possible to surreptitiously blur the "good" eye with trial lenses and the patient reads better because he thinks both eyes are being used.
- If normal vision and visual fields cannot be ultimately demonstrated, then neuroimaging, electroretinogram, or visual-evoked potential testing should be considered to elucidate a cause.
- Differential includes cerebral blindness, amblyopia, traumatic, or Leber hereditary optic neuropathy.

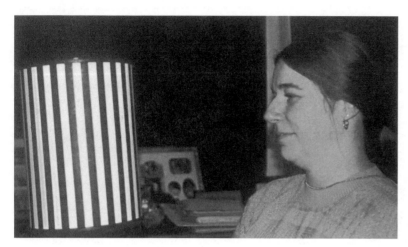

FIGURE 11-24 An optokinetic nystagmus (OKN) drum is rotated slowly in front of a patient claiming poor vision.

TREATMENT

- Patients with functional vision loss should not be confronted or threatened. Instead, reassurance of normal eye examination results should be emphasized. Often patients will return with normally documented visual acuity.
- Psychiatric referral is rarely indicated.

OCULAR MOTILITY

- In the approach to double vision, one must distinguish between monocular (second image disappears only when *affected* eye is covered) and binocular (second image disappears when *either* eye is covered) diplopia.
- Monocular diplopia is an optical phenomenon (cataract, refractive error, retinal disease, corneal changes) and not a neurologic issue.
- Binocular diplopia represents misalignment between the eyes (nerve palsy, extraocular muscle dysfunction or restriction, central nervous system lesions).

TREATMENT

- Simplest treatment of binocular diplopia is to occlude one eye (patch, opaque contact lens, tape on one eyeglass lens)
- Prisms can be used to optically shift the second image to achieve single binocular vision.
- Strabismus surgery should be considered if the above fails and involves adjusting the relative position of eye muscles to restore alignment.

- Although not often used, botulinum toxin injection can temporarily weaken certain extraocular muscles to correct misalignment and diplopia.

CRANIAL NERVE PALSY

SIXTH NERVE (ABDUCENS) PALSY

CASE 15

The parents of an 8-year-old boy presented, having noted crossing of his eyes for the past 6 hours. The boy admitted to double vision that was binocular, horizontal, and worse when he looked to the right. He had a right face-turn. His visual acuities were 20/25 in each eye. He had an esotropia in primary gaze that worsened in right gaze and improved in left. He was able to abduct his right eye only 20° from primary position. A head MRI revealed a posterior fossa tumor.

PATHOPHYSIOLOGY

- The course of the 6th nerve is illustrated in Fig. 11-25. A lesion anywhere along its course from the nucleus to the orbit can cause a palsy.
- The 6th nerve innervates the ipsilateral lateral rectus muscle.
- The 6th nerve ascends the clivus before it enters Dorello's canal. Stretching occurs at this juncture with increased intracranial pressure.

CLINICAL FEATURES

- Horizontal, binocular diplopia is worse at distance and in ipsilateral gaze. Patient may have face-turn to ipsilateral side.

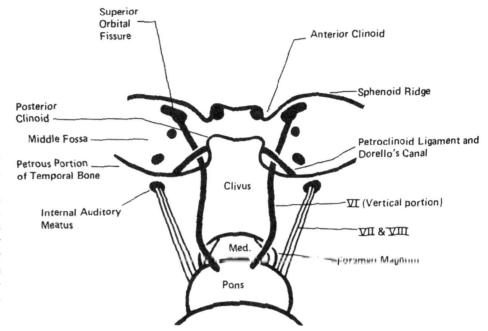

FIGURE 11-25 Anatomy of the 6th nerve. The 6th nerve nucleus lies in the pons and exits ventrally. It ascends the clivus and enters Dorello's canal. The 6th nerve travels freely in the cavernous sinus and then through the superior orbital fissure before innervating the lateral rectus. (Reprinted from Kline LB, Bajandas EJ, *Neuro-Ophthalmology Review Manual.* Thorofare, NJ, Slack, 1996.)

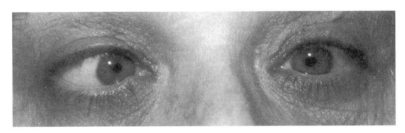

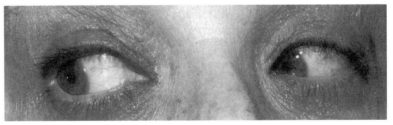

FIGURE 11-26 Left 6th nerve palsy. The patient is unable to abduct the left eye fully (*top*) compared to the right (*bottom*).

- Ischemic palsies may present with pain.
- When looking far laterally, the sclera is normally hidden by the lateral canthus. Patients with 6th nerve palsy are unable to "bury the sclera" on abduction (Fig. 11-26). Esotropia may be present, which worsens in ipsilateral gaze.
- Children under 7–9 years of age may develop amblyopia (see Strabismus section).

DIAGNOSIS AND DIFFERENTIAL

- Common causes of 6th nerve palsy include ischemia, intracranial tumor, increased intracranial pressure from any cause, trauma, and idiopathic.

- Less common causes include infection, inflammation, congenital, demyelination, and giant cell arteritis.
- Myasthenia gravis, thyroid eye disease, and restrictive orbital lesions can mimic 6th nerve palsy and may warrant edrophonium testing or CT of the orbits.
- Ischemia is presumed in an older patient with vasculopathic risk factors and an isolated 6th nerve palsy. MRI should be performed if it fails to improve after 6–8 weeks.
- Younger adults and children may warrant neuroimaging because of the high risk of intracranial neoplasm.

TREATMENT

- The underlying cause should be treated.

- Otherwise, diplopia is treated with occlusion, prisms, and surgery.

THIRD NERVE (OCULOMOTOR) PALSY

CASE 16

A previously healthy 57-year-old man complained of acute headache, left-sided ptosis, and binocular diplopia. His visual acuities were 20/20 in both eyes. His right eye was normal. His left lid was completely closed. The left pupil was 5.5 mm in diameter and unreactive to light or near stimulus. He could not elevate, depress, or adduct his right eye, but abduction was normal (Fig. 11-27). MRI/MRA revealed an aneurysm at the junction of the left posterior communicating and carotid arteries. The aneurysm was coiled by interventional neuroradiology, and the 3rd nerve palsy completely resolved over the next 6 months.

PATHOPHYSIOLOGY

- The course of the 3rd nerve is shown in Fig. 11-28.
- The 3rd nerve innervates the ipsilateral superior rectus, levator palpebrae, medial rectus, and inferior rectus, and inferior oblique muscles.
- 3rd nerve dysfunction can be secondary to compression (uncal herniation, aneurysms, tumors), trauma, or microvascular ischemia.
- Parasympathetic pupil fibers travel along the outside of the 3rd nerve. Damage to these fibers from compression results in a dilated, poorly reactive pupil.
- Microvascular ischemia occurs in the deeper substance of the 3rd nerve, and peripheral pupil fibers may be spared.
- Traumatic 3rd nerve palsy is usually associated with severe blunt head trauma causing shearing or penetrating injuries.

CLINICAL FEATURES

- 3rd nerve palsy results in poor elevation, adduction, and depression of the eye and ptosis.
- Pain is a common feature of ischemic and aneurysmal 3rd nerve palsies and cannot be used to distinguish etiology.
- Vasculopathic risk factors in ischemic palsies include diabetes, hypertension, age, high cholesterol, and smoking.

DIAGNOSIS AND DIFFERENTIAL

- It is important to determine whether the pupil is equal in size and reactivity to the fellow eye (pupil spared) or larger and poorly reactive (pupil involved).
- The extent of muscle and lid involvement (complete vs. incomplete) needs to be delineated.
- Pupil *involvement* with either complete or incomplete 3rd nerve palsy is a posterior communicating artery aneurysm until proven otherwise. MRI/MRA is mandatory, and if negative, angiography is recommended.
- Pupil sparing with *complete* 3rd nerve palsy: Older patient with vascular risk factors (diabetes, hypertension, etc.) can be observed. MRI is warranted if there has been no improvement in 6 weeks.
  - The patient who is younger than 50 years or has no vascular risk factors needs glucose, cholesterol, and blood pressure check. If negative, then an MRI is necessary.
- Pupil sparing with *incomplete* 3rd nerve palsy can be observed every other day for one week. Treat as above if pupil becomes involved or remains spared.
- The main differential in adults is aneurysm, ischemia, and compressive lesion. In children, congenital, trauma, and compressive tumors are more likely causes.

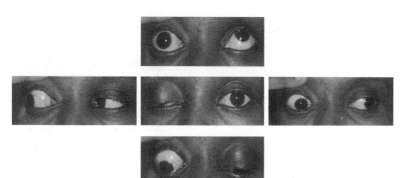

FIGURE 11-27 Third nerve palsy. Significant ptosis of the upper lid is present. The eye cannot adduct, elevate, or depress fully. Abduction is intact.

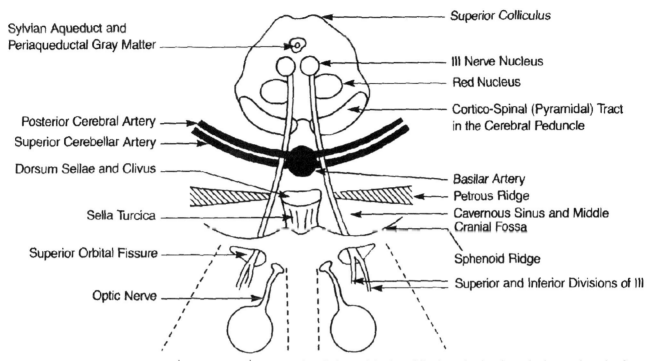

FIGURE 11-28 Anatomy of the 3ʳᵈ nerve. The 3ʳᵈ nerve nucleus is located in the midbrain and exits along the interpeduncular fossa between the posterior cerebral artery and the superior cerebellar artery. It travels through the cavernous sinus where it divides into a superior and inferior division and the superior orbital fissure before reaching the extraocular muscles. (Reprinted from Kline LB, Bajandas EJ, *Neuro-Ophthalmology Review Manual*. Thorofare, NJ, Slack, 1996.)

TREATMENT

- Diplopia: initially the eyelid may occlude vision and auto-patch. Otherwise, treat with occlusion, prisms, and surgery.
- Ischemic 3ʳᵈ nerve palsies are observed. Most resolve in 3 months.
- Aneurysms can be occluded by interventional neuro-radiology or treated neurosurgically.

FOURTH NERVE (TROCHLEAR) PALSY

CASE 17

A 28-year-old man slipped and fell down the stairs. He struck the left side of his head but did not lose consciousness. Upon sitting up, he noted binocular double vision. The images were separated diagonally and more so at near. He had a left head tilt. His visual acuities were 20/15 both eyes. Cover testing revealed a right hypertropia which worsened in left gaze and right head tilt.

PATHOPHYSIOLOGY

- The course of the 4ᵗʰ nerve is illustrated in Fig. 11-29.
- The 4ᵗʰ nerve has the longest intracranial course and is the only cranial nerve to exit dorsally from the brain stem. It innervates the ipsilateral superior oblique muscle.
- Blunt head trauma damages the 4ᵗʰ nerve as it travels in the anterior medullary velum.
- Congenital 4ᵗʰ nerve palsies decompensate when the ability to fuse the two images breaks down.

CLINICAL FEATURES

- Vertical or oblique binocular diplopia is worse at near, in contralateral gaze, and with ipsilateral head tilt. Often presents with contralateral head tilt.
- Depression of the eye in adduction may be limited, but the motility almost always appears grossly normal.
- In bilateral 4ᵗʰ nerve palsies, the left eye is higher in right gaze and left head tilt and the right eye is higher in left gaze and right head tilt.

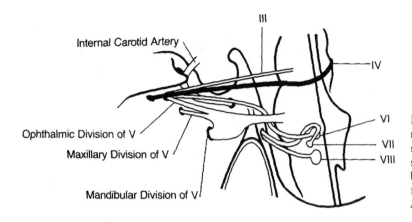

FIGURE 11-29 Anatomy of the 4th nerve. The 4th nerve exits dorsally from the midbrain and decussates. It travels through the cavernous sinus, then the superior orbital fissure outside the annulus of Zinn, before innervating the superior oblique. (Reprinted from Kline LB, Bajandas EJ, *Neuro-Ophthalmology Review Manual*. Thorofare, NJ, Slack, 1996.)

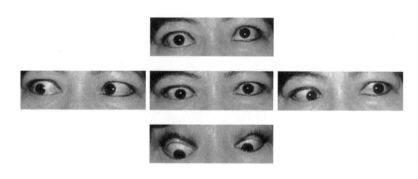

FIGURE 11-30 Thyroid eye disease limits the ability for the eyes to look in all directions except downgaze. Note the upper and lower lid retraction.

DIAGNOSIS AND DIFFERENTIAL

- Common causes of 4th nerve palsy include trauma, ischemia, decompensation of a congenital palsy, and idiopathic.
- Intracranial neoplasms, primary schwannomas of the trochlear nerve, dolichoectasia of the basilar artery, and MS are less common.
- Patients with decompensated congenital 4th nerve palsies often have a longstanding head tilt evident in old photographs. These patients also can fuse a larger amount of vertical prism than normal.
- Patients with vasculopathic risk factors and an isolated 4th nerve palsy are observed. MRI is warranted if no improvement occurs in 6–8 weeks.
- Skew deviation, myasthenia, and thyroid eye disease may mimic 4th nerve palsy.

TREATMENT

- Treatment is directed at any underlying cause.

- Otherwise, treat diplopia with occlusion, prisms, and surgery.

RESTRICTIVE LESIONS

CASE 18

A 35-year-old woman complained of progressive painless, binocular, vertical double vision over the past 2 months. The diplopia was worse in upgaze and better in downgaze. She also noted bilateral eye redness that was worse in the morning. Her visual acuities were 20/20 in each eye. Her upper and lower eyelids were retracted above and below the limbus, respectively, in both eyes. She had injection of both conjunctivae. She had limited motility in all directions with the left eye. The right eye could depress fully but otherwise could not move completely. See Fig. 11-30. Findings from the rest of her examination were normal. CT scan of the orbits revealed bilateral, enlarged extraocular muscles. See Fig. 11-31. Forced ductions were positive (see Clinical Features section).

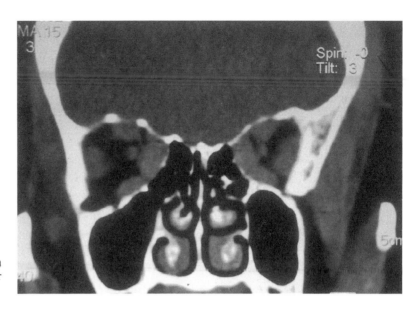

FIGURE 11-31 Orbital CT scan of the patient in Fig. 11-30 demonstrates enlarged extraocular muscles.

PATHOPHYSIOLOGY

- Tethering occurs when the patient attempts to look in the direction opposite to the restricted muscle.
- Interference of the eye may occur as it attempts to look in the direction of an orbital mass.

CLINICAL FEATURES

- Inability to move the eye.
- May have anomalous head posture to eliminate diplopia (typically chin up in thyroid eye disease).
- Lid retraction and proptosis may be present in thyroid eye disease.
- History of previous blunt trauma or ophthalmic surgery.
- After instilling a topical anesthetic into the eye, forced ductions are performed with a cotton swab or toothed forcep to push or pull the eye, respectively. With the patient looking in the abnormal direction, the eye should move easily if no mechanical restriction is present. Otherwise, this is called positive forced ductions.

DIAGNOSIS AND DIFFERENTIAL

- Diagnosis of restrictive lesion confirmed with positive forced duction test.
- Thyroid eye disease and blow-out fractures, most common in adults.
- Previous ocular surgery with a scleral buckle or periocular injection.
- Orbital tumors or orbital cellulitis.
- Rarely, metastasis to an extraocular muscle (lung, breast, lymphoma).

- Poor movement of superior oblique muscle through the trochlea, (Brown syndrome) in children and congenital fibrosis of extraocular muscles.

TREATMENT

- Occlusion, prisms, and surgery. But surgery is more common in restrictive lesions.

INTERNUCLEAR OPHTHALMOPLEGIA

CASE 19

A 65-year-old diabetic noted acute, horizontal binocular diplopia, worse in left gaze while driving. He denied any pain or other neurologic deficit. His visual acuities were 20/20 in each eye. In primary gaze, his right eye was deviated laterally. He was unable to adduct his right eye past the midline (Fig. 11-32). Otherwise his eye motility was full. Forced ductions were negative. MRI of the head was found to be normal.

PATHOPHYSIOLOGY

- The anatomy of the horizontal gaze pathways is shown in Fig. 11-33.
- Interruption of the medial longitudinal fasciculus (MLF) results in an ipsilateral internuclear ophthalmoplegia (INO).
- Increased attempt to innervate the adducting eye causes contralateral abducting nystagmus.

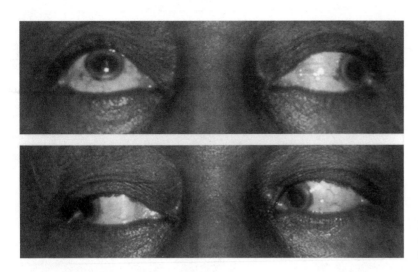

FIGURE 11-32 Internuclear ophthalmoplegia secondary to lacunar infarction. The right eye cannot adduct past the midline.

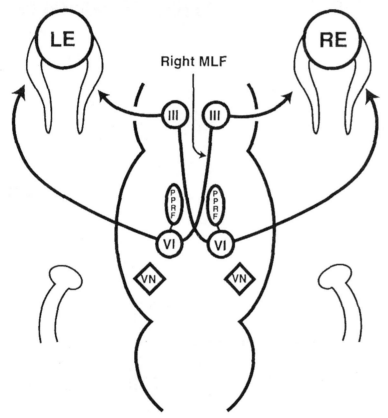

**Internuclear Connections of
PPRF and Nuclei of Nerves III and VI**

FIGURE 11-33 Anatomy of the horizontal gaze pathways. Input from higher centers is conducted to the paramedian pontine reticular formation (center for lateral gaze). From there it crosses the midline and ascends the contralateral medial longitudinal fasciculus to the oculomotor subnucleus responsible for the medial rectus. (Reprinted from Kline LB, Bajandas EJ, *Neuro-Ophthalmology Review Manual*. Thorofare, NJ, Slack, 1996.)

CLINICAL FEATURES

- The ipsilateral eye cannot adduct and the contralateral abducting eye develops horizontal nystagmus. In milder cases, the ipsilateral eye may have only slow adducting saccades.

- The eye may converge to near stimulus.
- A vertical deviation may be present with unilateral INO, and upbeat nystagmus in upgaze occurs with bilateral INO.
- Bilateral defects may present with a very large exotropia.

DIAGNOSIS AND DIFFERENTIAL

- Diagnosis is made based on the clinical features. MRI is necessary to establish underlying cause.
- In young adults, usually MS (often bilateral) is the cause.
- In older patients, brain stem strokes are common causes.
- Less commonly, brain stem masses, trauma, or drugs may cause an INO.
- Myasthenia gravis or a restrictive lesion may cause an adduction deficit (pseudo-INO).

TREATMENT

- Occlusion, prism, and surgery.
- Discontinuation of drugs, if medically possible, should be considered.

GAZE PALSY

CASE 20

A 71-year-old woman complained, "I can't move my eyes to the left." She was walking down the aisle of the grocery store when she noted this inability. Her visual acuities were 20/20 in each eye. Her visual fields were full. Extraocular motility revealed a complete adduction deficit in the right eye and a complete abduction deficit in the left. Otherwise, motility was intact.

PATHOPHYSIOLOGY

- The anatomy of the horizontal gaze pathways is shown in Fig. 11-33.
- Horizontal saccades are initiated in the contralateral frontal eye field (FEF). Input is relayed to the paramedian pontine reticular formation (PPRF) and on to the ipsilateral 6th nerve nucleus. An interneuron then leaves the 6th nerve nucleus and crosses the midline and ascends in the contralateral MLF to synapse with the contralateral medial rectus subnucleus.
- Vertical saccades require bilateral input from the FEF. These pathways are not well understood but information is relayed to the rostral interstitial nucleus of the MLF, which then innervates the 3rd and 4th nerve nuclei to coordinate vertical gaze.

CLINICAL FEATURES

- Conjugate impairment of the eyes to look in a certain direction from a supranuclear disturbance. Can be either horizontal or vertical.
- Diplopia is uncommon since both eyes tend to be equally affected.
- If a conjugate horizontal gaze palsy is accompanied by an inability to adduct the ipsilateral eye, then it is called the one-and-a-half syndrome. For example, a patient may have a left-gaze palsy and an adduction deficit of the left eye. This is caused by a lesion of the PPRF and the ipsilateral MLF.
- Lesions of the contralateral frontal eye field may be associated with contralateral motor deficits.
- A conjugate upgaze paresis is the predominant feature of dorsal midbrain syndrome. Lid retraction and light near dissociation may be associated.

DIAGNOSIS AND DIFFERENTIAL

- In the pons, lacunar strokes of the ipsilateral PPRF or the ipsilateral 6th nerve nucleus may be responsible.
- Causes of dorsal midbrain syndrome include hydrocephalus and tumors.
- Less common causes of gaze palsies include generalized neurologic diseases such as spinocerebellar ataxia, Parkinson's, Wernicke's encephalopathy, and progressive supranuclear palsy (tends to affect vertical before horizontal).
- Chronic progressive supranuclear palsy is typically associated with ptosis and orbicularis weakness.

TREATMENT

- Wernicke's encephalopathy can be treated with thiamine (vitamin B_{12}).
- Patients with downgaze paresis have difficulty with bifocals and may benefit from single-vision reading glasses.

NYSTAGMUS

- Nystagmus is a repetitive oscillation of the eyes as a result of a defect in the slow eye movement system (vestibular, optokinetic, and pursuit) or the neural integrator (allows eccentric positions of gaze to be held).

- Jerk nystagmus: slow drift of the eyes in one direction followed by a quick corrective opposite movement. The fast phase defines the direction of nystagmus.
- Pendular nystagmus: rhythmic, smooth oscillations of the eyes (no fast component).
- Most nystagmus occurs in the horizontal or vertical planes, but a torsional component may be evident. It is often described as clockwise or counterclockwise from either the patient's or physician's perspective.
- Patients may be asymptomatic or experience movement of the visual environment (oscillopsia).

CONGENITAL NYSTAGMUS

CASE 21

A mother presents with her 7-month-old son because "his eyes have been shaking" for the past 3–4 weeks. He was the product of a full-term, uncomplicated pregnancy via spontaneous vaginal delivery. His Apgar scores were 10 and 10. He sat at 4 months and was just beginning to crawl. On examination, he did not appear to fixate on or follow small objects. He had horizontal pendular nystagmus in all gazes. When the lights were dimmed, his pupils paradoxically constricted. Otherwise his examination revealed nothing remarkable in both eyes. Electroretinogram (ERG) testing revealed markedly reduced responses. Congenital nystagmus secondary to vision loss from the retinal degeneration (Leber's congenital amaurosis) was diagnosed.

PATHOPHYSIOLOGY

- Significant visual loss results in a lack of visual calibration of a neural integrator for gaze holding leading to nystagmus.
- Some patients do not have vision loss or a structural lesion and it is not clearly understood why they develop congenital nystagmus.

CLINICAL FEATURES

- Usually sporadic, but can be inherited as autosomal recessive, dominant, or X-linked.
- Congenital nystagmus can begin at birth; however, more commonly it begins at 4–6 months of age. (Parents often state that it has been there since birth.)
- Horizontal, pendular nystagmus that remains horizontal in upgaze.
- May worsen when patient attempts to fixate.

- Patients may have a face turn or a head tilt to orient the eyes at the null point (position where the eyes are still or almost still), because vision is better there.
- Convergence can dampen the nystagmus.
- Strabismus is not uncommon (30%).
- Patients do not complain of oscillopsia.

DIAGNOSIS AND DIFFERENTIAL

- Most often no structural abnormality can be found.
- MRI can rule out structural lesions of the brain.
- ERG and visual-evoked potential should be considered in cases of vision loss not due to high refractive error. See Table 11-4 for causes of early vision loss leading to congenital nystagmus. Typically, cortical vision loss does not cause nystagmus.
- Delayed visual maturation can rarely cause congenital nystagmus that resolves.

TREATMENT

- Prisms can induce convergence or shift the null point to the primary position.
- Eye muscle surgery can adjust eye position so that the null point is straight ahead.
- Patching may be necessary if amblyopia is present.

DOWNBEAT NYSTAGMUS

CASE 22

A 54-year-old man with no significant past medical history complains of blurry vision when he looks to the left or the right but feels his vision is clear in primary gaze. Acuities are 20/20 both eyes. His eyes are straight and steady in primary gaze. Gazes left and right produce downbeat nystagmus; his eyes beat quickly downward and slowly upward. This is also evident in downgaze but dampens in upgaze. Thin-section, saggital MRI through the foramen magnum reveals an Arnold Chiari malformation (Fig. 11-34).

TABLE 11-4   Causes of Congenital Nystagmus from Vision Loss

Albinism
Achromatopsia
Colobomas of optic nerve and retina
Congenital cataracts
Congenital stationary night blindness
Leber's congenital amaurosis
Optic nerve hypoplasia

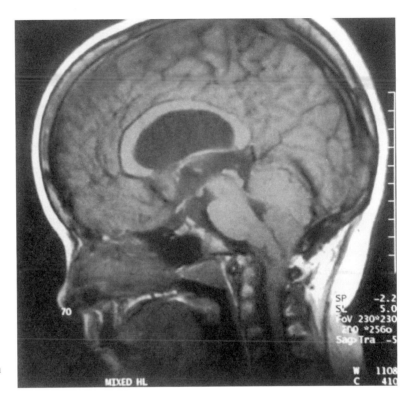

FIGURE 11-34 Saggital MRI through the foramen magnum shows an Arnold Chiari malformation.

PATHOPHYSIOLOGY

- It is theorized that posterior semicircular canal projections are damaged, causing unopposed input from the anterior canals with slow upward drift.
- Cerebellar lesions may play a role with loss of inhibition on anterior semicircular canal input or with imbalance to the vertical neural integrators.

CLINICAL FEATURES

- Conjugate, jerk nystagmus with slow phase upward and compensatory fast phase downward.
- Most evident in lateral and downgaze. May dampen in upgaze. May accentuate with convergence.

DIAGNOSIS AND DIFFERENTIAL

- The most common causes include Arnold Chiari malformation, mass at the cervicomedullary junction, and idiopathic. MRI with thin sagittal views through the foramen magnum is necessary.
- Other causes include lithium, carbamazepine, phenytoin, and alcohol. Thiamine and magnesium deficiency should also be considered.
- Familial spinocerebellar degenerations and MS may also cause downbeat nystagmus.

TREATMENT

- Clonazepam may be helpful. Second line agents include baclofen and gabapentin.
- Removal of lesion at cervicomedullary junction or decompression of foramen magnum may not relieve nystagmus.
- Withdrawal of lithium may not resolve nystagmus.

END-GAZE NYSTAGMUS

CASE 23

A 38-year-old healthy woman was referred for nystagmus by her internist. She had been complaining of pain behind her eyes. While examining her eye movements, he noted nystagmus when she looked to the far left and right. Her visual acuities were 20/15 in each eye. Her eye examination was normal. In far left, sustained gaze, she had a leftward beating horizontal nystagmus, and in right gaze a symmetric response.

PATHOPHYSIOLOGY

- Presumably, fatigue or breakdown in the neural integrator is responsible for end-gaze nystagmus.

CLINICAL FEATURES

- Most normal individuals develop horizontal or torsional jerk nystagmus with extreme or prolonged lateral gaze.
- The amplitude is typically small and symmetric between the two eyes.
- It is poorly sustained secondary to fatigue.

DIAGNOSIS AND DIFFERENTIAL

- End-gaze nystagmus is a common finding in normal individuals.
- There is a need to differentiate this from *pathologic* gaze–evoked nystagmus.
  - It is asymmetric on right and left gaze and has moderate amplitude.
  - It occurs before the patient reaches the extremes of gaze.
  - After prolonged eccentric gaze and return to primary position, a transient nystagmus in the opposite direction may occur (rebound nystagmus).
  - Causes include cerebellopontine angle tumors, vestibular nerve damage, and cerebellar lesions.

TREATMENT

- Reassurance.

OTHER TYPES

Oculopalatal Nystagmus
- Pendular nystagmus associated with rhythmic movement (1–3 per second) of upper palate or facial muscles that is unabated during sleep.
- Typically begins several months after brain stem stroke interrupting connections between the inferior olive, red nucleus, and dentate nucleus.

Periodic Alternating Nystagmus
- This is horizontal nystagmus that changes direction in cycles. It beats in one direction for 60–90 seconds, halts for 5–10 seconds, and changes direction for 60–90 seconds.
- Can be congenital or acquired (drugs, trauma, cerebellar lesions).
- Baclofen is often helpful in acquired cases.

Seesaw Nystagmus
- As one eye elevates and intorts, the other eye depresses and extorts. This is followed by a reversal of torsion and vertical movements for both eyes.
- Associated with tumors near the sella turcica and midbrain strokes.

Opsoclonus
- Involuntary, omnidirectional, back-to-back saccades without an intersaccadic interval. If the saccades are limited to the horizontal plane, then it is called ocular flutter.
- Opsoclonus in a child is highly associated with neuroblastoma. Screening for urine catecholamines (homovanillic and vanillymandelic acid) and for tumors of the adrenal gland and thoracic sympathetic chain should be performed.

Superior Oblique Myokymia (not a nystagmus)
- Idiopathic, intermittent, *monocular* oscillation.
- Magnification is often necessary to observe movements.
- Diagnosis is often made by history alone if the patient is not observed by the clinician. Movements can be elicited by asking the patient to look down and nasal, then back to primary position.
- It can be treated with carbamazepine or occasionally eye muscle surgery.

BIBLIOGRAPHY

Ischemic Optic Neuropathy Decompression Trial Study Group. Characteristics of patients with non-arteritic anterior ischemic optic neuropathy eligible for the Ischemic Optic Neuropathy Decompression Trial. *Arch Ophthalmol* 1996;114:1366–74.

Leigh RJ, Zee DS. *The Neurology of Eye Movements*, 3rd ed. New York: Oxford University Press, 1999.

Miller NR, Newman NJ: *Walsh and Hoyt's Clinical Neuro-ophthalmology*, 5th ed. Baltimore: Williams & Wilkins, 1998.

Optic Neuritis Study Group. Visual function five years after optic neuritis: experience of the Optic Neuritis Treatment Trial. *Arch Ophthalmol* 1997;115:1545–1552.

Thompson HS. Functional visual loss, *Am J Ophthalmol* 1985; 100:209–13.

Thompson HS, Pilley SFJ: Unequal pupils. A flow chart for sorting out the anisocorias. *Surv Ophthalmol* 1976; 21:45–48.

Wall M. Idiopathic intracranial hypertension. *Neurol Clin* 1991;9:73–95.

INDEX

Page numbers followed by an "f" indicate figures; numbers followed by a "t" indicate tables. The letters CP indicate that the figure(s) also appears in the color plate section.

237

Ulcerative keratitis, in contact lens wearers, 20
Uveitis, 131–133, 132f, 133f
    cytomegalovirus, 200, 200f, CP
    histoplasmosis, 200–201, 201f, CP
    posterior, 198–201
    sarcoid, 199–200, 199f, CP

Vasoconstrictors, topical ophthalmic, 102t
Vergence, 41
Vergence formulas, 11, 13f
Version, 41
Verticillata, 122
Virtual image, 8, 9f
Vision
    abnormal binocular, 38–39
    fusion in, 37
    nonphysiologic loss of, 225–226, 226f

    normal binocular, 37–38, 37f, 38f
Visual acuity, 1–2
Visual field
    defects of, 2, 221–226, 222f, 223f
    definition of, 2
    examples of, 2
    in glaucoma, 153–157
    measurement of, 160–161, 161f, 161t, 162f, 163f
    normal, 153, 153f, 153t
Visual function, 1
Vitamin B_{12}, deficiency of, 220–221, 220f
Vitrectomy, for retinal detachment, 197
Vitreous
    degeneration of, 202, 203f, CP
    detachment of, 180, 180f
    floaters, 179, 179f
    hemorrhage of, 181–182, 181f, CP

Vogt's striae, 118
Vortex keratopathy, 122

Waardenburg's syndrome, 140
Warts, on eyelid, 68–69, 68f
Wavelength, of light, 7, 7f
Weill-Marchesani syndrome, 142–143
Weiss ring, 180
Wilms' tumor, aniridia with, 135
Wilson's disease, corneal complications of, 122–123, 123f, CP

Xanthelasma, 71, 71f

Zeiss, gland of, 64